WEIGHT LOSS BY GINA

SPRING/SUMMER 2023 PROGRAM

POSTS AND GUIDELINES

ISBN: 9798390720448

Weight Loss By Gina is committed to making weight loss as easy as possible. In doing so, we have put together this book containing the instructional information which will be posted in the Livy Method App and Spring/Summer 2023 Facebook Support Group week to week. Please keep in mind this booklet does not contain all of the information and posts, so you will still need to check into the Facebook Group or the Livy Method App day to day to review any newly added information and to watch the videos that go along with these posts.

At the end of this workbook you will find additional resources that may help with your journey. Included is the science guide, which contains additional articles that go more in depth into the science behind the program and the process, some sample recipes that you can try, and tracking sheets that you can use to track your progress.

I want to acknowledge and thank Tony An, Sonya Cholakov, Odette Ropchan, Megan Corbett, Kim Turnbull and Rebecca Ross-Zaiontz for contributing content that is included in this booklet. Special thanks also goes out to Terry-Ann Pighin, Kim Johnstone and Drew Dafoe for their help in bringing it all together, and Chrissy Hobbs from Indie Publishing Group, who helped with all the editing and formatting. Thank you so much for all your efforts and this booklet wouldn't be possible without your help.

- Gina

Disclaimer: These documents do not contain medical/health advice. The information is provided for general informational and educational purposes only and is not a substitute for professional advice. Please speak to your healthcare provider if you have any concerns before starting and/or during the Program.

CONTENTS

WEIGHT LOSS BY GINA

SPRING/SUMMER 2023 PROGRAM

WELCOME TO GINA'S SPRING/SUMMER 2023 WEIGHT LOSS PROGRAM

LET'S GET STARTED WITH PREP WEEK!

If you are new to the Program, Prep Week is all about introducing and implementing the Food Plan. This is where you can start reviewing the information, like the Food Plan you are to follow, how the Program works, as well as gather anything you might need and ask any questions you have.

Day 1 of Prep Week is where you start to implement the changes you need to make and start following the Program. If you are using the Livy Method App you can start tracking your progress right away. Keeping in mind it's not about being perfect, it's about progress over perfection.

If you are a returning member, Prep Week is all about getting back at it and setting yourself up for success as you continue your weight loss journey on the road to Finally & Forever.

WHAT IS THE LIVY METHOD:

- The Livy Method is about losing weight in a way that is healthy for the body and equally healthy for the mind, so your weight loss is easier to maintain.

- The approach is to systematically lower your setpoint. Your setpoint is the weight your body is used to functioning at – also known as homeostasis – where all the regulatory systems in your body work together to maintain balance for the purpose of helping the body survive and work at the most optimal level.

- Each week the Program addresses weight loss from a variety of different angles, physically and mentally. You will work through issues and associations when it comes to food and beliefs, while working through old habits and creating new ones.

- There is a basic Food Plan you will need to follow, where each week will have a different focus, so keep in mind what you eat and when you eat will change and evolve week to week.

HOW THE PROGRAM WORKS:

- This Program is designed to be followed day by day, week by week, for the full 91 days, regardless of how much weight you have to lose or how long it takes you to follow through and finish.

- The Program can also accommodate any time off or off day, and can be done on your own timeline. If you stop following for any reason, you will simply pick up from where you left off.

- You can use the Livy Method App to help guide you through the Program and track your progress along the way.

- The Program is broken down into a week-by-week and day-by-day process where each week will have a different focus and each day we will be presenting and discussing the information you need to be successful.

- The best way to follow the Program is to check into the Facebook Support Group or use the Livy Method App each day to watch the Daily Check In Video and review the accompanying posts for a detailed explanation of the changes you are advised to make.

- The Facebook Support Group is also where you can ask any questions and have them answered by Gina and her team of Program Specialists.

- You can also use the SEARCH feature in your Livy Method App to access the extensive database of frequently asked questions.

- Gina will be going Live in the Facebook Group Monday - Friday at 9AM EST and Saturday at 10AM EST.

- The Live segments are saved in GUIDES in the Facebook Support Group to be viewed later and will be linked from the Livy Method App. The lives will also be available on the Weigh In with Gina podcast found on all podcast platforms and also accessible in the Livy Method App.

- The Live segments are not mandatory. All the information you need will be posted in the Facebook Support Group or in the Livy Method App.

DAILY CHECKLIST:

1. Check into the Facebook Support Group or the Livy Method App.

2. Watch the Daily Check In Video.

3. Watch/Review any additional support videos or posts.

4. Ask any questions you have.

5. Implement the changes you need to make.

6. Watch/participate in the Facebook Lives. (Suggested but not Required.)

Check out the Table of Contents to review all of the topics that we will be discussing week to week.

Please take the time to head over to the Facebook Group or the Livy Method App and watch the quick video that accompanies this post.

FAQS - ABOUT THE PROGRAM

Here are some of the most popular questions asked about the Program:

1. **Is the Program low carb?**

    - No, the Program is more about eating the right carbs at the right time. It is suggested to take out or minimize breads, pastas, baked goods and obvious sugars. However, the Food Plan includes a variety of carbohydrates like grains such as quinoa and rice, starchy vegetables like potatoes and squash for example, along with fruits.

2. **Do we have to count, weigh, or measure or food?**

    - No need to count, weigh, or measure your food. The Livy Method has a unique way of addressing portions where the focus is on being in tune with your body's needs. In the first few weeks of the Program, the key is to follow the Food Plan consistently and eat to satisfaction after each meal and snack. We start to address portions in Weeks 3 and 4.

3. **What kind of results can I expect?**

    - Although the goal is to lose as much weight as possible, in the healthiest way possible in the timeframe we have, each person's journey is unique.

    - Depending on the amount of weight you have to lose, it is not unreasonable to expect upwards of 60 lbs.+ loss for men and 40 lbs.+ loss for women, but that would depend on the state of your body when you started, along with other variables.

    - Based on our survey results, the weight lost per 91 day Program averages between 12 - 16 lbs. The Livy Method is not a quick fix program, the focus is on losing weight Finally & Forever and the time that takes can vary person to person.

    - Because the Program is focused around losing weight in a healthy way, both physically and mentally, many members also experience improvements with their overall health. Some examples are reduction of medications, improved digestion, better sleep, and increased energy, just to name a few.

    - The Program is focused on improving the mind-body connection, so members also often experience better relationships with themselves, their food choices and a decrease in cravings.

4. **What can I expect in the first week of the Program?**

    - In the first week (Prep Week) we start to post the information you will need day to day to follow the Program, including the Food Plan, which outlines what to eat and when.

    - The Program starts on Day 1, where you start to implement the changes you need to make. You can use your Livy Method App to guide you through the process and to track your progress.

- Don't expect to be perfect from Day 1. The focus is on progress over perfection, so it is not about how strong you start or how perfectly you start, it is about progressing day-to-day, week-to-week and following through and finishing all 91 days of the Program.

- While some may start losing weight in the first week, some might not. How quickly you lose in the beginning is not an indication of how successful you will be in the end. If you do not lose weight in the first few weeks, there is nothing to be concerned about as the focus is more about allowing your body to adjust to the changes that you are making that will eventually lead to the scale moving.

- Everyone's body will respond differently, so be mindful not to rush the process or compare what is happening with you to what someone else is experiencing.

5.   **What is "detox"?**

- Detox is a very loose term used to describe when the body is about to, or in a state of releasing fat while following The Livy Method.

- Detox happens naturally in the body so things like detox kits, teas, juices or any type of cleanses are simply not needed.

- With The Livy Method, you are piggybacking the body's natural detox response by focusing on helping to support the body and its needs, so it can better focus on fat loss.

- When it comes to detox and helping the body release fat, there is nothing you need to do other than follow the Program as designed.

- The topic of detox will be discussed in further detail throughout the Program. More information is available in our Science Guide, accessible on the Livy Method App, in the book, and on our website.

6.   **What if I have health issues? How will they affect me while following the Program and is there anything I need to do to compensate or adjust?**

- If you have any concerns about your individual health needs while following the Program, be sure to discuss them with your healthcare provider.

- Because the Program is based on losing weight in a healthy way, physically and mentally, the suggestions made while following are beneficial to everyone.

7.   **Do I have to watch every Facebook Live video?**

- Although they are beneficial and informative, they are not a mandatory part of the process. You can choose to participate and/or watch some, all, or none of the Live segments. They are posted in the group under GUIDES and are available for you to access at any time.

- The Lives can be found across all podcasts platforms and linked directly in the Livy Method App.

8.   **What if I have a question about the Program or Plan?**

- Once the Program starts, if you have any questions, you can ask in the Facebook support group where we have a full team of Program Specialists who are ready and happy to help. Or you can search the database within the Livy Method App.

- If you need any administrative assistance, you can reach out to our team by way of email at weightloss@ginalivy.com.

- If you require technical support with the Livy Method App, contact techsupport@ginalivy.com.

THE FOOD PLAN

The Food Plan is designed to stimulate your digestive system, increase nutrient absorption, decrease the amount of insulin that your body is accustomed to using, and give the body the resources it needs to make change.

You are to follow the Food Plan as is outlined in this post for the next few weeks. As we progress, you will be making slight changes where what you eat and when, along with what you focus on each week will change and evolve as you go.

The goal is to be as consistent as possible in following the Food Plan to allow the body to react and adjust to the changes you are making. It is important to eat all of the meals and snacks as outlined below.

If you are not hungry, you should still eat a small token amount (4-5 bites with chewing in between) and be mindful not to skip any meals and snacks.

THE BASIC FOOD PLAN AT A GLANCE:

FIRST THING – Lemon water and/or apple cider vinegar

BREAKFAST – Protein is the focus

SNACK #1 – Fruit on its own

LUNCH – Vegetables are the focus with added protein, leafy greens, and healthy fats. Add in starchy carbs and grains as needed.

SNACK #2 – Vegetables, with or without added protein and fat

SNACK #3 – Nuts and/or seeds on their own

DINNER – Protein is the focus with added vegetables, leafy greens, and healthy fats

TIMING - The time between all meals and snacks should be anywhere from 30 mins to no more than 3.5 hours. It's important to keep the order of the food, but the timing between meals and snacks can change day to day.

See the individual posts that break down each meal and snack for more information, meal ideas and frequently asked questions.

THE GOAL:

Keep things simple and routine. Don't overthink it. It is about progress over perfection as everything will come together in time.

There is no need to be concerned about portion sizes. You will find as you move along through the Program and you are consistently following the Food Plan and eating to satisfaction, your portions will naturally adjust as you become more and more in tune with your body's needs.

Try to be as consistent as possible with this basic Food Plan in these next few weeks, as the goal is to build a strong foundation. In the weeks to come, what you eat and when will change and evolve.

This first week is all about taking the time to understand the process and making the changes you need to make. Be sure to ask any questions you have along the way!

FREQUENTLY ASKED QUESTIONS

1. **Do I need to follow the plan exactly and do I need to eat all the meals and snacks even if I'm not hungry?**

   Yes. This is super key. For best results do not deviate, improvise, or skip any meals or snacks. They are all equally important and for a rhyme and a reason. The only meal you don't need to eat is breakfast as outlined in the Food Plan.

2. **How far apart should my meals and snacks be?**

   Ideally no sooner than 30 minutes from when you are done eating your previous meal or snack, and no longer than 3.5 hours between meals and snacks. The order is important, but the timing between meals and snacks can change day to day.

3. **Can I add in green powders, pre-workout drinks, BCAAs, etc.?**

   You can add in these types of supplements if you feel you need. Keep in mind that they are not to replace your meals and snacks. Just be sure to look for ones with all natural ingredients, with no artificial additives. Also, be mindful of sugar content.

4. **Can I switch out the snacks for other things or change the order?**

   No. For optimal results, eat the suggested snacks in the order they appear in the Food Plan.

Please take the time to head over to the Facebook Group or the Livy Method App and watch the quick video that accompanies this post.

LET'S TALK LEMON WATER AND APPLE CIDER VINEGAR

Lemon water is enzyme-based while apple cider vinegar is bacterial based. Both can be beneficial when it comes to your morning routine. You can take one or the other or both. This is not "make or break" but can be a benefit if you choose to add in.

Lemon water first thing in the morning promotes hydration, helps to stimulate your digestive system and cleanses your palate.

Apple Cider Vinegar can be beneficial if you suffer from acid reflux and/or other digestive issues. It can also aid in digestion for anyone who has had their gallbladder removed.

Lemon Water - Juice of half a lemon or 2 tbsp juice in as much water as you need and at any temperature you prefer. You can use fresh lemons or bottled lemon juice as long as it is all-natural.

Apple Cider Vinegar - 1 tablespoon in as much water as you need. If you are just starting out, you may want to start with 1 tsp and work your way up. Choose ACV containing "the mother" (a good bacteria), which would be listed on the product.

Please note: It is recommended to wait 5-10 minutes before you have any other beverage or eat your breakfast.

FREQUENTLY ASKED QUESTIONS

1. **Should I have both lemon water and apple cider vinegar?**

   You can have one or the other, or both, and that can change day to day as they both have their benefits.

2. **Can I use lime instead of lemon in my morning drink?**

   Yes, you can.

3. **Can I use apple cider vinegar gummies instead of the liquid?**

   Supplements in gummy form do not provide the same benefits. When it comes to apple cider vinegar, we recommend the liquid with the "mother" (good bacteria) in it.

4. **Can I use bottled lemon juice for my morning lemon water?**

   Yes, you can, as long as it's made with all-natural ingredients.

5. **Can I drink water before my morning apple cider vinegar or lemon water?**

   Yes. Water is fine to have before your morning ACV and/or lemon water.

6. **Can I take my medications with my apple cider vinegar or lemon water?**

   Best to speak with your healthcare provider when it comes to timing of your medications. If you need to take your medication on an empty stomach, you can take it before your ACV or lemon water.

7. **Can I swap lemons for lemon essential oil in my lemon water?**

Best to use lemons or lemon juice. If you choose to use essential oils, be sure it is food grade and safe for consumption.

Please take the time to head over to the Facebook Group or the Livy Method App and watch the quick video that accompanies this post.

LET'S TALK BREAKFAST

Having a higher protein breakfast is a great way to maximize your efforts when trying to lose weight. However, contrary to popular belief, it is not the most important meal of the day.

When you wake up, you are already full of energy from what you ate the day before. So you do not need to rely on breakfast to give you energy. That is why you have the option of skipping breakfast. However, eating it can be very beneficial when it comes to maximizing your efforts while losing weight.

BREAKFAST - PROTEIN IS THE FOCUS

Starting your day with a high protein breakfast is a great way to "break the fast" and get your body working harder from the get go.

It pains me to say it…but that means burning more calories throughout your day! (And NO, we still don't count calories!)

It is ideal to eat breakfast within 2.5 hours of waking, regardless of when you wake up. However, this is not a hard and fast rule. For example, if you wake up at 5 am and you are not active, you can still eat breakfast as late as 9 am. If you get up later, that gives you less time to have breakfast before your morning snack, so you might choose to skip breakfast and go straight to your fruit snack.

Whether you eat breakfast or not, you will still need to have your fruit snack mid-morning.

Please note: Next week, we will be introducing Bonus Snacks which are extra snacks that you can add in to help fill in the blanks for those of you who are up extra early, are more active in your day, or do shift work where you are waking up at odd hours, working overnight, or extended hours.

When it comes to portions, there is no need to count, weigh or measure! You want to eat enough to feel satisfied in the moment. If you are not hungry, it is still important to have a few token amounts of your snack (4-5 bites with chewing in between).

BREAKFAST MEAL IDEAS

Examples of higher protein breakfast (keep in mind these are not your only options, just some examples to get you started):

Eggs – Have them on their own, cooked any way you like. You can also add sautéed veggies, meat or other proteins, cheese, some greens, a small amount of fruit, nuts and seeds, avocado etc. to make your meal more nutrient rich.

Leftovers - Breakfast doesn't always have to be breakfast-type food. You can also use leftovers from lunch or dinner. For example, meat or fish, a soup, stew, or even chili.

Tofu Or Tempeh – Any way you like. If using plant protein as your main source, be sure to combine a variety of proteins to ensure you are getting enough to feel satisfied.

High Protein Cereal - Made with whole grains and seeds like buckwheat, chia seeds, hemp hearts, to name a few. Buy pre-made or make your own. Check out our WLBG Special Blend Cereal in the Recipe Guide.

Yogurt Or Cottage Cheese – Breakfast is the one place that you could use dairy as your main protein source. When doing so, try adding in hemp hearts, nuts, nut butter and/or seeds to bump up the protein and make your meal more nutrient rich. Avoid low or no fat as they tend to contain added fillers. You can have yogurt plain or flavoured as long as it is made with natural ingredients. Adding a small amount of fruit is okay, just be mindful to keep protein as the focus.

Non-dairy Options – When choosing non-dairy options, be sure to add in extra toppings to bump up the protein and healthy fat.

Chia Seed Pudding - Try adding in hemp hearts, nuts, seeds etc. to bump up the protein. Keep any added sugar to a minimum.

Oatmeal - Oatmeal can work as a breakfast option when adding in extra protein. For example, add in hemp hearts, nuts, nut butter and/or seeds along with higher fat yogurt or other dairy. Fruit and sweeteners like honey or maple syrup are fine in small amounts, but best kept to a minimum.

High Protein Pancakes – Fine to have on occasion. If buying pre-packaged, look for quality ingredients and try adding in hemp hearts, nuts, seeds, etc. to bump up the protein or try making your own. Regardless, be mindful of what you are topping them with and keep the focus on protein.

A NOTE ABOUT BREAD:

You can still lose weight while eating bread, however it can slow the process. If you choose to have it, look for sprouted grain breads or darker denser breads that are higher in protein and fiber and made with all-natural ingredients. Read the ingredients list rather than the nutritional label to make the best choice. Keep bread to a minimum and have it at breakfast OR lunch. Not both.

FREQUENTLY ASKED QUESTIONS

1. **Can I drink coffee or tea?**

   Yes, coffee and tea are totally fine to have.

2. **Does coffee and tea count towards water intake?**

   Yes, all beverages except for alcohol count towards water intake.

3. **Can I have cream and sugar in my coffee?**

Yes, you can have cream or creamers. Look for ones that contain all-natural ingredients. Sugar is fine, you can also use honey or maple syrup.

4. **Can I have stevia or monk fruit sweetener?**

It's best to keep artificial sweeteners to a minimum. Stevia and monk fruit are better quality options if you do choose to use them.

5. **Do I have to be consistent with eating or not eating breakfast?**

No, you can eat breakfast some days and choose to not have it other days. Although it is still a benefit to start your day with a higher protein breakfast.

6. **Can I have protein shakes?**

When trying to lose weight, you want your body to work hard to digest and process its food. It is hard to gauge satiety levels with liquid nutrients, so it is best to avoid protein shakes in the first few weeks of the Program. If you choose to keep them in, be sure to use protein powder that contains all-natural ingredients and is low in sugar. Add little to no fruit and add in some healthy fat like avocado, nut butter, coconut oil etc.

Please take the time to head over to the Facebook Group or the Livy Method App and watch the quick video that accompanies this post.

LET'S TALK FRUIT SNACK

Why you need to have it and why you cannot add anything to it.

SNACK #1: FRUIT ON ITS OWN

Normally, it is a good idea to combine carbohydrates with a protein and fat which feed into your satiety hormones and help minimize the amount of insulin needed to convert the food you eat into energy.

Which may have you wondering why you are eating the fruit on its own?

Why fruit and why on its own?

Whether you have breakfast or not, by mid-morning, your glycogen (energy) reserves start to deplete. The goal is to replenish those energy stores as quickly as possible, before your body needs to utilize your fat reserves, which is something you are trying to avoid. So by having fruit on its own, you are able to replenish those stores easily.

In the weeks to come, you will be making changes to your morning snack, but for now, you want to stick to having fruit on its own.

When it comes to what fruit is best, that's up to you; no fruit is off limits. You can have one or any combination of fruits. Fruit cups, frozen fruit, and applesauce are fine as long as they have no added sugar. Bananas are a little higher in sugar but are a great addition for anyone who is more active.

When it comes to portions, there is no need to count, weigh or measure! You want to eat enough to feel satisfied in the moment. If you are not hungry, it is still important to have a few token amounts of your snack (4-5 bites with chewing in between).

FREQUENTLY ASKED QUESTIONS

1. **Can I eat frozen or canned fruit for the fruit snack?**

    Yes. If you choose canned or frozen, look for all natural with no added sugar.

2. **If I have fruit with breakfast, do I still need to eat fruit for the morning snack?**

    Yes. Fruit should be eaten on its own, mid-morning, regardless of whether or not you had some at breakfast.

3. **Can I have dried fruit for the fruit snack?**

    It's not ideal but if you are in a pinch, such as on the road and stuck without any other option, it's fine once in a while.

4. **Can I have more than one type of fruit, like a fruit salad?**

    Yes, any combination of fruit is fine.

Please take the time to head over to the Facebook Group or the Livy Method App and watch the quick video that accompanies this post.

LET'S TALK LUNCH

Where vegetables are the star of the show and why it's not about having salads every day.

Think of vegetables as being the focus of the meal and build your lunch around them. Follow the guidelines of vegetables, protein, leafy greens, healthy fats, and add starchy vegetables and grains if needed. You can do this by way of soups, stews, stir-fry, curries, straight up or in a salad. If you choose to have salad, be sure to load it up with vegetables and make it as nutrient rich as possible.

LUNCH: VEGETABLES ARE THE FOCUS WITH PROTEIN, LEAFY GREENS, HEALTHY FATS AND HEAVIER CARBS IF YOU FEEL THE NEED FOR THEM.

Vegetables: The focus of the meal. You will want to make sure that there are more vegetables than anything else on your plate. Any vegetables will work, cooked or raw.

Side note: Leafy greens do not count as vegetables on this plan, so if you are having a salad be sure to load up on vegetables.

Protein: The source of protein is your choice, for example, you can have meat, eggs, fish or seafood, or any vegetable protein you wish (see the Let's Talk Groceries post for more options). If using plant protein as your main source, be sure to combine a variety of proteins to ensure you are getting enough to feel satisfied.

Leafy Greens: Packed with nutrients and beneficial to the detoxification process, when it comes to leafy greens, you can have them raw or cooked and choose from a wide variety (see Let's Talk Groceries for options).

Healthy Fats: Add healthy fats to your lunch at will to bump up the nutrient value and give you more sustaining energy throughout the day by feeding into your satiety hormones (see Let's Talk Groceries for options).

Heavier Carbohydrates: If you feel you need a little more "oomph", this is also when you might want to add in some heavier carbohydrates such as whole grains like rice or quinoa or starchy vegetables like potatoes or squash. These carbohydrates are better eaten at lunch so your body has the day to utilize the energy from them.

When it comes to portions, there is no need to count, weigh or measure! You want to eat enough to feel satisfied in the moment. If you are not hungry, it is still important to have a few token amounts of your lunch. (4-5 bites with chewing in between).

LUNCH MEAL IDEAS

Salad – When having a salad, make sure it is as nutrient rich as possible and includes the components you need. Load up your salads with lots of veggies, proteins of your choice and healthy fats.

Soup, Stew, Chili, Curry, Stir Fry – These one-pot wonders can be a life saver! You can make big batches and freeze for quick and easy meals.

Lettuce Wraps – Use large lettuce leaves, collard greens or other leafy greens to wrap up your fave sandwich fillings. Perfect for on the go!

Leftovers From Dinner – Use your leftovers for a quick and easy lunch.

Keep it Simple – You can toss some snack-like things into a container or onto a plate. Mix and match veggies and dip, pickles or fermented foods, proteins of your choice like meat, boiled eggs, beans, and healthy fats such as avocados or olives. Add a few green leaves and you're all set!

Don't Like to Cook or Don't Have Time? – There are lots of prepared foods that can work with the Program. Check for quality ingredients, avoiding things like partially/hydrogenated oil, artificial flavours and colours. Check the freezer section, the soup aisle, and the ready-made foods for some good options.

FREQUENTLY ASKED QUESTIONS

1. **Do I have to have salad every day?**

   Definitely not. You can have a vegetable heavy lunch prepared any way you like. Soup, stir fry, roasted vegetables, raw vegetables etc. with added protein, leafy greens and healthy fats.

2. **Can I add fruit at lunch?**

   Yes, you can. Just keep it minimal, for example, berries on a salad. Also, avoid using fruit as a dessert.

3. **What if I'm on the road and have to stop at a fast food restaurant?**

   Most fast food places have healthier options such as salads, soups, chilis, etc. These are your best bets. Make the best choice based on what is available.

4. **Can I use rice paper wrappers or rice noodles?**

   Rice paper wrappers are fine to use. However, we suggest keeping rice noodles to a minimum.

Please take the time to head over to the Facebook Group or the Livy Method App and watch the quick video that accompanies this post.

LET'S TALK VEGETABLE SNACK

Vegetables can be hard to digest, which makes them the perfect food for stimulating your digestive system, especially after eating a larger meal at lunch.

SNACK #2: VEGETABLE SNACK

Although it is ideal to eat them raw, if you find you get bloated or have a hard time digesting them, you can cook or steam your vegetables.

You can have any vegetables, in any combination. You do not need to worry about getting in a huge variety. You can also have pickles or fermented foods like kimchi or sauerkraut for your vegetable snack.

You could also do a salad and use leafy greens as long as it is loaded up with vegetables. If you add vegetables to lunch, you will still need to have them for your afternoon snack.

As a compliment and to bump up the nutrient value of your vegetables, you can add protein and fat by way of natural dressings, dips like hummus or guacamole, cheese, olives or nut butter. Keep in mind that vegetables should be the focus.

When it comes to portions, there is no need to count, weigh or measure! You want to eat enough to feel satisfied in the moment. If you are not hungry, it is still important to have a few token amounts of your snack. (4-5 bites with chewing in between.)

FREQUENTLY ASKED QUESTIONS

1. **Do I have to eat my vegetable snack if I'm still full from lunch?**

   Yes, it is key to get in all meals and snacks. If you are not hungry, you still want to eat a token amount, 4-5 bites to stimulate digestion.

2. **Can I have a dip with my veggies?**

   Yes, you can use dips or have with cheese, nut butter, olives, or any type of healthy fat.

3. **Can I have sauerkraut or kimchi for my vegetable snack?**

   Yes, fermented foods are excellent for gut health and considered a raw vegetable on plan.

4. **Can I have pickles for the vegetable snack?**

   Yes, any kind of pickled vegetables work for the vegetable snack.

Please take the time to head over to the Facebook Group or the Livy Method App and watch the quick video that accompanies this post.

LET'S TALK NUTS AND SEEDS SNACK

Nuts and seeds can be very hard to digest, even harder than raw vegetables, which is why they make the perfect second afternoon snack.

SNACK #3: NUTS AND/OR SEEDS

Around 3-4pm, the body is naturally wired to take a dip in energy. Because most of us can't just take a nap during the day, this is where people go looking for sugar or caffeine as a pick-me-up.

By adding in the nuts and or seeds, you are keeping your digestive system stimulated and working hard, which helps to keep your energy up. The protein and fat from the nuts and seeds will feed into your satiety hormones, providing you with sustaining energy, which will leave you feeling more satisfied and help prevent you from overeating your dinner.

You can have nuts or seeds or a combination of both. Keep the number of nuts you eat to approximately 25 pieces and seeds to one shot glass full, give or take. Nuts and seeds can be very hard to digest and eating too many can lead to digestive upset. However, if you need to add more to feel satisfied, feel free to add more.

Nuts and seeds are ideally eaten with no added ingredients, such as added oils or sugars. You could have them roasted or raw, and ideally you want to avoid any added oil. If you find them hard to digest, you can soak them.

You can also add nuts and/or seeds to your meals. If you do, keep in mind you will still need to eat your nut and seed snack.

The nut and seed snack does not have an equal alternative, so it is best to make a point of eating it unless you are allergic. If this is the case, you can substitute with olives, beans, or dairy.

FREQUENTLY ASKED QUESTIONS

1.   **What if I have problems digesting nuts and seeds?**

     If you have trouble digesting nuts and seeds you can soak and/or roast them to make them easier to digest.

2.   **What if I'm allergic to nuts?**

     If you can't eat nuts due to allergies, you can stick to seeds. If you can't have either due to allergies or preparation for a procedure, the alternatives are dairy, such as cheese or yogurt, olives, or beans like chickpeas, edamame, black beans etc.

     Please Note: these alternatives are to be used as a last resort as nuts and/or seeds are the best choice.

3. **Do I eat both nuts and seeds or just one?**

You can have one or the other, or both.

Please take the time to head over to the Facebook Group or the Livy Method App and watch the quick video that accompanies this post.

LET'S TALK DINNER

Given that it's at the end of the day, try to think of dinner as more of a top-up rather than a need for fuel which is why the goal is to minimize any heavier carbohydrates, like grains and starchy vegetables, and focus on protein.

Use the guideline of protein being the star of the show, with vegetables, leafy greens, and healthy fats. Protein being the focus of this meal along with added fat, will feed into your satiety hormones, keeping you more satisfied throughout the evening and into the night.

DINNER: PROTEIN IS THE FOCUS WITH VEGETABLES, LEAFY GREENS, AND HEALTHY FATS.

If you find yourself extra hungry for dinner, make sure that you are eating breakfast, along with all of your other meals and snacks and making them as nutrient rich as possible. Alternatively, if you are not hungry for dinner, it is still best to have a small portion of it.

Dinner can be in any combination like soup, stew, stir fry, chili, salad etc. You can use sauces, dressings, gravy, condiments, and spices and can be used at will; just look for natural ingredients and avoid anything artificial. You can also use flour in your recipes and use it for things like breading.

Avoid using things like yogurts and oatmeal for dinner but you can still use breakfast foods like eggs, making sure to incorporate the vegetables and greens.

If using plant protein as your main source, be sure to combine a variety of proteins to ensure you are getting enough to feel satisfied.

You can add heavier carbohydrates, like rice and quinoa, or starchy vegetables, like potatoes or squash to dinner if you feel you need them. For example, if you are very active in the evening (ie. playing a sport or going to the gym). Otherwise, it's best to keep them to a minimum.

In terms of the timing of dinner, it is best to eat as early in your evening as possible. Eating too late will prevent the body from following through on its wind-down process, which can mess with your body's ability to get the deep and REM sleep it needs to make change.

When it comes to portions, there is no need to count, weigh or measure! You want to eat enough to feel satisfied in the moment. If you are not hungry, it is still important to have a few token amounts of your dinner (4-5 bites with chewing in between).

After dinner snack: It is best to avoid snacking after dinner. If you need something to take the edge off as the body adjusts to the new Food Plan, an option is to have some air popped popcorn with butter and sea salt if you like. We suggest eliminating this altogether by Week 2.

You can also try having herbal teas in the evening which can be helpful when breaking the nighttime snacking habit.

DINNER MEAL IDEAS

Meat, Poultry, Fish or Seafood – Grill it, bake it, bread it (yes you can use breading!), fry it (yes you can fry it too!). Add your favourite vegetables on the side with some leafy greens (cooked or raw) and don't forget to add in some healthy fats.

Tofu, Tempeh, Beans and Lentils – If you are looking for plant-based protein, there are a lot of great options. Marinated tofu or tempeh can be grilled, baked, or fried. Try sautéing some beans or lentils with veggies or make soup or chili.

Eggs – Eggs make for a quick and easy dinner. Prepare them the way you like, with some sautéed vegetables and a salad on the side. For example, an omelet with leafy greens and vegetables covers all the bases.

Curry, Chili, Soup, Stew, Stir Fry – Keep them protein and vegetable based and minimize any heavier carbs. So, if you are used to having rice with your curries and stir fries, try using cauliflower rice instead.

Spaghetti Sauce – Have on top of zucchini noodles, cauliflower rice or spaghetti squash instead of pasta and be sure to make protein the focus.

Tacos – Put all your favourite taco fillings on a bed of leafy greens or in a lettuce or collard green wrap instead of a taco shell or tortilla.

Rotisserie Chicken – It's an easy and convenient option. Add veggies and greens and you're good to go!.

Don't Like to Cook or Don't Have Time? – When buying prepared foods or ordering in, look for good quality and foods that fit into the Food Plan.

FREQUENTLY ASKED QUESTIONS

1. **Can I use frozen vegetables?**

   Yes, they are great for convenience. Canned ones are also fine.

2. **What about plant-based meat substitutes like Beyond Meat?**

   You can but be mindful that many contain processed ingredients. Whole foods are best.

3. **Can I cook with oil?**

   Yes, you can use butter and/or oil. Choose higher quality oils such as olive oil, avocado oil, and coconut oil.

4. **Can I have potatoes or rice with dinner?**

   You can if you feel you need them, although these starchy carbohydrates are best eaten at lunch.

5. **Can I have pasta made with konjac, black beans, quinoa etc.**

Best to avoid any kind of pasta. Even when made with other ingredients it is still a processed product and not a whole food.

6. **Can I have breakfast foods for dinner?**

When it comes to eggs or things like tofu or beans then yes. But things like yogurt, cereals and oatmeal are not the best options for dinner.

7. **Can I have wine with dinner?**

Yes, alcohol is totally fine to have. Drink extra water to compensate for dehydration.

8. **Can I use flour to thicken a sauce?**

Yes, a small amount of flour for thickening is totally fine.

9. **Can I eat breaded meats, vegetables etc.?**

Yes, breading is fine.

10. **When is the best time to eat dinner?**

You want to eat dinner as early in the evening as possible and ideally before it starts getting dark or soon after.

11. **What if I'm not hungry for dinner?**

You still want to have a token amount of food, even if you are not hungry.

Please take the time to head over to the Facebook Group or the Livy Method App and watch the quick video that accompanies this post.

LUNCH AND DINNER VISUAL GUIDELINE

Do not take this too literally. Keep in mind that this is meant as a visual guideline. You don't want you to start counting, weighing, or measuring your food.

This is to help you put your meals together when it comes to the components you need, like proteins and vegetables, depending on the focus of the meal, along with leafy greens, healthy fats and any heavier carbs while following the basic Food Plan.

Keep in mind that your body's needs change day to day. The goal is to be in tune to that, so when it comes to portions, they are always based on what they feel like and never what they look like.

There are times that this visual guideline will not apply, for example when eating chili, stew, soup or stir fry. Just be sure to include the components required at each meal.

Note About "Grains as Needed" - This will become easier to gauge as you progress through the Program. If you are feeling like you need a little more "oomph" to your meal, be sure to make your foods as nutrient rich as possible and add in any heavier carbs or starchy vegetables as needed.

Note About "Healthy Fats at Will" - Healthy fats like added oils, avocado, nuts, seeds, dairy and dressings should be added to meals as they help to bump up the nutrient value and feed into your satiety hormones, which will have you feeling more satisfied.

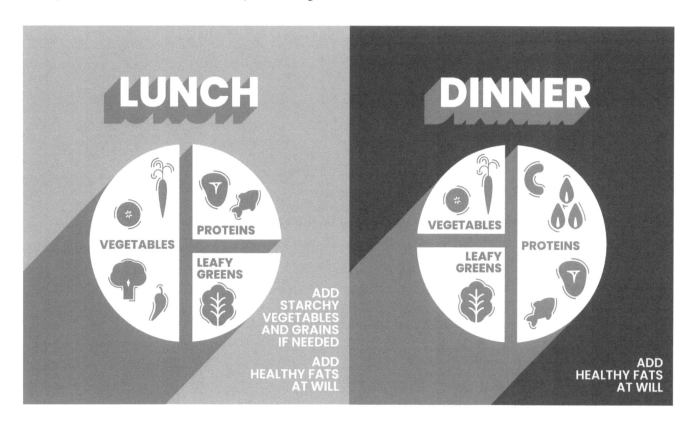

LET'S TALK PROTEINS CARBS AND FATS

Here is a brief outline and breakdown of proteins, carbs and fats.

Please note: You do not need to worry about percentages or serving sizes while following the Program. This is just to give you examples of what foods fall under each category.

SOURCES OF CARBOHYDRATES (foods that break down into energy)

- Fruits
- Vegetables
- Starchy vegetables like potatoes, squash, cassava, plantain
- Naturally occurring sugar, found in things like beans and lentils and chickpeas
- Rice and grains like black rice, quinoa, barley, and buckwheat
- Oatmeal and cereals
- High fiber crackers and dark, dense, or sprouted grain breads

SOURCES OF PROTEIN (feeds the muscles helping to repair and rebuild along with maintaining and building muscle mass)

- Meat (Any kind, including organ meat)
- Eggs
- Fish
- Seafood
- Beans, lentils, legumes
- Nuts (all)
- Seeds (all, including hemp hearts and chia seeds)
- Dairy - cheese, yogurt, milk products (not to be used as a main source)
- Tofu

PLANT PROTEIN

As you can see below, there is protein found in lots of things besides animal sources.

- Broccoli - 2.6g per 1 cup
- Asparagus - 2.4g per 1 cup
- Peas - 9g per 1 cup
- Cauliflower - 2g per 1 cup

- Brussels - 3g per 1 cup

- Bok choy-1g per 1 cup

- Spinach, collard greens - 1g per 1 cup

- Mung bean sprouts - 2.5g per 1 cup

- Beans (kidney, pinto, black beans, chickpeas etc.) - 7.5g per 1/2 cup

- Lentils - 9g per 1/2 cup

- Quinoa - 4g per 1/2 cup

- Tempeh - 11g per 1/2 cup

- Tofu - 7g per 1/2 cup

- Buckwheat - 6g per 1 cup

- Soybeans/Edamame - 10g per 1/2 cup

- Rice - 7g per 1 cup

- Hemp seeds - 10g per 3 tbsp

- Pumpkin seeds - 5g per oz

- Chia - 4g per 2 tbsp

- Nut butter -15g per 2 tbsp

- Hummus - 7g per 2 tbsp

- Spirulina - 4g per 1 tbsp

Keep in mind you DO NOT need to worry about these measurements. They are for reference only and to point out the fact that some proteins have carbs in them, some vegetables have protein in them, and that protein adds up.

As long as you are following the Program as outlined, you are getting enough and the right mix of everything you need.

SOURCES OF FATS (essential for cellular function, providing alternative energy and brain fuel)

- Fish/Fish oil

- Omega 3 and or 369

- Oils like olive oil, coconut oil, avocado oil, grape seed oil, flax and hemp oil

- Salad dressings made with good quality oils

- Olives

- Avocado

- Nuts (all)

- Seeds (all, including hemp hearts and chia seeds)
- Dairy

This is not a complete list, it is just to give you an idea of the kind of foods suggested when talking about incorporating proteins, carbs and fats to your meals.

Please take the time to head over to the Facebook Group or the Livy Method App and watch the quick video that accompanies this post.

LET'S TALK LEAFY GREENS

With all of the changes you are making in your diet, leafy greens are an ideal addition to meals as they provide the roughage your body needs to process food through your digestive system.

Leafy greens are also packed with tons of nutrients that are great for your health and cellular function and an excellent source of fiber. They also help to increase the Glucagon-like-Peptide-1 hormone that keeps blood sugar more stable and can help keep you more satisfied.

Leafy greens can be added to meals raw, like in a salad, but also cooked or sautéed and/or added to soups, stews and stir fry.

Tips for Adding in Leafy Greens:

- Have a side salad.

- Add any leafy green to your bowl or plate and add the rest (such as a soup) on top.

- Add leafy greens to the recipe such as in a soup, stew, chili or stir fry that doesn't include it. A handful of baby spinach and you are done!

- Simply pop a handful into your mouth and away you go!

- Use them as a wrap.

- Sauté a bunch of heartier greens such as kale, collard greens, Swiss chard, bok choy, etc. with some butter and garlic and keep in the fridge to add to any meal.

If you are not a fan of eating your leafy greens, it is still key to get them in. You don't have to be fancy about it or get in a huge variety. It's also not a big deal if you are a bit hit and miss getting them in, as long as you are mindful to be as consistent as possible.

Although they are suggested at lunch and dinner, leafy greens can also be added to breakfast or to the afternoon vegetable snack.

Please note: Leafy greens are not considered a vegetable on plan. An exception would be Brussels sprouts, cabbage and bok choy, among others which are listed in the Let's Talk Groceries post, that are also classified as veg and can be used as one or the other or both in your meals.

Please take the time to head over to the Facebook Group or the Livy Method App and watch the quick video that accompanies this post.

LET'S TALK GROCERIES

This is just to give you an idea of the types of foods you can incorporate into your meals and snacks while following the Food Plan.

Keep in mind that this is not an exhaustive list. This list does not include condiments or spices, which you are free to use.

PROTEIN

Protein is needed at breakfast, lunch and dinner so consider each meal when making your shopping list.

ANIMAL

- Beef (all cuts)
- Canned meat/fish
- Chicken (all cuts, with or without skin)
- Eggs
- Fish (all types)
- Game Meats
- Pork (all cuts)
- Turkey (all cuts, with or without skin)
- Seafood (all types)

PLANT BASED

If using plant protein as your main source, be sure to combine a variety of proteins to ensure you are getting enough to feel satisfied.

- Beans/Chickpeas
- Edamame Beans (higher protein veg)
- Lentils
- Nut Butters (all)
- Nutritional Yeast
- Nuts (all)
- Seeds (all, including hemp hearts and chia seeds)
- Sprouts (higher protein veg)
- Tempeh
- Tofu

KEEP TO A MINIMUM

- Bacon (any kind)
- Deli Meats
- Sausages

If consuming processed meat, look for quality ingredients.

FRUIT

Literally ANY kind of fruit will work while following the Program. Fresh fruit is best but frozen and canned are fine as well. Canned fruit should be without added sugar.

- Apples
- Apricots
- Bananas
- Berries (all)
- Cherries
- Cranberries (fresh)
- Dates (fresh & Medjool)
- Fresh figs
- Grapefruit
- Grapes
- Kiwi
- Lemons
- Limes
- Mango
- Melons (all)
- Nectarines
- Oranges (all types)
- Papaya
- Peaches
- Pears
- Pineapple
- Plums
- Pomelo
- Pomegranate

VEGETABLES

Any and all vegetables are on plan. Here are just a few examples.

- Artichokes
- Asparagus
- Beets
- Bell Peppers
- Bok Choy
- Broccoli
- Broccoli Rabe/ Rapini
- Brussels sprouts
- Cabbage
- Carrots
- Cauliflower
- Celeriac/Celery Root
- Celery
- Corn
- Cucumber
- Edamame Beans
- Eggplant
- Fennel
- Fiddleheads
- Green beans
- Green Peas (all types)
- Hearts of palm
- Hot Peppers (all)
- Jicama
- Kimchi
- Kohlrabi
- Leeks/Scallions
- Mushrooms (all)
- Onions (all)
- Pickled Vegetables (all)
- Radishes
- Rhubarb
- Sauerkraut
- Split Peas
- Sprouts
- Summer Squash (For example, zucchini, crookneck, pattypan and yellow)
- Tomatoes
- Turnip & Rutabaga
- Water Chestnuts

STARCHY VEGETABLES (IDEALLY ADDED AT LUNCH WHEN NEEDED)

- Cassava
- Parsnips
- Plantain
- Potatoes
- Sweet potatoes/Yams
- Winter squash (For example, butternut, acorn, pumpkin, spaghetti squash)
- Yucca

VEGETABLES THAT ALSO DOUBLE AS LEAFY GREENS

Some vegetables can work as the veg and leafy green component in your meals.

- Bok Choy
- Brussels sprouts
- Cabbage
- Chinese Broccoli
- Fiddleheads
- Kimchi
- Rapini
- Sauerkraut

LEAFY GREENS

Any leafy green works and can be eaten raw or cooked.

- Arugula
- Bok Choy
- Brussels Sprouts
- Cabbage
- Chinese Broccoli
- Collard Greens
- Endive
- Fiddleheads
- Iceberg lettuce
- Kale
- Leaf Lettuce
- Mustard Greens
- Radicchio
- Rapini
- Romaine lettuce
- Salad Mixes (all)
- Seaweed
- Spinach
- Spring Mix
- Swiss Chard
- Watercress

GRAINS

Whole Grains are best added to lunch if you feel the need to have a little more substance. You can have them at dinner as well but keep the portion size small. Only use as needed.

Oats and high protein grain cereals are fine to have at breakfast with added hemp hearts, nuts and seeds or quality protein powder, to boost protein.

- Amaranth
- Barley
- Buckwheat
- Bulgur (cracked wheat)
- Farro
- Millet
- Oats - Add extra protein when having for breakfast.
- Rice – black, red, wild, brown, white or brown basmati
- Sorghum
- Teff
- Quinoa

DAIRY

Avoid low or no-fat dairy products as these tend to have more additives. Best to avoid artificial flavours, colours, or sweeteners.

When it comes to percentage of milk fat, that is your personal preference.

Dairy can be used as a main source of protein at breakfast but not at lunch or dinner. However, it can be used to bump up the nutrient value of your meals and vegetable snack by ways of dips, dressings, added cheeses and such.

When it comes to cheese, there are far too many to list. All cheese is fine as long as it isn't processed or containing artificial colours or flavours.

- Blue cheese
- Bocconcini
- Brie
- Butter
- Camembert
- Cottage Cheese
- Cream (any fat %)
- Cream cheese (no artificial flavours)
- Feta
- Goat's cheese
- Gouda
- Havarti
- Kefir
- Manchego
- Milk (any fat %)
- Mozzarella
- Non-dairy milk (all)
- Non-dairy yogurts
- Parmesan
- Provolone
- Sour cream
- Swiss
- White cheddar
- Yogurt (any kind)

FATS

Healthy fats are important to incorporate into your meals. Here are some examples of healthy fats to have on hand.

- Avocados
- Avocado Oil
- Butter
- Coconut
- Coconut Oil
- Cold pressed canola oil
- Extra Virgin Olive Oil
- Flax Oil
- Ghee/Clarified Butter
- Hemp Oil
- Nut Butters (all natural)
- Nut Oils
- Nuts (all types)
- Olives
- Seeds (all types, including hemp hearts and chia seeds)
- Sesame Oil

A NOTE ABOUT BREAD

You can still lose weight while eating bread, but it can slow the process. If you choose to have it, look for Ezekiel bread in the freezer section at your grocery or health food store. If you can't find Ezekiel, look for other sprouted grain breads or darker denser breads that are high in protein and fiber and made with all-natural ingredients. Keep it to a minimum and have it at breakfast OR lunch. Not both.

LET'S TALK WATER

Making sure you are properly hydrated is one of the top things you can do to help maximize your efforts and support your body's needs while following the Program.

The Livy Method utilizes the body's natural detox process. Because the body releases fat when you poop, pee, breathe, and sweat, drinking enough water is key.

Recent studies suggest that the average person needs 2.7 - 3.5 litres of water at minimum for basic body functions like digestion, pumping blood through your veins, sweating, bowel movements etc. (Refer to original post in the Livy Method App or Facebook Support Group for source)

In order to optimize your body's ability to focus on fat loss while you are following The Livy Method, you will need to drink above and beyond what it needs for basic body functions.

Besides aiding in fat loss, being properly hydrated has many other health benefits such as:

- Increased energy and brain function
- Can help relieve constipation
- Increased cardiovascular health
- Increased function of muscles and joints
- Promotes healthy "glowing" skin
- Helps flush toxins from your organs
- Helps curb cravings, especially for sugar

SO HOW MUCH SHOULD YOU DRINK?

This is a simple question with no easy answer.

Everyone requires different amounts depending on individual needs. How much water you need day-to-day can also vary, depending on a variety of factors.

Start with the 2.7 – 3.5L suggested for basic body function and increase or decrease as needed. Play around with it to see what works for you, keeping in mind that your body's needs can change day-to-day.

Listed below are things to consider when assessing how much you need.

YOU NEED EXTRA WATER WHEN:

- You are taller than average (over 5'5" for women, 5'9" for men)
- You have weight to lose
- Your body is releasing fat

- When the scale is bouncing between the same 2 numbers
- You are fighting an illness
- You are menstruating
- You take medication that causes weight gain or dehydration
- You work or live in a dry environment
- You exercise or are active enough to sweat
- You drink alcohol
- You eat salty food

WHEN INCREASING WATER INTAKE:

- When increasing your water intake, be mindful to increase slowly. Start early and spread your water drinking throughout the day. Don't chug a large amount at once.
- To help achieve and maintain proper hydration levels, add a pinch of pink Himalayan, Celtic or Sea salt to your morning water, or add salt to your food. This will add in minerals and electrolytes as well as support hormone and adrenal function. Alternatively, you can purchase trace minerals to add to your water.

HOW DO YOU KNOW YOU ARE DRINKING ENOUGH?

- You no longer feel thirsty
- You no longer have a dry mouth or lips
- Your trips to the bathroom have decreased (they will increase until you are properly hydrated)
- Your sugar cravings are decreasing

DO YOU NEED TO WORRY ABOUT DRINKING TOO MUCH?

The goal when following the Program is to support your body's individual needs while focusing on fat loss. When it comes to water, it is about drinking enough, not just drinking more.

Overhydration and water intoxication happen when you drink more water than your kidneys can get rid of through urinating. You have a greater risk of developing water intoxication if you drink a lot of water in a short period of time. When you drink too much too fast, your kidneys have a hard time getting rid of the excess water.

Therefore, to avoid overhydration, you should not drink more than 1 litre of water per hour and be mindful to include salt in your diet or add in trace minerals to maintain proper sodium levels.

Refer to the post "Let's Talk Low Sodium" for more information. If you have any concerns, speak with your healthcare provider.

TIPS FOR GETTING IT IN:

- Have fun with it even though it can feel like work sometimes.

- Start drinking early in your day. Most people find it easier to get the majority of their water intake in the first half of the day.

- Sip, don't guzzle.

- Get a water bottle or cup that you enjoy drinking from.

- Track your water (and other fluids such as coffee, tea, bone broth) intake by using the Livy Method App.

- Set reminders to drink.

- Add fresh or frozen fruit, cucumber slices, and/or fresh herbs or ginger.

- Slow down your water intake in the evening if frequent trips to the bathroom tend to interrupt your sleep.

When it comes to how much water you need for your individual needs, beyond what is recommended, it is important to drink the amount that works best for you. Consult with your healthcare provider if you have any concerns.

On a final note: Tea, coffee, soups, and essentially any other liquid (except for alcohol) counts towards your water intake, although the majority of your fluid count should be water.

FREQUENTLY ASKED QUESTIONS

Here are some of our most popular questions asked about water.

1. **Why so much water?**

    Because of the nature of the Food Plan and eating so often in the first few weeks of the Program, along with the process of piggy-backing the body's natural detox response, making sure you are drinking enough water is essential in supporting your body's needs.

2. **Can I drink too much?**

    Yes, although you would have to drink an extreme amount of water in a very short period of time for there to be any detrimental side effects. Avoid drinking more than 1 litre per hour and sip instead of guzzling.

    When increasing your water intake, be sure to include enough salt to your diet or add trace minerals to your water to maintain proper fluid and electrolyte balance.

    When it comes to drinking water, it's not about drinking more and more, it's about drinking enough for your individual needs.

3. **Does it matter when I drink the water?**

    No, however it is best to start early and spread it out throughout the day.

4. **Will I always have to drink this much water?**

    Drinking enough water is necessary while you are trying to lose weight. When maintaining your weight, you can scale back to basic requirements. The amount of water you need will fluctuate from day-to-day both during and after weight loss.

5. **Can I add anything to my water?**

    Yes, you can add fresh or frozen fruit or vegetables, like cucumber slices, fresh herbs etc. Anything that is all natural, with no sugar or sweeteners added. Naturally flavoured teas can also be used.

6. **How should I keep track of my water intake?**

    There are many methods, so experiment to find out what works best for you. It's a great idea to use the Livy Method App to record your water intake. Some people use elastic bands on a water bottle or glass to keep track or fill a large container and pour their glasses from that each day.

7. **Do other drinks count towards water intake?**

    Yes, all drinks except alcohol count towards water intake.

8. **Should I buy a water filter?**

    This is a personal choice. It's up to you whether or not you want to use a filter or drink filtered water.

9. **Can I have carbonated or sparkling water?**

    Yes, although you want to avoid any added ingredients, like artificial flavours and sweeteners. Keep in mind that carbonated water can cause bloating and gassiness in some people, which can cause discomfort and interfere with hunger cues.

10. **Why am I thirsty and have dry lips and a pasty mouth even though I'm drinking more water than ever before?**

    This can be your body's way of communicating that you are not fully hydrated and still need to drink more water. It can also be a sign your weight is about to drop, so try increasing your water slightly by adding in a cup or two which can make all the difference. Keep in mind this can also be due to medications or underlying health issues.

Please take the time to head over to the Facebook Group or the Livy Method App and watch the quick video that accompanies this post.

LET'S TALK COFFEE

Coffee is totally fine to have while following the Program.

Here are a few things to note:

- You can drink as much coffee as you like, whenever you like, but try to avoid drinking it later in the day if it messes with your sleep.

- Best to wait 5-10 min to drink your coffee after your lemon water or apple cider vinegar, if you have added it to your morning routine.

- Even though it is a diuretic, coffee counts towards your fluid intake, just be sure not to use it as your main source.

- You can use any type of creamer you like, dairy or non-dairy. Look for naturally flavoured and be mindful of the amount of sugar that is added to some creamers.

- You can use sugar or natural sweeteners like honey or maple syrup.

- And when it comes to artificial sweeteners, stevia and monk fruit are the better quality ones on the market.

- Agave is super sweet and high in fructose, so if using use minimal amounts.

- For tea drinkers, the same rules apply.

It's worth noting that some coffees can be more like a dessert, but for the most part, you can enjoy your coffee any way you like; black, with cream, latte, cappuccino, espresso, Americano, etc., while keeping these things in mind.

Please take the time to head over to the Facebook Group or the Livy Method App and watch the quick video that accompanies this post.

LET'S TALK SHIFT WORK

Although it can be more challenging, it's key to note being a shift worker will not impact your ability to be successful in following the Program and reaching your goals.

HERE ARE SOME TIPS FOR WORKING OUT AN EATING SCHEDULE:

- The basic rule for shift workers when it comes to the Food Plan is to start your day from when you wake up, regardless of what time of day that might be.

- Even if it's 3am or 3pm, wake up and start your day with lemon water or ACV (if having), followed by your higher protein breakfast.

- If you are eating breakfast at 9pm you may be more inclined to have something like fish or chicken and vegetables as opposed to more "breakfast-y" type foods, and that's ok.

- Normally, you want to eat dinner shortly after it gets dark. However, if you are working the night shift, you ideally want to eat your last meal of the day at least 3 hours before you go to sleep.

LET'S TALK EXTENDED SHIFTS

If needed, you can extend your eating times by breaking your lunch and/or dinner portion into 2 servings. If you are working and awake for extended hours, it could look something like this:

- Breakfast
- Fruit
- 1/2 of lunch
- Other 1/2 of lunch
- Vegetable snack
- Nut/seeds snack
- 1/2 dinner
- Other 1/2 of dinner

This will have you eating 8 times a day so you can cover more hours.

Next week, we will be introducing Bonus Snacks that you can add in above and beyond the suggested meals and snacks to help with extending your day, instead of splitting up your meals. For now, follow the basic Food Plan as designed, as consistently as possible.

LET'S TALK NAPS

If your day is broken up by taking naps, you can insert them into your day and continue to follow the order of the Food Plan.

For example: If you get up at 9am but then go back to bed at 12pm, you can have breakfast and then fruit...then nap. Or just breakfast then nap, then fruit when you wake up. Regardless of when you wake up, continue with your day where you left off Food Plan wise.

This is how it can look:

- ACV/Lemon Water
- Breakfast
- Fruit Snack
- **Nap**
- Lunch
- Veg Snack
- Nuts/Seeds Snack
- **Nap**
- Dinner

Working shift work can throw off your body's natural circadian rhythm, which in turn can cause you to be extra tired.

When tired, the body looks for pick-me-ups like carbs, caffeine, and sugar. This is generally a sign the body is asking for more water. Making water your focus will not only help with your energy levels but will also help to decrease any cravings, helping you stay on track. The more routine you can be following the Food Plan and drinking enough water, the better.

As you progress through the Program, you will become more in-tune with your hunger levels, you will notice some days you will feel hungrier than others. When working the night shift, for example, you may find your appetite is much lighter compared to the day, which is normal. Just be sure to continue to have token amounts of each meal and snack if you are not hungry.

It might take you a while to find the right balance. Play around with the timing until you find what works best for you.

Please take the time to head over to the Facebook Group or the Livy Method App and watch the quick video that accompanies this post.

LET'S TALK NUTRIENT RICH MEALS

While following the Food Plan, the goal is to eat all your meals and snacks and make them nutrient rich. Let's talk about what that really means.

When it comes to making your food choices nutrient rich, it's about adding in nourishing whole foods that give the body what it needs in terms of vitamins, minerals and healthy fats.

For example, when having a salad you want to avoid having just lettuce with some chicken on it. Be mindful to add in other nutrient rich ingredients, like the ones listed below.

Let's break down a salad:

- Spring mix/leafy greens = roughage + vitamins + minerals
- Variety of vegetables = energy + fiber + vitamins
- Chicken = protein
- Avocado = energy + healthy fat + potassium + fiber
- Feta cheese = energy + healthy fat + protein
- Nuts and Seeds = energy + healthy fat + protein
- An all-natural vinaigrette or dressing = healthy fat when made with good quality oils

This salad loaded up with all the fixings, not only provides a variety of nutrients, but is also more sustaining as nutrient rich meals provide longer lasting energy.

Just adding in one or two extra things like a drizzle of olive oil, a different type of vegetable, or a few nuts can make all the difference. Keep in mind this can be applied to any meal, prepared in any way.

EASY THINGS TO HAVE ON HAND THAT CAN QUICKLY INCREASE THE NUTRIENT VALUE

Here are some great items to have on hand for quick and easy ways to level up your meals:

- Pickled and marinated vegetables like artichoke hearts, pickled beets, roasted red peppers, etc.
- Salsa
- Hemp hearts
- Nuts and/or seeds
- Nut butters
- Hummus
- Nutritional Yeast
- Protein powder

- Cheese or other dairy such as yogurt or cream

- Natural oils, dressings and dips

- Olives

- Coconut milk

- Avocados

- Condiments and spices

Bumping up the nutrient value of your meals is not only a great way to give the body what it needs, it can also help give you more sustaining energy which has you feeling more satisfied with smaller portions.

Please take the time to head over to the Facebook Group or the Livy Method App and watch the quick video that accompanies this post.

LET'S TALK PORTIONS

Because we don't count, weigh and measure our food, you may be wondering how we are going to address portions.

By following the Food Plan and spreading out the number of times you are eating each day and by focusing on giving your body what it needs by making your food choices nutrient rich, you will find your body will naturally start to adjust and reduce the amount of food it is used to consuming to feel satisfied.

Within days to a few weeks you will notice you will start to feel more satisfied with smaller portions and your cravings will reduce and even start to go away.

This is why being as consistent as possible when following the Food Plan is key. Be sure to eat all your meals and snacks and still have token amounts when you are not hungry, make your food choices as nutrient rich as possible and eat to satisfaction.

Portion wise the goal for the next few weeks is to follow the Food Plan as designed and eat to feel satisfied in the moment. If you are unsure of what that means or what eating to satisfaction feels like for you…just don't try to eat less right now.

With this process we measure portions by what they feel like and never what they look like. Your body's needs can change day to day which can affect your hunger levels, so one day you may feel you need more portion wise, and the next day less. As we move forward in the Program we are going to work to be more in-tune to your body's changing needs and hunger levels.

For example one day you may need one egg to feel satisfied for breakfast, and then the next day you might need to eat three eggs to feel satisfied.

There will also be times where you may find you are not hungry at all for some of your meals or snacks. This is normal, however, you will still want to have token amounts (4-5 bites) as your body adjusts to the Food Plan.

When it comes to portions, avoid the temptation of trying to eat less for the sake of losing like you may have done while following other diets. While the focus is on losing weight, right now it's important to consistently give the body what it needs to address its needs so it no longer feels the need to store fat.

You will also want to avoid trying to eat more to avoid feeling hungry later. The goal is to eat enough to feel satisfied in the moment. You may find you feel hungry in between meals and snacks, this is normal as your body adjusts.

With that said, if you are unsure of what eating to feel satisfied means to you, it's better to give your body more of what it needs rather than less. You will not gain weight while following the program. Rest assured while your body is adjusting to the food plan you may see fluctuations on the scale, but this is expected and normal.

The more consistent you can be, the quicker your body can adjust and the sooner you will start to see and feel results.

Moving forward in the weeks to come we will be working towards becoming more in-tune to portions and your body's needs. We will be addressing hunger levels and portion sizes in a variety of different ways by switching up the focus and making changes to the Food Plan week to week.

This will include bringing awareness to portions by asking 4 mindfulness questions in Week 3, down-sizing portions in Weeks 4 and 6, along with splitting up meals and snacks in Weeks 7 and 8. Week 9 has us revamping the Food Plan and then moving forward you will work to get even more in-tune to your body's needs.

The ultimate goal is to get you to a place where you are in tune with when to eat, what to eat and how much you need to eat to help your body focus on fat loss, so you can reach your goal weight and move on from losing weight Finally & Forever.

There will be much to cover, discuss and accomplish over the 3 Months. For now, focus on taking things day by day and being as consistent as possible with the changes you need to make in these first few weeks.

Please take the time to head over to the Facebook Group or the Livy Method App and watch the quick video that accompanies this post.

LET'S TALK BREAD, PASTA, FLOUR AND CRACKERS

It is important to note that this Program is not low carb. The focus is on eating the right carbs at the right time, which is why we include lots of energy foods like vegetables, fruits, grains and starchy vegetables while following the Food Plan.

However, when it comes to weight loss and this process, we consider bread, pasta, flour, and crackers to be processed foods. You can eat them, but it can slow down the process, so it is best to keep them to a minimum.

By following the Food Plan you are trying to decrease the amount of insulin your body is used to using. Bread, pasta, flour and crackers in general, require more insulin than whole foods when the body breaks them down, regardless of the type or source. While trying to lose weight, you want to decrease and balance out blood sugar levels, so adding them in can be counterproductive.

BREAD

If you are going to have bread, it is best eaten at breakfast or lunch, but not both.

The best choice is Ezekiel Bread which is a high quality, sprouted grain bread that does not contain any flour and is free of any preservatives and sugar. It is usually found in the fridge or freezer section of most grocery stores.

Ezekiel Bread ingredient list: *Organic Sprouted Wheat, Filtered Water, Organic Sprouted Barley, Organic Sprouted Millet, Organic Malted Barley, Organic Sprouted Lentils, Organic Sprouted Soybeans, Organic Sprouted Spelt, Fresh Yeast, Organic Wheat Gluten, Sea Salt.*

If you cannot find Ezekiel, and choose to keep bread in your diet, look for other sprouted grain options or breads that are dark, dense, grainy, and seedy. Go for high fiber and quality ingredients.

PASTA

When it comes to pasta, it is best to leave it out or keep it to a minimum. Although pastas made with alternative flours such as chickpea, black bean or konjak are better choices than ones made with wheat flour, it is still recommended to keep those to a minimum as well.

FLOUR

Small amounts of flour used for breading or thickening a soup or sauce is totally fine as a small quantity won't have the same effect on your blood sugar levels.

CRACKERS

When it comes to crackers, you also want to keep those to a minimum. If you choose to keep it in, we recommend having high fiber crackers, like Ryvita. These crackers have a short ingredient list, contain whole grains, and are high in fiber.

RYVITA MULTI-GRAIN CRISPBREAD INGREDIENTS:

Whole grain rye flour, Toasted grains and seeds (buckwheat, soy meal, sesame seeds, flaxseed, kibbled rye), Rye bran, Salt.

Mary's Super Seed Crackers are a good gluten free alternative for those of you who can't digest gluten. If you cannot find these brands specifically, look for crackers with similar ingredients.

Please note: Some people can continue to eat bread, pasta, flour and crackers and still lose weight, but if you are looking to maximize your efforts you might want to consider limiting or skipping them altogether. If you prefer to take a more relaxed approach and leave these things in, that is fine. However, if you find that your weight is not dropping, you may want to consider taking them out at some point.

We understand that bread and pasta are convenient, easy, and taste great and we know you might miss having them. Keep in mind that this Program is not a "lifestyle", it is about making a concentrated effort to lose as much weight as possible in the healthiest way possible in the time frame we have.

The goal here is to lose weight in a way that is going to be easy to maintain where you will be able to enjoy all of the foods you love after you reach your goal.

LET'S TALK CONDIMENTS

Condiments can be a great way to not only add flavour, but also add in nutrient value to your meals and snacks.

For the most part, condiments are fine to use. Be mindful to look for natural ingredients and avoid the following:

- Artificial flavour
- Artificial colour
- Partially/hydrogenated oil

This applies to sauces, dressing, gravies, dips, and all condiments in general. Use as you wish to flavour and enhance your foods.

Please take the time to head over to the Facebook Group or the Livy Method App and watch the quick video that accompanies this post.

LET'S TALK DAIRY

If you don't consume dairy, that's okay. You do not need to eat it or add it in. If you do, here are a few things to keep in mind.

LET'S TALK ABOUT CHEESE

When can you have it?

- You can have cheese with any of your meals. It can also be added to your veg snack, just make sure vegetables are the main component.

How much can you have?

- As with all meals and snacks you are to eat to satisfaction. So, when adding cheese to your meal, eat to feel satisfied.

What kinds of cheese can you have?

- White cheeses are great, especially old white cheddar.

- Always look for all natural ingredients.

- Avoid any processed cheeses with anything artificial in them including artificial colours. Some examples are; Velveeta, Cheese Whiz, American Cheese, Kraft Cheese Slices, Cheese Strings, any cheese that comes in a tube or jar.

- Pre-shredded cheese has some questionable anti-caking agents, so it is fine to have occasionally, but it is best kept to a minimum.

- Avoid "light" or low-fat cheeses as they often contain additives to compensate for the fat removed.

If you are concerned about cholesterol:

Cheese is a saturated fat and you should be mindful about how much saturated fat you consume. Saturated fat is a good fat, but it is important to make sure you are getting enough great fat like omega 3 and omega 6, which you will do by following the Food Plan.

When it comes to avoiding high cholesterol, it's all about the kind of fats you are consuming. To review a list of good fats, check out the Let's Talk Proteins Carbs and Fats post and Let's Talk Groceries. If you have any concerns, be sure to check in with your healthcare provider.

LET'S TALK ABOUT YOGURT

When can you have it?

For the first part of the Program, yogurt is eaten mostly at breakfast with added protein such as hemp hearts, nuts, seeds, nut butters and/or protein powder.

It can also be added to meals and vegetable snack as an added dip, dressing, sauce, or condiment.

What kinds can you have?

Plain, unsweetened yogurt is the best option. Look for options like Greek yogurt that are higher in protein and lower in carbs. This is because of the straining process used to make it where they remove the excess liquid whey and lactose (natural sugars) making it a better choice.

It is best to avoid low or no-fat yogurts because they usually contain additives to compensate for the lack of fat and have added artificial flavours and sugars. There are some low and no-fat yogurts that do not contain any additives, but you want the fat and protein for more sustaining energy, especially at breakfast.

Can you have flavoured or sweetened yogurt?

Yes, you can. Be sure to look for all-natural ingredients.

A better alternative to sweetened yogurt is to use plain and add a touch of honey or maple syrup instead. Or mix your favourite sweetened yogurt with plain yogurt. That way you have control over the amount of sugar added and can slowly reduce it as your taste buds adjust.

What about non-dairy or plant-based yogurts?

Non-dairy and plant-based yogurts tend to be higher in sugar and lower in protein and fat. If you are having, be sure to bump up the nutrient value with added protein and fat.

LET'S TALK ABOUT MILK AND CREAM

When can you have it?

Milk and cream can be used at any time. You can have a glass of milk whenever you like, and it counts towards your fluid intake. Milk and cream can also be added to coffee, tea, high protein cereal, oatmeal, soup, sauces, and such at will.

What kinds can you have?

When it comes to milk and dairy you do not have to avoid low or no fat. The removal of fat here does not require additives to compensate for taste or texture. The fat is simply removed. So, you can enjoy anything from skim to full fat when it comes to milk and cream.

What about lactose free, dairy free and plant-based milk options?

These are fine to have, just be sure they are made with all natural ingredients, nothing artificial and be mindful of any added sugar.

Can you use flavoured creamers?

When it comes to flavoured creamers, whether they are dairy or non-dairy, make sure they are made with all natural ingredients, nothing artificial, and watch the amount of sugar added as some can be very high in sugar.

Please note: Although dairy products contain protein, they are not a good stand-alone option for your main source of protein when it comes to meals while following the Program.

Please take the time to head over to the Facebook Group or the Livy Method App and watch the quick video that accompanies this post.

LET'S TALK DETOX

How we use the body's natural detox process to lose weight.

It is key to note the body does not need any help when it comes to detoxing. This is something the body does naturally every day. This is why I'm not a fan of detox kits, teas, juices or cleanses.

When it comes to detox and helping the body release fat, there is nothing you need to do other than follow the Program as it's designed to do all the work for you.

When your weight is about to drop and your body is focused on releasing fat, it is normal to experience some signs and symptoms related to the detox process.

Some typical responses include:

- Feeling rundown
- Flu-like symptoms
- Runny nose
- Dizzy as hormones balance
- Headaches, chills, night sweats, aches and pains (nothing severe)
- Feeling tired
- Feeling bloated
- Metallic taste in your mouth
- Being thirsty and having dry lips even though you are drinking lots of water
- Waking up around 3-4 am to pee
- Loose bowel movements and/or constipation
- Itchy skin or mild rashes (nothing severe)
- Night sweats
- Leg cramps

Keep in mind not everyone will experience detox symptoms. If you don't, that doesn't mean your body is not detoxing. You can be just as successful losing weight without experiencing any detox symptoms as someone who experiences strong detox symptoms.

If you are someone who experiences stronger detox symptoms, there is no need for concern. There is nothing you will do on this Program that will cause, or lead to, any detrimental effects in the body. However, if you feel something is off, or you are experiencing something out of the norm, please make sure to always check in with your healthcare provider with any concerns.

Keep in mind, all you are doing is eating healthy food and drinking enough water to be hydrated. It's the changes in your food choices, the design of the Food Plan, and the process of releasing the fat that causes the body to react. You can't expect your body to make significant changes without noticing.

In fact, noticing detox symptoms can give you insight into where your body is at and can be a sign your weight is about to drop. Keeping a journal or using the Livy Method App to track how your body is responding to the changes you are making can help you pick up on patterns of behavior to recognize what weight loss looks like and feels like to you.

This can be an advantage when it comes to helping the body focus on fat loss by supporting its needs to help maximize your efforts when it comes to getting and keeping the scale moving.

Please take the time to head over to the Facebook Group or the Livy Method App and watch the quick video that accompanies this post.

LET'S TALK THE SCALE

Let's take a moment and talk about the Scale.

You may not be a fan of stepping on the scale every day and for some it can be downright frustrating. Which is why it is ultimately up to you if you are going to use it while following the Program.

While focused on weight loss, the scale is a tool. When used every day, it can help indicate where your body is at in the process based on the changes you are making and how your body is responding. For example, the foods you are eating, the water you are drinking, and any supplements you are taking along with how you are feeling day to day.

Trying to lose weight without using a scale is like trying to build a house without a hammer. It can be done, but it is so much easier when you use the right tools. This is why it is suggested that you step on the scale every day during this process.

THINGS TO KEEP IN MIND:

- The scale is not a measure of success. It is just a tool to help you in your weight loss journey.
- The best time to weigh yourself is in the morning after you go to the bathroom. For shift workers, weigh yourself when you wake up and start your day.
- A digital scale is ideal as you can see the small fluctuations, which can be helpful.

If you choose not to step on the scale, you can always take measurements, record your non-scale victories or go by how your clothes feel.

HERE IS HOW TO USE IT SO YOU CAN LOSE IT!

Using the scale makes it easier to pick up on any fluctuations so you can make the necessary adjustments day to day. It's normal for the scale to go up and down and to experience plateaus throughout this process. When it comes to the scale, it's all about the downward trend.

WHEN THE SCALE IS UP:

When following The Livy Method, the scale can be up for a variety of different reasons, none of which have anything to do with actual weight gain. You will not gain weight while following the Program.

Reasons why the scale can be up:

- Your weight is about to drop
- Stress
- Lack of sleep
- Salty food

- Hard to digest food

- Dehydration

- Body fighting an illness

- Body sore from a workout

- Body reacting to change in routine

- Body reacting to change in food

- Body reacting to new medication

- Body reacting to introducing supplements

- Deficiencies like being low in iron

- Hormones fluctuating

- PMS

- Your scale needing new batteries

What to do when the scale is up:

- Keep showing up!

- Keep following the Food Plan

- Make sure you are properly hydrated

- Be as consistent as possible with the changes that you are supposed to make

- Don't stress! The scale will come back down

So, when you say, "I gained weight last night" or "Why is my weight up even though I'm doing everything right?!," understand that even though your weight is showing as up, it is not actual weight gain.

WHEN THE SCALE IS DOWN:

When it comes to the scale, while following The Livy Method, a drop is always a drop. When the scale moves down, you can count on it being because of actual fat loss. Whereas when the scale is up, it is always a superficial increase based on what you did or didn't eat or drink the day before.

Things to keep in mind when your weight is dropping:

- It's normal to feel extra hungry the evening before a drop.

- It's normal to wake up around 3 or 4 in the morning before a drop.

- It's normal for weight to go up before a drop.

- It's normal for weight to go back up after it drops to a new low.

- It's normal for some to see the scale go down over a few days.
- It's normal for some to see a big drop in one day.

Once the scale starts to move, assume it is moving for the next 3-5 days, even though you may see a slight increase. Keep following the Food Plan as consistently as possible. Make sure you are properly hydrated to support the body in detox.

WHEN THE SCALE IS BOUNCING UP AND DOWN:

If the scale is bouncing up and down, it usually means your body needs more water because it is trying to focus on releasing fat. It can also mean that your weight is dropping but simultaneously up for other reasons (see list above).

When this happens, increase your water slightly and be as consistent as possible following the Food Plan and the changes that you are advised to make.

WHEN YOU ARE ON A PLATEAU:

Plateaus are NOT a sign that things aren't working. They are needed and wanted to help the body adjust to the changes that you are making and solidify the weight you have lost. Plateaus are your body's way of adjusting to your new lower weight, so your new weight becomes your new norm.

- Plateaus can last days, weeks and even months for some people, depending on where they are at in their weight loss process.
- You can speed up the time spent on a plateau by being as consistent as possible when it comes to following the Program.

It is key to understand that weight loss is based on momentum, not on how you ate the day before. Learn to embrace the ups, the downs, and the plateaus as they are all a normal part of the process.

It's a great idea to use the Livy Method App to track your weight every day so that you can pick up on patterns of response and what weight loss looks like to you.

The scale is just another tool in your toolbox. Ultimately, it's about the downward trend from the beginning of your journey to the end, as you work towards your Finally & Forever goal weight.

Please take the time to head over to the Facebook Group or the Livy Method App and watch the quick video that accompanies this post.

LET'S TALK GOAL WEIGHT

What is a good goal weight and how do you know what is right for you?

It is not about a number, it's about feeling confident and comfortable in your own skin. With that said though, a good baseline to start with is the lowest weight you weighed after the age of 21 that you were able to easily maintain.

That does not mean if you have carried extra weight since childhood, that you can't weigh less than you ever have as an adult. Once you address why your body is feeling the need to store fat (as we do with this process), the body will be happy to release it, regardless of when you gained it or how long you have carried the extra weight.

Things to Keep in Mind:

- Genetics can play a role but will not stop you from reaching your goal. People who have genetically more fat cells may have the capacity to gain more when they do gain, but that doesn't mean it's harder for them to lose.

- When it comes to the number on the scale, it's best to ditch the BMI charts and the old archaic means of measuring what your weight should be. There are so many variables they do not account for. Instead, go by how you feel and aim to be as healthy as possible, regardless of the number on the scale.

- It can be good to set a target weight as a goal, but it can also just add more stress. Visualizing looking and feeling your best can be just as, if not more, effective.

- It may be easier said than done to focus on the positive changes and non-scale victories that come with losing weight on The Livy Method. However, that can be more motivating than aiming for a certain number on the scale when it comes to reaching your goals.

When it comes down to setting a goal weight, some people overestimate, and some people underestimate and that is okay. It is normal to find yourself adjusting and setting new goals along the way. Only you will know when you get there.

Please take the time to head over to the Facebook Group or the Livy Method App and watch the quick video that accompanies this post.

LET'S TALK WEIGHT LOSS

And get real about it.

Losing weight can be unnerving at times, as the Program is designed to bring up all the feels while you work through issues and associations. The feelings and emotions you have about weight loss are real, valid and all part of the process. Take it day by day and as long as you keep showing up, you can't mess it up.

When it comes to numbers on the scale, be sure to review the Let's Talk The Scale post and understand that your weight is going to fluctuate, even when you are focused on losing. This is not only normal - in most cases, it is to be expected.

Let's Review the Reasons Why the Scale Can Be Up:

- Your weight is about to drop
- Stress
- Lack of sleep
- Salty food
- Hard to digest food
- Dehydration
- Body fighting an illness
- Body sore from a workout
- Body reacting to change in routine
- Body reacting to change in food
- Body reacting to new medication
- Body reacting to introducing supplements
- Deficiencies like being low in iron
- Hormones fluctuating
- PMS
- Your scale needing new batteries

The sooner you understand that the body is not trying to make you fat, the less stressed you are going to be throughout this process. Your body converting the food you eat into fat that makes you fat is a complicated and complex process and takes longer than you think. Even though the scale can fluctuate, you are not going to gain weight while following the Program.

THIS IS NOT ABOUT A QUICK FIX:

The Livy Method is about healthy, sustainable weight loss. It is about losing weight in a way that is healthy for your body and equally healthy for your mind. The focus is being as consistent as possible by giving your body what it needs in the first few weeks, not on the numbers on the scale. If the scale moves in the first few weeks, great! And if it doesn't, no need to be concerned. This is normal and expected for some.

How much you lose in the beginning or how quickly you lose, is not an indication of how successful you will be in the end. You will be successful if you show up every day and do the work for as long as it takes to reach your goal.

The goal is to be here at the end of 91 days.

Please take the time to head over to the Facebook Group or the Livy Method App and watch the quick video that accompanies this post.

LET'S TALK ABOUT EXERCISE

How to incorporate it into the Program and tweak it so it is more conducive to fat loss to maximize your efforts while losing weight.

Before we get into talking about exercise, it is important to note that although there are many beneficial reasons to exercise, it is not a mandatory requirement while following the Program.

However, it is important to move your body. As you move forward in this process and continue to put the time and energy into giving your body what it needs, your body is going to start giving you access to more energy. After a few weeks on the Program, you may be surprised that you will naturally start to be more active and will want to move your body more.

Let's talk about the best way to implement exercises that will fall in line with your weight loss goals.

HOW TO AMPLIFY YOUR FITNESS FOR FAT LOSS:

If you are new to exercise, you can start by simply being more active. It may sound cliché, but things like taking the stairs and parking further away when getting groceries, going for walks or doing some push-ups or squats in your kitchen, can add up and have a big impact.

If you are looking for something more intense, there are a lot of great home workout options. It is best to start slow to minimize the stress on the body and build up to it. Whatever you choose to do, it should be something you enjoy so you make a positive association to exercise moving forward and it becomes something you look forward to doing.

In terms of intensity, you want to walk away from any exercise feeling good and energized, not tired, taxed, or drained.

THIS BRINGS US TO THE TOPIC OF REST:

If you choose, you can incorporate intense workouts and challenge your body. However, if you are going to work out to the point of being sore, you need to make sure you are giving your body adequate rest time to repair and rebuild, or you will run the risk of overtraining.

Overtraining happens when the body cannot catch up to the damage that's been done, leaving your body feeling weak and in a deficit, which in turn can cause the body to feel the need to hold on to fat or store more fat for easy energy.

Be mindful of taking rest days, making sure to drink enough water, and getting good quality sleep to help the body recover.

CARDIO AND GETTING YOUR HEART RATE UP:

When it comes to exercise and weight loss, it is all about the message you are sending to the body. Your physical brain that runs your body does not see what you are doing for exercise, it only interprets what you are doing based on your movements and heart rate. This is where you can use the body's natural fight or flight response to maximize your results.

Getting your heart rate up as high as you can for as long as you can, even if just for a few minutes, evokes the fight or flight response in the body and immediately sends a message for the body to work to make you stronger.

The body's sole responsibility is to keep you alive, so if you repeatedly evoke the fight or flight response, your body will look to make you as strong and efficient as possible. In wanting to be as efficient as possible, your body will look to get rid of any extra fat that could be slowing you down. This makes cardio (exercise that gets your heart rate up) very effective for fat loss.

Cardio does not have to be running, it can be walking fast, skipping, swimming, dancing, lifting lighter weights with higher reps, resistance training, sports activities, and anything else that helps get your heart rate up.

With cardio you are basically taking the muscle you already have in your body and using it to move your body, which will get your heart rate up without creating damage, making it a complement to the Program.

Alternatively, there is also a benefit in adding in some endurance training. Where the goal is more extending the length of time or distance you are moving, as opposed to how high your heart rate gets or how intense the workout is.

An example of this would be a longer bike ride, hiking, walking, jogging and swimming for 40 mins or longer at a more moderate pace.

LIFTING WEIGHTS:

Lifting weight can be a great complement to the Program. Weight lifting is great for bone density, building muscle and shaping your body.

However, it's important to keep in mind that when you lift weight, the goal is to purposely create damage in the body. This causes the body to have to repair the damage, which makes the muscle stronger. Which is why it's important to make sure to get adequate rest in between workouts.

With that said, if you want to lift heavier weight you can. And if you are already exercising there is no reason why you can't continue to follow through on your routine.

MY EXERCISE FAVES FOR FAT LOSS:

- **Walking:** It is conducive to healing and the least stressful type of exercise you can do.

- **Anything outside**: It stimulates the brain and works the body while communing with nature and relieving stress.

- **Dance:** Moving the body in different ways other than side to side and up and down strengthens the mind-body connection.

- **Boxing/martial arts type classes:** Effective for evoking the fight response.

- **Biking or spinning:** Great for getting your heart rate up and evoking the flight response.

- **Resistance training:** Exercises like pilates and aquafit use your own body weight to get your heart rate up.

- **Meditative:** Yoga and stretching help with healing and lowering stress levels.

Regardless of the type of exercise you choose, you want to avoid using exercise as a punishment, or for burning off or offsetting any indulgences you have.

You should look at exercise as a complement to the Program and a way to help your body level up your health and wellness. Focus on all of the amazing benefits that come with moving your body.

Be sure to check in with your healthcare provider before starting, or if for any reason you are feeling apprehensive about adding exercise into your routine.

Please take the time to head over to the Facebook Group or the Livy Method App and watch the quick video that accompanies this post.

LET'S TALK ALCOHOL

Let's discuss drinking alcohol when following the Program.

Generally, consuming alcohol is not the reason your body is feeling the need to store fat. With that said, there are benefits to limiting your intake, so it's good to be mindful of what you are drinking when looking to lose weight.

If you like to enjoy an alcoholic beverage every now and then, following these tips can help minimize the impact on your body and the scale.

- The most important tip is to add in extra water to compensate for the dehydration that alcohol can cause. We recommend a minimum extra cup (250 mL) of water per drink, regardless of the type or size of drink.

WINE

- There are benefits in choosing red wine over white. Although both are fine, red has more antioxidants and is slightly better for you. That isn't a reason to give up your white if that's what you prefer.

ROSE & CHAMPAGNES

- A little higher in sugar, so don't be surprised if you wake up with a headache, but it is totally fine to have.

BEER/CIDERS

- Darker beers like Guinness are higher in nutrient value but any of your regular, all-natural ales, lagers, pilsners etc. are totally fine.

- When it comes to ciders, be mindful of added sugars and artificial ingredients. Otherwise enjoy!

- Avoid added ingredients and preservatives when drinking "light" or "low-cal" beer. Some are better quality than others.

- When it comes to non-alcoholic beverages, be mindful of artificial ingredients and added sugar.

HARD LIQUOR

- When it comes to the hard stuff, be mindful about what you are using as a mix. Try to avoid pop/soda, including diet versions and artificially flavoured juice.

- If you enjoy something like rye and coke, or gin and tonic once every now and then it's no big deal.

- When it comes to coolers and premixed drinks, look for natural ingredients and avoid anything artificial.

When it comes to losing weight, the issue with alcohol is less about the kind you are drinking and more about the food you are eating with it. If you are following the Food Plan this is a non-issue.

Here are a couple of things to keep in mind if you find yourself drinking and indulging:

- Drinking alcohol slows down the metabolism and your digestive system, so you want to avoid any heavy carbs like bread and pasta and stick to more protein, fats (like cheese and nuts) and vegetables.

- Keep in mind alcohol can affect weight loss in other ways. For example, interrupting your sleep, messing with estrogen levels, and causing dehydration, to name a few.

- Alcohol increases the production of galanin, a neuropeptide in the brain, which causes you to crave greasy food. Pair that with the effects of dehydration that can cause you to crave sugar, and you are ready to eat your face off the next day!

- Increasing your water, having a banana (which is high in potassium), along with bumping up good fats like oils, nuts, seeds, and avocados the next day, will help the body metabolize the alcohol and reduce the galanin.

- Drinking can also affect the good bacteria in your digestive system, so if your stomach always feels off the next day, try adding in digestive bitters. Digestive bitters will be discussed in more detail in Week 2.

REMEMBER:

Besides keeping these tips in mind, the best thing you can do to offset any negative effects of alcohol consumption is to add in that one cup of extra water per drink, regardless of the drink or mix you are using.

Cheers, enjoy your beverages!

Please take the time to head over to the Facebook Group or the Livy Method App and watch the quick video that accompanies this post.

LET'S TALK CHOCOLATE

Dark chocolate can be a source of magnesium and when it's good quality it can be low in sugar. However, it is advised to skip it while you are following the Program and here is why.

In the early weeks of the Program, the focus is on becoming more in tune to your body's needs over your wants, so you want to avoid using food for anything other than nutritional requirements right now. If you find yourself craving chocolate, you want to ask yourself why as every craving is a message from your body.

You do not want to be feeding into cravings or trying to manage or mask them. You want to address them, so you don't have them anymore. Down the road you will be able to add chocolate back in, but for now, if you are looking to maximize your results, it is best to keep it out.

If you are concerned about sugar cravings, then simply follow the Food Plan, as it is designed to address them. Focus on eating all of your meals and snacks, making your food choices nutrient rich, eating to satisfaction, and drinking your water.

With that said, having a few pieces of chocolate here and there is not going to stop you from reaching your goal. If you do end up eating some or indulging in any treats, all you need to do is keep moving forward and get back at it.

Please take the time to head over to the Facebook Group or the Livy Method App and watch the quick video that accompanies this post.

LET'S TALK ABOUT GUM

Can you chew it while following the Program?

It is not advised and here is why.

Digestion starts in the mouth, technically with smell first and then by chewing. Chewing gum artificially stimulates your digestive system. Without following through and eating food, it can affect hunger cues and suppress your appetite.

When following the Program, you want to be in-tune to your body's needs, not suppress them, so in no way is chewing gum a benefit.

IF YOU CHOOSE TO CHEW:

- Be mindful of gum that is high in sugar.
- Look for all natural ingredients, avoiding anything artificial.
- Best to chew natural gum which can be found online or at health food stores.
- Try to chew directly after a meal as opposed to in between.

PLEASE NOTE: Mints have the same effect.

Please take the time to head over to the Facebook Group or the Livy Method App and watch the quick video that accompanies this post.

LET'S TALK WEEKENDS

Why they are nothing to be concerned about and how to make the most of them.

When it comes to weight loss, it can seem like there is always something getting in the way and throwing you off track; birthdays, holidays, vacation days, let alone just your average weekend.

Lack of routine, travel, eating salty food, hard to digest food, high sugar content foods, lack of water, and even lack of sleep can easily have you feeling off and your weight up.

Good thing it's not as easy as you think to gain weight, and it takes a lot longer than you think for your body to convert the food you eat into actual fat. So, when you find the scale creeping up after a little indulging, chances are it's not real weight gain.

Which is why I always say there is nothing you can do on a weekend that can't be undone by getting right back at it!

TIPS FOR STAYING ON TRACK:

- Make a plan for your weekend.
- Start your day with a higher protein breakfast.
- Be prepared and pack some snacks if you are going to be out and about.
- Try to be as consistent as possible with the Food Plan leading up to any events/meals. (Don't not eat in anticipation.)
- Try to get in your water where you can.
- Don't blow off your whole day because of one indulgent meal or snack.

Indulging on the weekend is going to happen. For the sake of weight loss, you want to keep those days to a minimum. But with that said, there is also nothing to stress about. This Program is very forward moving where one week leads into the next, so you don't want to go back and repeat steps. It's all about progress over perfection. As long as you keep showing up, you can't mess it up. So, if you find yourself going off track, simply keep moving forward and no harm done.

Staying as consistent as possible is key, but if you get off track just get right back on track, because as long as you keep showing up, you can't mess it up. There is a lot to be learned in not being perfect and having a few indulgences here and there. It is all part of the process.

Please take the time to head over to the Facebook Group or the Livy Method App and watch the quick video that accompanies this post.

LET'S TALK TRAVEL

How to navigate it and make the most of it.

Whether traveling for vacation or traveling for work, there is no reason that you can't still work towards your weight loss goals.

LET'S START WITH VACATIONS:

Vacations can do wonders for weight loss. Change in environment, less stress, abundance of fresh food, and some decent sleep can be exactly what the body needs to get the scale moving. So, don't stress if you can't follow the Food Plan perfectly while away. It's ok to have your food choices be off routine if your schedule is off from your normal weekly routine.

No one is expecting you to deprive yourself of any of the joys that come with being on vacation to be successful. Feel free to indulge, just be mindful to balance it out. Focus on your water and try to get in fresh fruits, vegetables, and leafy greens when you can.

One of the biggest challenges while vacationing is flying. Here are some tips:

- Resist the urge to indulge in treats before you fly. Flying is super dehydrating and combined with high sugar is a recipe for craving carbs, serious bloating, and constipation once you land.
- Spend the money on healthy snacks so you are not inclined to eat the crackers and cookies or heavily salted meal they serve during the flight.
- HYDRATE! The altitude when flying is very dehydrating. So, before, during and after you land, focus on getting your water in.

While it's not unusual to lose weight while away on holiday, most people will find their weight will go up. This can be due for a variety of reasons. Have faith that after a few days of getting back at it and following the Program, your weight will drop right back down again. Have fun and focus on making choices that make you feel good and you can't go wrong.

LET'S TALK TRAVELING FOR WORK:

Traveling for work can have you here, there and everywhere while making a lot of stops along the way. This can make it challenging when it comes to following the Food Plan. Whether you are hitting the road for long hours, or just driving to and from work, having a plan and being prepared can make all the difference.

One of the biggest challenges while traveling for work is the inconsistencies of being on the road. Here are some tips:

- Assess your day before it starts and make a plan.

- Be prepared with extra snacks and keep water on hand.

- Look for quick and easy snacks that work on the go.

- Try to keep the routine of the Food Plan the best you can.

- Set timers and alarms to help keep you on track.

- Don't worry about a few off meals or snacks.

- Stop at grocery stores instead of fast food restaurants.

- Make the best choices you can when you can if the choices are limited.

- Focus on the water.

- Bathroom visits can be inconvenient. Get the water in when you can and hold off when you need to.

Traveling for work is not as fun but can be just as effective, as travel in general is very stimulating for the body. Try to stay on plan the best you can and don't stress. It's all about being mindful, planning ahead, and making choices that fall in line with your goals to set yourself up for success.

Please take the time to head over to the Facebook Group or the Livy Method App and watch the quick video that accompanies this post.

LET'S TALK FRESH EYES

Fresh eyes are key when redoing the Program to continue to reach your goal.

Redoing the Program is a very effective method for continued weight loss. Each time you do the Program, it works just as well, if not better. Not only are you more in tune with your body's needs, but it is also working at more optimal levels.

With that said, even though you absolutely have the advantage, there are some things that you may struggle with when repeating the process that are good to keep in mind. For example:

1. **You have done it before, and you know you can do it again.**

   Sometimes rather than this being an advantage or a motivator, it can be used as an excuse to allow in bites of bits that you didn't add in the first time around.

   With knowing how to get Back on Track and what's to come, you give yourself more wiggle room to indulge. This is an issue because you end up spending more of the process getting Back on Track and never gain the momentum you need to see the results you expect.

2. **You know what's coming next and expect your body to respond the same way.**

   This can be an issue because you end up focusing on the things you did the last time and not on the things you need to do this time. You may assume the process is not working simply because your experience is different from your last group. Your body is different each time around and you should expect and want it to respond differently.

   What your body connected with the first time around will be different the second, third and fourth time around. By assuming how it will respond, you end up missing out on capitalizing on the areas that actually need work. Be mindful of getting in the way of your body making progress because you are trying to control what it is focusing on and how it responds.

3. **Your motivation has changed.**

   This happens a lot when people try to use the motivation they had last time to lose weight this time. Chances are what motivated you last time is not what is motivating you this time. Re-evaluating your "why" can make all the difference.

4. **You do not see an end-game.**

   You need to see an end to the process. Leaving things open ended is not motivating and can keep you stuck in the cycle of trying to lose. Have a realistic time frame and make a plan for crossing the finish line. Not only when, but also how that will feel and what it will look like.

5. **Not understanding that you have the advantage subsequent times around.**

   If you are repeating the process then you want to be all in, stepping up your game, and using your past knowledge to challenge yourself along the way, especially when it comes to maximizing. Be mindful of holding yourself back. Fear of being successful or fear of not following through tend to pop up the closer you get to your goal.

To reiterate, when re-doing the Program, you are absolutely at an advantage. So, if you find yourself struggling, chances are it is because you are getting in your own way. Take a step back and assess what you need to do to step up your game, be all in and follow through and finish!

Please take the time to head over to the Facebook Group or the Livy Method App and watch the quick video that accompanies this post.

WEEK 1 GUIDELINES: FINE TUNING AND ADJUSTING

This week is about fine tuning and adjusting the changes you made during Prep Week, focusing on being as consistent as possible and paying attention to how your body is responding. This is also where we introduce Bonus Snacks if needed.

THE GOAL FOR WEEK 1:

- Continue to follow the Food Plan.
- Eat ALL meals and snacks.
- Make food choices as nutrient rich as possible.
- Eat to satisfaction, meaning do NOT try to eat less.
- Add in Bonus Snacks if needed.
- Continue to work on getting your water in.

You want to be as consistent as possible when implementing the changes you need to make.

This week you are looking to fine tune and adjust the changes you have made so far, and to be in tune to how your body is responding and make any adjustments as needed.

For example, if you are hungry at the end of your day, be sure to eat all of your meals and snacks, having token amounts even if you are not hungry. Be mindful not to skip breakfast, make your foods as nutrient rich as possible, and use Bonus Snacks if needed. (See post on Let's Talk About Bonus Snacks)

Bonus snacks are extra snacks that you can add in if you feel you need more food than the Food Plan provides. Keep in mind Bonus Snacks are to be added in ONLY if needed.

Bonus Snacks are NOT meant to replace your regular snacks so you will still need to keep those in.

Alternatively, if you are feeling overly full at the end of your day, you want to pay attention to your portions the next day. Although you are not counting, weighing, or measuring food, there is a lot to be learned by bringing awareness to the portions you are consuming and how your body is responding.

You will find as you progress through the Program your portions will naturally start to decrease and adjust to be more in tune to your body's needs.

For now you want you eat to feel satisfied in the moment. Keeping in mind when it comes to portions, it's what they feel like, not what they look like. So you may find each day might be a bit different.

For example, one day you might not be hungry at all, although it's still important to have all your meals and snacks. And then the next day, you might be extra hungry and need to add in bonus snacks.

Although this is a Weight Loss Program, the focus is NOT on the scale right now. Focus on the basics while fine tuning and adjusting and be as consistent as possible. It's the quickest way to start feeling and seeing results.

Keep in mind that it's progress over perfection. As long as you keep showing up, you can't mess it up. It is not about how strong you start; it's about following through, finishing strong and being here at the end.

FREQUENTLY ASKED QUESTIONS

1. **Is it normal for the scale to fluctuate?**

    Yes it is totally normal for the scale to fluctuate and you should expect it. The scale will fluctuate for a number of reasons, none of which have anything to do with actual weight gain. Some reasons the scale can be up include your body reacting to a change in foods, your body being sore from a workout, poor quality sleep, medications, and dehydration to name a few. It is also normal for your weight to be up right before it drops.

    If the scale is bouncing up and down between the same numbers that is usually an indication your body is about to release fat and that you need to add a bit more water.

2. **Is bloating and constipation normal?**

    You can experience bloating and constipation as your body adjusts to any changes in your diet. Being consistent with following the Food Plan and making sure you are drinking enough water will help as everything comes together. It is also normal to feel constipated and bloated before your weight drops. If you feel that something more is going on, be sure to check in with your healthcare provider.

3. **I have esophageal reflux (GERD) and am concerned about taking lemon or apple cider vinegar (ACV). What do you suggest?**

Following the Program and Food Plan can naturally help with your reflux. Adding in ACV and lemon water can be very beneficial for this. Feel free to dilute the lemon or ACV in as much water as you need. You can always leave it out or if you have any concerns, speak with your healthcare provider.

4. **Can I have a shot of apple cider vinegar (ACV) followed by a glass of water?**

You are welcome to have ACV on its own followed by water if this is the way you like it. You can also dilute the ACV in as much water as you need to get it down. There is some benefit to having your ACV in water as it is fairly acidic and some people find it can be gentler on their system.

5. **Does it matter what time of day I have my coffee/tea?**

You can have coffee and tea as you like at any time throughout the day. They would count towards your water intake. That said, if drinking caffeinated beverages affects your ability to sleep at night, avoid drinking them too late into the evening.

6. **Are smoothies and/or shakes okay to have while following the Program?**

At this point of the Program, while we are preparing our body for weight loss, we want our bodies to work hard to digest and process its food, which is why it's important to chew our food. There will come a time later in the Program that you can add them in.

If you do choose to keep them in, it's best to use a protein powder that contains all natural ingredients, without artificial sweeteners that are low in sugar. Add little to no fruit and add in healthy fat like avocados, nut butters and coconut oil, to name a few.

7. **Does skipping breakfast on some days and eating it on others have adverse effects? Should it be one or the other consistently?**

Starting your day with a higher protein breakfast is always a benefit when following the Program. It is a great way to "break the fast" and get your body working harder from the get-go. However, skipping breakfast does not have any adverse effects. You can assess how you feel day to day, one day you may want to have breakfast and the next day you may want to skip it. You do not have to be consistent either way.

8. **If I am busy in the morning, is it better to skip breakfast and go straight to the fruit? Or eat breakfast late and schedule my other meals for later in the day?**

It's always best to start your day with a high protein breakfast, and breakfast is ideally eaten within 2.5 hours of waking. However if you are up at 5am and not active or exercising you can still eat breakfast as late as 9am. If you get up later that gives you less time for both breakfast and fruit snack so you might skip breakfast and go straight to fruit snack. Keep in mind you have between 30 min and 3.5 hours for your next meal or snack so you can still fit in all your meals and snacks into your day. Whether you have breakfast or not, you still want to have your fruit snack mid morning.

9. **If something counts as a vegetable and a leafy green, does it cover both purposes in a meal?**

   Yes, if a vegetable also counts as a leafy green, it would count towards both the vegetable and leafy green component of your meal. Some great examples are cabbage, bok choy and Brussels sprouts.

10. **What nuts can I have?**

    Any type of nuts and seeds are great. You can have them raw or roasted. It is best to avoid nuts and seeds that have added oil.

11. **Do I still include the other snacks if I am adding in Bonus Snacks?**

    Bonus Snacks are not meant to replace your regular snacks, so you cannot switch out your regularly scheduled snacks for Bonus Snacks. Bonus Snacks are extra snacks that can be used by those who are up very early, are more physically active during the day, or those that have long shift turnarounds. Bonus Snacks are to be added only if needed for nutritional requirements because you feel like you need more above the basic Food Plan. They do not need to be added every day.

12. **What foods can be used for the Bonus Snacks?**

    Here are some options:

    - Yogurt or other dairy products, such as cottage cheese or other cheeses
    - Fruit with nuts, seeds, nut butter, cheese or any protein and fat
    - Vegetables raw or cooked and you can add dip or cheese
    - Boiled egg or any other protein
    - Half of your lunch eaten early or half later
    - High fiber cracker with protein and fat (only if not used at breakfast)
    - Protein shake with vegetables or fruit and added fat (be mindful of portion size)

Refer to the Let's Talk About Bonus Snack post for more information.

Please take the time to head over to the Facebook Group or the Livy Method App and watch the quick video that accompanies this post.

LET'S TALK ABOUT BONUS SNACKS

What they are, if you need them and when to add them in.

The focus for Prep Week was introducing and implementing the Food Plan and the changes you needed to make to get started. For example, eating all of your meals and snacks, making food choices as nutrient rich as possible, all while eating to satisfaction. This week the focus is on fine tuning and adjusting which is where Bonus Snacks come in.

Bonus snacks are extra snacks that can be used if you feel you need more than the Food Plan provides. For example, if you are up extra early, are more physical in your day (super active job) or have long shift turnarounds where you are awake for 24 hrs or more.

It is key to note that Bonus Snacks are not meant to replace your regular snacks, so you will still need to follow the Food Plan as designed and only use Bonus Snacks as extra.

Please note: If you are continually skipping breakfast and find yourself in need of adding in Bonus Snacks, then you should consider having it, along with making sure that all of your food choices are as nutrient rich as possible and you are eating to satisfaction.

THE TIMING OF THE BONUS SNACKS IS VERY SPECIFIC:

1.   They can be added in between your morning fruit snack and lunch.

2.   They can be added in between your lunch and afternoon vegetable snack.

For example:

- Breakfast
- Fruit snack
- **BONUS SNACK**
- Lunch
- **BONUS SNACK**
- Vegetable snack
- Nuts/seeds snack
- Dinner

The timing between meals and snacks remains the same; 30 minutes to 3.5 hours.

WHAT YOU CAN HAVE FOR BONUS SNACKS:

MORNING BONUS SNACK:

- Yogurt or other dairy products, such as cottage cheese or other cheeses
- More fruit with nuts, seeds, nut butter, cheese or any protein and fat
- Vegetables raw or cooked and you can add dip or cheese
- Boiled egg or any other protein
- Half of your lunch eaten early
- Ryvita/high fiber cracker with spread (only if not used at breakfast)
- Shake with protein, vegetables or fruit and added fat (be mindful of portion size)

AFTERNOON BONUS SNACK:

- Can be any of the above, except nuts and seeds because you are already having these at your second afternoon snack while following the Food Plan.

Keep in mind, if you add in the Bonus Snacks and find yourself not hungry for your regular snacks, you still need to eat them even if you keep the portion small.

It may seem counterintuitive to eat more when trying to lose weight, but right now it is key to address why your body is feeling a need to store fat and support its needs.

Depending on how early you get up or how active you are, or the hours you work, you may need to add in Bonus Snacks more often, while others may not need to utilize them at all.

Please take the time to head over to the Facebook Group or the Livy Method App and watch the quick video that accompanies this post.

LET'S TALK SELF-SABOTAGE

This is the point in the Program where self-sabotage can start to pop up. Rest assured, it is perfectly normal and very common.

WHAT IS SELF-SABOTAGE?

Self-sabotage is choosing (consciously or unconsciously) to do something that undermines your success and gets in the way of you reaching your goal. The two main reasons people sabotage their weight loss goals are lack of self-esteem and fear.

Lack of self-esteem can lead to negative thinking, self-talk and doubt. These feelings can come on and take over without you even realizing it. This internal dialogue can feed into your fears, which is another reason for self-sabotage.

Not all fears are obvious and may be subconscious. Have a look at this list and see if any of these resonate with you:

- **Fear of change** - You feel more comfortable with what is familiar. It can be hard to step outside of your comfort zone into the unknown. You may have no idea what losing weight will feel like physically or emotionally and that can be unnerving. Will you be able to trust the changes you are making?

- **Failure and embarrassment** - Are you afraid of failing at another attempt at weight loss so might as well just give up? Are you worried you will be embarrassed if you fail again, leading to you giving up before you reach your goals?

- **Changing body type** - Are you afraid of what your body might look like once you have lost the weight? A body you aren't familiar with?

- **Losing your comfort foods** - Are you nervous of losing your old coping mechanisms? Thinking, "What am I going to do without my comfort foods? I can't handle stress without them."

- **New clothes** - Are you concerned about having to buy a new wardrobe? Not knowing how to shop for clothes to suit your new body. Being unsure of stepping out of your comfort zone. Finances can also be a concern.

- **Relationships** - Perhaps you are worried people will think differently of you or how losing weight might change the relationships with those around you. Thinking, "Will people be jealous or uncomfortable around me if they have weight to lose? Will my friends and family look at me differently or treat me differently?"

- **Fear of your abilities** - Not believing in yourself is a big one. This plays into the negative self-talk; "I can't do this", "I'm just a failure". It can be easier said than done to trust in yourself and be your own cheerleader.

- **Fear of the new you** - Getting to know and trusting the new you can be exciting but can also bring up all the feels. Asking, "Who am I without the weight?" or feeling afraid of becoming someone you don't recognize. Even though you are happy with the change, you may not feel comfortable with it at first.

Some self-sabotaging behaviours are obvious, like indulging, overeating, not drinking enough water, skipping meals and snacks etc. However, there are other behaviours that can also get in the way of reaching your goals that aren't as obvious. For example:

- **Focusing on the end result instead of the journey** - Are you so focused on your goal weight that you aren't paying attention to all the other positive changes that are happening?

- **Procrastinating** - Are you avoiding doing the things you know you need to do?

- **Trying to rush results** - Are you frustrated all the time because the scale isn't moving as fast as you want it to?

- **Focusing on the scale** - Is the number on the scale going down the only thing you are thinking about? Are you stressing every time it goes up or doesn't come down as fast as you want?

- **Overthinking things and becoming overwhelmed** - Overthinking things causes unnecessary stress and can have you feeling overwhelmed.

- **Avoiding accountability** - Are you avoiding showing up every day and being real with yourself about what you are or are not doing?

- **Not taking responsibility and blaming other factors** - Are you blaming your behaviours on your family? ("I'm a busy mom"), work? ("I'm just too busy"), on the Program? ("It's too much information" or "I don't have time").

- **Comparing yourself to everyone else** - "Everyone else is losing weight and I'm not, so obviously this doesn't work for me," "It's hard to watch other people lose when I'm not".

- **Perfectionism** - Are you focused so much on doing everything perfectly that it's stressing you out? Are you hard on yourself every time you feel like you are not perfect, leading to negative self-talk?

- **Not asking for help** - Are you avoiding asking for help, whether it's from the group or family or friends? Maybe you need extra support from your family but are afraid to ask.

Being self-aware is the first step when it comes to working through self-sabotage. It is all part of your weight loss journey as you work towards strengthening your mind-body connection, understanding your body's needs and wants, and all of the things you need to do and work through to reach your goals.

Here are some questions that can help bring awareness and give you a better understanding of where you are at and what you are working through if you feel self-sabotage is an issue for you.

1. **Ask yourself "What am I afraid of?"**

   Make a list of your fears, writing them down in your own words helps to bring awareness to them.

2. **What are my triggers?**

   What is causing me to have these thoughts and feelings of self-doubt? What makes you turn to food for reasons other than nutritional requirements? What emotions are coming up? Angry, sad, stressed, bored, happy? Write them down to understand how you are feeling, or what is happening when you feel the urge to sabotage.

3. **How does it make you feel when you are not doing the things you know you need to do?**

   What you learn by not doing the things you need to do, can be just as insightful and of value as when you are doing everything perfectly. Does indulging make you feel better? Maybe it does in the moment, but how do you feel after?

4. **Make a list of things you can do instead of turning to food.**

   Maybe it's taking a walk, cuddling with your pet, taking a bath, having a nice soothing tea, or listening to a podcast. Perhaps it's deep breathing, meditation, yoga, listening to your favourite music and dancing it out. Give yourself a few options. This will help you create new habits and healthier coping mechanisms.

5. **Make a list of positive self-talk/affirmations.**

   Thoughts are habits and even if you don't believe them at first, practicing positive self-talk and affirmations can make all the difference when it comes to a more positive outlook and internal dialogue. "I've got this!" "I am doing a great job," and "I am proud of myself for showing up every day". Make a point to say these things to yourself each morning, throughout the day, and before you go to bed.

6. **What is your WHY?**

   Write down all the reasons why you want to lose weight. Why is reaching your goal important to you? What will it mean to you? How will you feel when you reach your goal? Refer to it when you are in need of motivation along the way.

Increasing awareness of your triggers and changing your internal dialogue to be more supportive is a solid first step in changing your patterns. Making change doesn't happen overnight, and some issues and beliefs are so deeply rooted that it might take more than a few lists to undo. In time, your efforts will add up, to not only strengthen your mind-body connection, and bring awareness to your needs, but also ultimately help you reach your weight loss goals.

LET'S TALK SETTING INTENTIONS

Setting intentions can help you stay more focused and motivated while working towards your weight loss goals by keeping all of the things you need to do and work through at the forefront of your mind. They can also help to keep you on track if you find yourself dealing with self-sabotage along the way.

Setting your intentions in the morning is like making a declaration that you are still working towards your goal, and to remind yourself of all of the things you need to do to reach it. You can take a few minutes to think about them, meditate on them, or jot them down in the Livy Method App or your journal.

Visualization is also helpful. It can work like a blueprint or a guide in your mind. It can be done on a small-scale, day-to-day by visualizing and harmonizing your daily tasks. It can also be done on a larger scale in terms of visualizing reaching your goals, and how that will look and feel.

Setting your intentions first thing in the morning, along with checking in on yourself mid-day, and then reflecting on the choices you made at the end of the day, can help to keep you accountable to yourself. Especially in today's world with all the extra stress you can find yourself dealing with day to day, your goal of trying to lose weight can sometimes end up on the back burner.

Please take the time to head over to the Facebook Group or the Livy Method App and watch the quick video that accompanies this post.

LET'S TALK ABOUT HUNGER

What it means to be hungry and how your hunger levels will change throughout this process as well as the difference between true hunger vs. various other factors.

Because your body's needs change day to day, your hunger levels can change day to day. As we will be making changes to the Food Plan week to week, you will also notice changes in your hunger levels and cues along the way.

THE MOST IMPORTANT THINGS YOU NEED TO UNDERSTAND ABOUT HUNGER:

- Hunger is not an immediate need for food. The body knows that it can take time for you to find and prepare food and that some foods can take hours to process and digest through your system. Therefore, it takes that into account when giving you a heads up on when you need to eat.

- Hunger is the way your body checks in with you and lets you know where it is at in terms of energy reserves and what it needs throughout the day.

- It is normal for your hunger levels to be all over the place as your body adjusts to the Food Plan.

HUNGER VS. CRAVINGS:

- When you are dehydrated, you may crave carbohydrates and sugar as the body looks for high water content foods. This can often be mistaken for hunger. If you drink a glass of water and no longer feel hungry, you were probably just thirsty.

- If you are craving salty foods, this can be a sign that your body is looking for more good fat.

- Check out the Let's Talk Cravings post for more information.

HUNGER IN DETOX:

- Typically late in the evening, you may feel extra hungry, even after eating all of your nutrient rich meals and snacks. This can be a sign of detox and your body is about to release fat.

- You may find that once your body is in detox and the scale is moving, it is normal to feel extra hungry as your body is working extra hard. Alternatively, it is also normal to not feel hungry when the scale is moving as your body is focused on fat loss. Everyone is different.

HUNGER VS. MIGRATING MOTOR COMPLEX (MMC):

- The MMC is the body's self-cleaning mechanism where in between meals and snacks, it works to clear bacteria and food particles out of the stomach and small intestine.

- There is a difference between true hunger and your tummy rumbling. If you notice your tummy rumbling after eating to satisfaction, this is typically your migrating motor complex kicking in.

- If you wake up in the middle of the night and notice your tummy making noises, chances are you are picking up on your MMC at work.

HUNGER VS. RESIDUAL CRAVINGS:

- If you have a habit of eating after dinner, you may feel the need to snack after dinner. This is based more on habit than actual need.

- If you had a routine of eating certain foods at certain times, for example snacking while watching your favourite T.V. show, or having something to eat before bed you may continue to crave those foods at that time, until new habits are formed.

The more consistent you are with the Food Plan and implementing the changes you need to make, the more in tune with your hunger levels you will be. For now, focus on eating all of your meals and snacks, making them as nutrient rich as possible and be sure to eat to satisfaction.

Please take the time to head over to the Facebook Group or the Livy Method App and watch the quick video that accompanies this post.

LET'S TALK CRAVINGS

Cravings are usually a sign that your body is trying to communicate its needs by associating the foods that can help it get what it wants.

If you are consistently following the Food Plan any cravings you have should be few and far between. And if they do pop up, it's usually just a matter of making a few tweaks.

LET'S TALK SUGAR:

The key to addressing sugar cravings is in understanding that it's not actually sugar your body wants. It is the increase in insulin as a result of having it that has your body asking for more.

Insulin is the hormone that allows your body to use glucose for energy. Glucose is a type of sugar found in carbs like fruits, vegetables, and naturally occurring sugar that your body uses for energy. After you eat food and your digestive system breaks it down, your pancreas releases insulin to help regulate your blood sugar.

When you reach for sweets or foods with high sugar content, your body increases insulin production, which can cause your blood glucose levels to drop. This can create a dip in energy and a desire for even more sugar.

REASONS WHY WE CRAVE SUGAR:

1. **More is more.**

When you have sugar, your body tends to want more sugar. These cravings can be so intense that if you create a habit of having sugar at the same time every day, your body will begin to crave and expect it at that same time each day. This is also the reason you end up eating that whole box of cookies in one sitting!

THE FIX:

- Making sure to add in healthy fats to your meals along with protein, which will help feed into your satiety hormones, and have you feeling more satisfied and prevent any cravings along the way.

- If you do find yourself indulging, you can decrease sugar cravings by having some protein and fat with your sweet treat. For example, if you indulge in a cookie, you can minimize the desire to eat another cookie by having a slice of cheese, a handful of nuts, or a glass of milk.

2. **Dehydration is a factor.**

When you are dehydrated and not picking up on the cues from your body to drink enough water, your body's next best bet is to crave foods with a high water content, like fruit. Fruits are also sweet, so you may mistake your body's cue to consume more water and instead find yourself reaching for processed carbs and sugar.

This is why you may hear the advice to drink a glass of water before you eat to satisfy your appetite. Drinking water doesn't actually satisfy your appetite. So if you drink it and feel satisfied, chances are you were never hungry and didn't need that sweet treat in the first place.

THE FIX:

- Drink more water.
- Sip water throughout the day, aiming for a minimum of 2.7 - 3.5 L a day and even more on days you exercise, are more active, sweating a lot or when the climate is hot and/or dry.

3.   You are tired.

When you are tired, your body goes looking for a pick-me-up so you may find yourself reaching for something sweet.

The same thing happens around 3 or 4 p.m. each afternoon when the body is wired to take a dip in energy and slows your circadian rhythm. What your body is really looking for is a nap. (There are places in the world that do just that: think of the siesta.) In our fast-paced, high-stress world, it's not always possible to have an afternoon nap, so the body goes looking for easy energy by way of higher sugar to pick it up and keep it going.

THE FIX:

- Make sure to eat all your meals and especially your snacks. This will help to avoid energy levels that dip when you go for long periods of time without eating.
- Your mid-morning snack of fresh fruit will top up your energy reserves in the morning and your vegetables, nuts and seeds in the afternoon will keep your body working hard throughout the afternoon.
- These foods have a high nutrient value and are harder to digest, which will keep your digestion stimulated and your body awake and functioning when it's craving a nap.

With a few adjustments, you can easily beat the need for sweets and stay on track to reach your goals and not be held captive by sugar cravings anymore.

LET'S TALK SALT:

REASONS WHY WE CRAVE SALT:

1.   You need more salt.

Salt is one of the electrolytes quickest to deplete through sweating. When exercising, living in a hot climate or taking some medications that can cause dehydration, sometimes in extreme cases, when you crave salt, it means you need salt.

THE FIX:

- Add salt to your diet
- Add trace minerals to your water
- Check out the Let's Talk Low Sodium post for more information

2.   You need more good fat.

When you crave salt, it generally means that the body is asking for more good fat. When you are stressed, your body is revving high, you burn lots of calories, your brain works really hard and your body quickly gets depleted of its nutrients. Periods of high stress can rapidly deplete your vitamin and mineral reserves. So, when you are stressed, your body is looking for more sustaining energy by way of good fat. You don't have to be stressed for the body to need more good fat. Fat is essential for cellular function as well as brain and heart health.

THE FIX:

- Your body would rather get that fat from the foods you eat than to utilize its emergency reserve. Without enough good fat coming in, your body will be reluctant to release fat. So, one way you can speed up that fat loss process is to make sure you are adding healthy fats to your meals. It's also beneficial to add in an omega 3 or 3-6-9 supplement, which we will be talking more about in Week 2.

LET'S TALK TUMMY RUMBLINGS & HUNGER PAINS:

We are taught to believe if your tummy rumbles you must be hungry, when in fact that's not what the noise and rumblings are about. It's actually your body's natural MMC or Migrating Motor Complex, a self-cleaning mechanism where in between meals and snacks, it works to clear bacteria and food particles out of the stomach and small intestine.

Because we are eating so often during the day, the body is doing most of this work at night. As we move through the Program, we will be phasing you into more natural patterns of eating which will be more in tune to your body's needs, which include the downtime it needs in between meals to self-regulate.

TO RECAP:

Cravings are nothing to stress about. They can give you great insight into your body's needs. Usually, the smallest tweak or adjustments can make all the difference.

It's important to note it's not about controlling your cravings; it's about being in tune to them. As you progress through the Program, you will become more in tune and able to differentiate between the body's needs and your wants.

Please take the time to head over to the Facebook Group or the Livy Method App and watch the quick video that accompanies this post.

LET'S TALK WHAT TO DO IF YOU ARE NOT HUNGRY

With all the changes the body is making in the first few weeks, it's normal to feel hungrier. However, it is also normal to not feel hungry.

Over the last few weeks, you have been working hard to give your body everything it needs so that it no longer feels the need to store fat. By being consistent and following the Food Plan, you are also addressing your cravings and naturally helping the body reduce portion sizes without even trying.

This will lead to a change in your appetite as the body will be working hard to regulate your metabolism and blood sugar, as well as making internal and external changes.

As your body works hard to make change and works hard to find balance, these changes will have your hunger levels changing day to day and week to week. Which is why it is normal to not feel hungry for some meals and snacks. One day you might be hungry every 5 mins and then the next day, a few hours can go by and you won't be hungry at all.

Why do you have to eat when you are not hungry?

- Consistency helps to maintain and reinforce the routine of the Food Plan. This will play a key role moving forward with addressing the body's needs while you focus on fat loss.

- We are still in the early stages of making the body feel confident it is going to get what it needs so it doesn't feel the need to store fat. Therefore you need to eat, even if just a small token amount.

- There are many benefits to eating a token amount of your meals and snacks even if you are not hungry. Having a small token amount of food stimulates your digestive system, regulates blood sugar and helps to keep you more satisfied leading into your next meal or snack, which can prevent overeating.

- Along with reinforcing the routine, following the Food Plan as designed also helps to prevent the urge to snack after dinner/before bed.

You are going to notice that some days you will be hungrier than others, which is totally normal and why the focus right now is to eat all meals and snacks, make your food choices nutrient rich, and eat to satisfaction regardless of what that portion looks like.

Bottom line: if you are not hungry, you still need to eat a small token amount. Token amounts means just enough food to stimulate your digestive system so at least 4-5 bites of food with chewing in between, give or take.

Please take the time to head over to the Facebook Group or the Livy Method App and watch the quick video that accompanies this post.

LET'S TALK SICKNESS

How to manage following the Program while you are sick and still stay on track.

Being sick is never fun and it can be very discouraging when you are trying your best to follow the Program. It is important to focus on feeling better, taking the time to recover, then you can resume the Program from where you left off.

If you follow the sickness protocol, it can actually work to your advantage when it comes to helping your body release fat.

WHAT TO DO WHEN YOU ARE SICK

1. **Drink extra water, especially if you are craving sugar and carbs.**

    - Resist the urge to go for crackers, white rice, bread products or sugar to settle your stomach. Chances are what you really need is water.

    - Water is essential for your body to detox out the virus, so stay hydrated and utilize teas and soups to increase your liquid intake.

2. **Don't force the food.**

    - Chances are you will not be hungry when you are sick and that is for a reason.

    - The body is not interested in processing and digesting food, it would much rather stay focused on getting the virus out. This is a natural process that allows the body to divert all its resources into healing you.

    - The body stores a certain amount of fat for emergency purposes to use when you are sick. Your body using fat reserves for energy when you are sick is not the same as when you ignore hunger signals and purposely do not eat to force your body to burn fat.

    - Keep the food light and go for food that is easily digested, like soup. Be in the moment with your food choices and don't be afraid to keep it light. Once your appetite comes back, you can pick up where you left off.

    - Don't be surprised if you find your portions are naturally smaller when you resume eating. This is just your body resetting, so go with it and be in tune moving forward.

3. **Ignore the scale.**

    - Chances are your weight will be up while you are sick, even if you are not eating. This is normal and happens because your body is retaining water it needs to detox the virus out.

    - Antibiotics and medications can also have your weight up. This is not real weight gain so it is nothing to be concerned about.

4. **Get lots of rest.**

   - There is no benefit in powering through. Give your body the time it needs to recover.
   - Taking naps and getting lots of rest will have your body bouncing back sooner than later, whereas powering through can just end up prolonging the sickness.

5. **Don't worry.**

   - Getting sick can feel like a major sidetrack, but it can work to your advantage. Your first priority is to feel better.
   - Your body will look to rid you of the virus and make you stronger. This leads to your body working harder and fast tracking the repair and rebuild process, which will only work to your advantage while working to lose weight.
   - Once your appetite comes back, get back on track and re-establish the routine and then you can pick up where you left off and keep moving forward.

TO RECAP:

- Drink extra water and stay hydrated.
- Keep the food light and easy to digest, don't force the Food Plan.
- Avoid eating later in the evening which can mess with sleep.
- Have a hot Epsom salt bath to help with detox.
- Take any medication needed to help.
- Get lots of rest.
- Once you feel better, pick up where you left off and keep moving forward.

Please note: The sickness protocol can be used any time you are unwell, physically, mentally, and emotionally. Really, any time your appetite is affected. Use it for as long as you need until your appetite comes back and you feel like you are able to move forward.

Please take the time to head over to the Facebook Group or the Livy Method App and watch the quick video that accompanies this post.

WONDERING WHY YOUR WEIGHT IS UP?

While following the Program, your weight might go up for various reasons, none of which will have anything to do with actual weight gain.

When following the Food Plan, consistently eating all the meals and snacks, making foods nutrient rich and eating to satisfaction, you are NOT going to gain weight.

The body is not inclined to want to store fat, in fact it's quite the opposite. The body wants your fat gone just as much as you do! It's important to understand that throughout this Program, your weight is going to naturally fluctuate, no matter what you do.

Reasons your weight can be up:

- Stress
- Lack of sleep
- Salty food
- Hard to digest food
- Dehydration
- Body fighting an illness
- Body sore from a workout
- Body reacting to change in routine
- Body reacting to change in food
- Body reacting to new medication or change in medications
- Body reacting to any new supplements or change in supplements
- Deficiencies like being low in iron
- Hormones fluctuating
- PMS
- Your scale needing new batteries

And the last, and most important reason, is that your body is detoxing and your weight is about to drop.

If you need to, review the Let's Talk The Scale post as it's important to get comfortable with what real weight loss looks like on the scale.

If you stick around and keep showing up, you are going to be successful and lose your weight regardless of the little ups along the way. So, keep in mind, the ups are normal and to be expected and nothing to stress about. Remember, even with all of the ups, it is all about the downward trend.

Please take the time to head over to the Facebook Group or the Livy Method App and watch the quick video that accompanies this post.

MANAGING THE PLAN WITH DIABETES?

Here is a share from one of our Program Specialists, Kim Turnbull, who has been successful on the Program while having diabetes and managing her needs.

The Program works well for those with diabetes regardless of issues. The focus is on decreasing and regulating insulin while giving the body the resources and time it needs to become as healthy as possible. It's a safe and effective Program not only for weight loss but also helping your body heal and address any and all health issues.

With that said, we know that some of you may be nervous about making changes to your diet and lifestyle. Follow the Program the best you can and be sure to make any adjustments that you need along the way.

Please note: This is Kim's personal story. To make sure you're making the most of yours, be sure to check in with your healthcare provider along the way if you have any questions or concerns.

Hi all!

I would like to share a bit about myself. I have Type 1 diabetes. I have been on insulin for 31 years and an insulin pump for 21 years. In 2016 I was diagnosed with rheumatoid arthritis (RA).

I cannot imagine where my life would be without Gina and The Livy Method, it has been a game changer. My health and well-being have been forever changed!

Lowering the amount of insulin your body needs is the key with weight loss. The more sugar/carbs you eat the more insulin your body needs to break it down. The more insulin in your system, the more you crave sugar and the more weight you gain. They feed into one another.

We all need carbs, and we have some great options on the Food Plan. I was just not having the right types. I was gaining weight and my sugar levels were on a roller coaster ride some days. Whether your body is making its own insulin or you are giving it insulin, the response is the same. Before I started the program, I was taking upwards of 38-50 units a day along with Metformin as my body was becoming resistant to insulin. My A1C was 8.9.

Fast forward to today, I am off the Metformin and take 23-28 units of insulin daily and my A1C is 6.5, however I have had it as low as 5.8 and lost weight! My doctors could not believe the change in my weight, sugars and insulin levels. Not to mention how I feel everyday, more energy, more in tune with the foods my body is looking for, better sleep and the list goes on.

I still have carbs, just better ones like sweet potatoes, quinoa, Ryvita crackers, fruits and vegetables. I make better food choices and enjoy more nutrient rich foods. As soon as I add in something I shouldn't, I know it by the way I feel. My weight is up, not to mention my sugars. I was a huge Diet Coke drinker and I struggled to cut it out, but did because as Gina says, it can mess with your hunger signals which we want to get in tune with and the artificial sweeteners and flavours can impact cravings.

As for my RA, I have reduced my meds. I was on 14 pills a week and now I take 3 a week. And again, if I go off with my food, I can feel it. I have not had a major flare in over 2 years. The minor ones I do have will resolve in a day or so, but they are few and far between.

Lowering the amount of insulin your body needs is real and has a direct impact on weight loss. If you do take insulin or medication for diabetes, make sure you test your levels and if you are making adjustments, talk to your doctor along the way. Share this program with them so they can support you along your journey.

I test a lot to know where I am sitting so I can minimize any high or low blood sugars. At times I had to manage low blood sugars and dealt with them with Dex-4 tablets or some juice as advised by my doctor. Once I knew the cause of the low sugar or saw a pattern, I would make the changes in my daily insulin levels. If my sugars run high, I look at what I am eating and watch to make sure it wasn't a rebound from a low.

Having diabetes isn't always about the food impacting sugars. It can be stress or illness, but food choices have the biggest impact on insulin levels.

Week 3 – Mindfulness is one of my favourite weeks. It allowed me to really focus on the choices I was making and being in tune with what my body was communicating to me. For me being boring or predictable and consistent helped me adjust the insulin my body needed for the food I was taking in. For those that like to change things up you are going to love the Recipe Guide!

This program allowed me to lose over 40lbs. I have had some ups and downs. Right now I am 5 lbs up from my lowest low but I know why and what I need to do to give my body what it needs to drop the weight. I would go weeks without my weight changing and then it would drop. Even though the scale wasn't always moving, I could see the changes in my body. Remember everyone's journey is their own and I can't wait to hear about yours. It is a journey but one that is worth the effort.

This is just my story and what has worked for me. Learn to love being bored - it works!

— with love, Kim Turnbull

Please note: *This inspirational post is not meant to replace your healthcare provider's advice. If ever you have concerns about managing the Program, always check in with your healthcare provider.*

LET'S TALK FERTILITY, PREGNANCY AND NURSING

The Program has many benefits if you are looking to conceive, looking to lose while pregnant, looking to lose after, or while nursing.

The Livy Method is about losing weight in a way that is healthy for your body and your mind. The Program has many benefits if you are looking to conceive, looking to lose while pregnant, or looking to lose after pregnancy or while nursing.

WHEN LOOKING TO CONCEIVE:

If you are dealing with fertility issues, you will find the Program falls in line with fertility protocols. It is based on healthy eating and allows for healing, repairing and rebuilding, and helps the body find internal balance.

Continue to take any supplements or medications advised by your healthcare provider or fertility expert and be sure to check in with them if you add in anything new.

WHEN PREGNANT:

When pregnant, there isn't any reason why you can't help the body focus on fat loss in a healthy way. Growing research suggests that losing weight during pregnancy is not only possible, it can actually be beneficial for women who are overweight or obese and doctors may even recommend it.

Being overweight and pregnant can come with its own set of issues you need to be mindful of. Having excess weight can cause problems during pregnancy and can lead to:

- Premature birth
- Stillbirth
- Cesarean delivery
- Heart defects in baby
- Gestational diabetes in mother (and type 2 diabetes later in life)
- High blood pressure in mother
- Preeclampsia: severe form of high blood pressure that can also affect other organs like the kidneys
- Sleep apnea
- Blood clots (especially in your legs)
- Infections in mother

Because the Program is based on helping the body become as healthy as possible and addressing the body's needs, you should be able to follow as designed.

However, as we move forward and start making changes to the Food Plan, here are some things to keep in mind:

- Check in with your doctor or healthcare provider along the way.

- Be in tune to your body's needs.

- Even when it comes to downsizing (Week 4), which is where you start to decrease portions, you will still be eating lots of nutrient rich foods (eating 6-8 times a day if using Bonus Snacks).

- Be sure to use Bonus Snacks as needed.

WHEN NURSING:

This Program is beneficial for milk supply due to all of the water you are drinking and the healthy foods you are consuming.

Even when we start to address portions (which we will discuss more in depth when the time comes), you will still be eating more than enough nutrient rich food to nourish both you and your baby.

When making changes in your diet, your baby may pick up on any new foods you add in. This is normal, and in time they should adjust. Implement any changes you need to make at a pace you are comfortable with.

When it comes to the supplements we will be introducing in the weeks to come, they are generally safe for everyone. However, check in with your healthcare provider as they may feel differently given your personal health history.

In fact, if you have any concerns along the way about pregnancy, fertility, nursing or any health issues, check in with your healthcare provider.

Please take the time to head over to the Facebook Group or the Livy Method App and watch the quick video that accompanies this post.

LET'S TALK BOWEL MOVEMENTS

During this process, because we piggyback the body's natural detox response when it comes to releasing fat, your bowel movements will be all over the place, meaning every shape, size and consistency.

You may experience bouts of constipation, which are normal before detox or when making changes in your diet. You may also experience episodes of diarrhea or loose bowel movements, which are a normal occurrence when the body is in detox and responding to the changes you are making along the way.

Your digestive health directly affects your bowel movements. Food goes in and the byproduct eventually needs to make its way out. If you have experienced constipation issues in the past, this could have played a role in your body's ability to focus on fat loss.

Here is what you can do, above and beyond following the Program, to help improve your bowel movements:

LET'S TALK CONSTIPATION:

Things to keep in mind if you are experiencing constipation:

- Drink enough water to be properly hydrated.
- Follow the Food Plan consistently and focus on making your meals and snacks as nutrient rich as possible to ensure you are getting enough fiber in your diet.
- Be sure to add leafy greens to meals for added roughage and to support detox.
- Taking a daily fiber supplement such as psyllium and inulin, can help prevent constipation.
- Consider adding in the suggested supplements that can aid in digestion (Vitamin D, Omega 3, Calm Magnesium, digestive bitters, probiotic and/or prebiotic).

In addition to what is listed above with regards to the basic supplements, the following can also be beneficial in addressing constipation:

VITAMIN C:

When taking higher doses of vitamin C, the extra or unabsorbed vitamin C pulls water into your intestines, which can help soften your stool.

- Take 30 mins before food in the morning, dose is dependent on the individual and can range from 90-2000 mg.

B COMPLEX:

Low levels of vitamin B, specifically B12, B1 and B5 may cause constipation. Adding in a B complex may help ease your symptoms.

You may prefer to eat more foods rich in this vitamin rather than take a supplement. For example:

Meat (red meat, poultry, fish)

- Beef
- Liver
- Trout
- Salmon
- Tuna fish
- Whole grains (brown rice, barley, millet)
- Eggs and dairy products (milk, cheese)
- Legumes (beans, lentils)
- Seeds and nuts (sunflower seeds, almonds)
- Dark, leafy vegetables (broccoli, spinach)
- Fruits (citrus fruits, avocados, bananas)

TRIPHALA:

Used in Ayurvedic medicine, it can help to support bowel health and aid digestion, detoxifying the body and supporting the immune system.

- Triphala is available as a pill, and in powder form. The powder is meant to be dissolved in warm water and consumed as tea. It can taste bitter but can be mixed with honey or lemon without diminishing its effects.

- Triphala supplements have varying daily dosages based upon the manufacturer. It's important to follow package directions exactly. Discuss with your healthcare provider.

EXERCISE/MOVE YOUR BODY:

Exercise can help with constipation by decreasing the time it takes food to move through the large intestine. This limits the amount of water your body absorbs from the stool.

- Cardio exercise speeds up your breathing and heart rate, helping to stimulate the natural contracting of muscles in your intestines which helps to move stool out quickly.

- Something as simple as going for a walk after dinner can make all the difference when it comes to improving digestion.

TIME AND CONSISTENCY:

It is important to note that in most cases the body just needs time to address and improve bowel movement issues, and to rewire how it has come to habitually function over the years.

- The foods you are eating, and the overall structure of the Program will help to address constipation issues.

- Be as consistent as possible and patient with the process.

With more extreme bouts of constipation, sometimes you may need to take something stronger like an over-the-counter laxative to help the body work through any backlog.

LET'S TALK LOOSE BOWEL MOVEMENTS:

Loose bowel movements are a normal and expected part of the process. All of the water you are drinking, the fiber rich foods like fruit, vegetables, and leafy greens you are eating, all contribute to your body's natural way of detoxing.

Things to keep in mind if you are experiencing loose bowel movements:

- Bowel movements are the number one way your body detoxes and releases fat, which can lead to loose bowel movements for some people, especially when the scale is moving.

- Keeping a journal and recording how you are feeling after eating meals and snacks can give you insight into food sensitivities that can cause loose bowel movements and discomfort. Dairy and gluten are the most common sensitivities. This can also include other types of foods and even spices used to prepare foods.

- If you are taking Calm Magnesium, try adjusting the dose. Although it is rarely the sole issue for loose BMs, decreasing it slightly may help.

Please note: Be sure to consult with your healthcare provider if you are concerned that your bowel movements are out of the ordinary.

While following the Program, your body will be working hard to address digestive and bowel movement issues. Some conditions including Crohn's disease, celiac disease, IBS, thyroid issues and medications can be the cause of loose bowel movements. However, if your changes in bowel movements go hand in hand with following the Program and the changes you are making, chances are there is nothing to be concerned about and given the time, the body will sort out and address it on its own.

Please take the time to head over to the Facebook Group or the Livy Method App and watch the quick video that accompanies this post.

LET'S TALK WEIGHT LOSS AND YOUR MENSTRUATION CYCLE

The menstrual cycle is another way the body detoxes. When you have it, you can capitalize on it when it comes to fat loss by supporting the body and its needs.

Here are some tips to help support the body during your menstrual cycle:

- Drink extra water to meet its increased need during this time.

- Be consistent with following the Food Plan.

- Go lighter on the carbs and heavier on the leafy greens at lunch and dinner for increased roughage to help support the body in detox.

- Eat as early as possible in the evening.

- Take warm Epsom salt baths.

- Focus on sleep quality and help the body get extra rest.

- Be consistent with supplements.

- Increase or add in Calm Magnesium.

Magnesium has many benefits like contributing to energy production, helping with digestion, relieving anxiety, boosting your mood by supporting serotonin production, and relaxing muscles which can help with cramping. It can also help relieve PMS symptoms and support hormonal function. Taking magnesium daily can aid in preventing menstrual migraines as your magnesium levels tend to be a lot lower on your period due to your hormones.

You can add an extra dose during the day or increase your dose at night. Taking it during the day will not cause drowsiness as your body is not producing Melatonin at that time.

THINGS TO KEEP IN MIND:

- Be mindful of iron issues. When blood is lost every month, the iron in red blood cells is also lost. If your monthly iron intake and absorption does not replace the iron lost during your period, you can end up with iron deficiency, which affects not only your energy, but your ability to lose weight. *If you think you might be low in iron, be sure to check in with your healthcare provider.*

- It is normal for your period to come early, late, or look and feel different than what you are used to while following the plan. Because of the holistic approach we are taking while following The Livy Method, cycle syncing (the practice of eating, exercising, and aligning your lifestyle choices according to your menstrual cycle) is something that happens naturally. Although this can be unnerving, rest assured your body is doing what's best to allow it to work at optimal levels.

- If you are concerned with changes in your cycle, it is always a good idea to check in with your healthcare provider.

- It is normal for your weight to go up right before and during your period. This is due to natural fluctuations like water retention, and is not real weight gain.

Please note: Although having your menstrual cycle can be beneficial with the weight loss process, if you do not have a period or you are in menopause, it will not affect your overall ability to lose weight and reach your Finally & Forever goals.

Please take the time to head over to the Facebook Group or the Livy Method App and watch the quick video that accompanies this post.

LET'S TALK LOW SODIUM

Sodium is the main component of salt and an essential electrolyte which helps with balancing water in the body, muscle function and nerve transmissions.

For years, health organizations have been warning people about the dangers of salt, linking too much sodium to high blood pressure and recommending people limit their intake. However, even though too much sodium can cause problems, consuming too little can be just as unhealthy. When following a healthy eating plan like The Livy Method, people tend to naturally reduce their salt intake.

Low sodium in your blood can occur when there is not enough sodium in your system to balance out fluid in the body. Symptoms of low blood sodium can vary from person to person and can cause serious issues if not addressed.

Common symptoms of low sodium include:

- Dizziness
- Weakness
- Fatigue or low energy
- Headache
- Nausea
- Vomiting
- Muscle cramps or spasms
- Confusion
- Irritability

Although it's worth noting, issues with low sodium levels while following the Program are few and far between. Unless you are excessively drinking way more water than you need, drinking more than 1 L per hour, sweating excessively, taking medication that can cause low sodium issues or avoiding salt, chances are there is nothing for you to be concerned about.

Keep in mind, there are other factors that can attribute to low sodium including:

- Taking certain medications, including antidepressants and pain medications
- Taking diuretics (water pills)
- Drinking too much water during exercise (this is very rare)
- Dehydration (please note low sodium can also be due to not enough water)
- Kidney disease or kidney failure
- Liver disease

- Heart problems, including congestive heart failure
- Adrenal gland disorders such as Addison's disease, which affects your adrenal gland's ability to regulate the balance of sodium, potassium, and water in your body
- Hypothyroidism (underactive thyroid)
- Primary polydipsia, a condition in which excess thirst makes you drink too much
- Using ecstasy or other hard-core drugs
- Syndrome of inappropriate antidiuretic hormone (SIADH), which makes your body retain water
- Diabetes insipidus, a rare condition in which the body doesn't make antidiuretic hormones
- Cushing's syndrome, which causes high cortisol levels (this is rare)
- Severe vomiting or diarrhea

(Sourced from Healthline)

WHO NEEDS TO BE MINDFUL OF LOW SODIUM?

- People who are older in age
- People who use diuretics
- If you use antidepressants
- If you are sweating a lot due to climate or exercise
- If eating a low-sodium diet
- If you have had heart failure, kidney disease, or other conditions

If you have any of these risk factors for low sodium, you may need to be more careful about your intake of water and be sure to add in salt or trace minerals as needed. A blood test can help your healthcare provider check for low sodium levels.

TIPS FOR PREVENTING LOW SODIUM IN YOUR BLOOD:

- Keeping your water and electrolyte levels in balance can help prevent low blood sodium.
- Including sodium in your diet by salting foods with pink Himalayan, Celtic or Sea salt, or adding in trace minerals with added sodium to your water is not only healthy for you, but an easy way to ensure you are getting the sodium you need.
- Working hand in hand with your healthcare provider while following the Program.

The moral of the story here:

Adding in salt or trace minerals as well as being properly hydrated is key to the process. Be mindful of your water intake to ensure you are drinking enough to meet your individual needs, and not just adding in more.

If you have any questions or concerns regarding your sodium levels, discuss them with your healthcare professional.

Please take the time to head over to the Facebook Group or the Livy Method App and watch the quick video that accompanies this post.

WEEK 2 GUIDELINES: CONSISTENCY AND MAXIMIZING

Week 2 has you focusing on consistency and maximizing your efforts, along with reviewing the suggested Supplements.

Prep Week was about introducing and implementing the Food Plan. Week 1 was focused on fine tuning and adjusting the changes you made. This week is about being as consistent as possible to help the body adjust while maximizing your efforts.

THE GOAL FOR THIS WEEK:

- Eat all meals and snacks
- Make all food choices as nutrient rich as possible
- Eat to satisfaction
- Add in Bonus Snacks if needed
- Stay hydrated
- Be as consistent as possible
- Look to maximize your efforts

The intention this week is to be as consistent as possible with the changes you have made so far, and to maximize your efforts while bringing awareness to how your body is responding.

Maximizing means focusing on all the other things you can do besides following the Food Plan, drinking water and adding in any supplements. For example, managing stress, trying to get better quality sleep, moving your body and working with your healthcare provider to address any health issues.

Be sure to check out the Let's Talk Maximizing Your Efforts Checklist post for more examples and areas you can focus on so you can be as proactive as possible when it comes to getting and keeping the scale moving.

WEEK 2 ALSO HAS US INTRODUCING SUPPLEMENTS THAT CAN PLAY A KEY ROLE IN THIS PROCESS.

Supplements are not mandatory, however; they can help where the body is deficient, which can make all the difference when it comes to addressing the body's needs and speeding up the weight loss process. Be sure to review the Let's Talk Supplements post (out this week) for more information, and if you have any questions, check in with your healthcare provider.

FREQUENTLY ASKED QUESTIONS

1. **What does Gina mean when she talks about consistency?**

    Consistency is when you are following the Program as it is laid out the best you can each day. Following the Food Plan and eating all of the nutrient rich meals and snacks to satisfaction, within the designated time frames and following the guidelines. It's also about being consistent with your hydration, getting good quality sleep, managing stress, getting in supplements and making as many choices as possible day to day that fall in line with your goals.

2. **How can I stay consistent on the weekends?**

    Weekends can be tricky because you are off of your regular routine which can lead to skipping meals and snacks, adding in extra bits and bites, not keeping up with your water, and lack of sleep. All things that can have your scale up. What's important to remember is that this is not real weight gain and there is nothing you can do on the weekend that cannot be undone by getting right back at it. As long as you keep showing up, you cannot mess it up. With that said, it is always a good idea to take a look at your social calendar and make a plan for yourself.

3. **I am still hungry at night, any tips?**

    It can be helpful to remember that hunger is not an immediate need for food, especially at night when your body is winding down and getting ready for sleep. Ways to help alleviate hunger at night are by starting your day with a high protein breakfast, eating all your meals and snacks to satisfaction, making your meals as nutrient rich as possible, and getting in your water throughout the day.

    Having herbal tea, taking a bath, going to bed earlier, or changing your evening routines are some things that may help as sometimes the desire to eat at night is based on habit.

4. **What does "eating to satisfaction" mean?**

The feelings of being satisfied can be very individual. As you continue to build your mind-body connection, these signals will become more clear and defined. Some people find they take a deep breath as soon as they are satisfied while others may put their utensils down and pause.

Once you slow down and tune in, your own satisfaction signals will become more and more apparent. This is something we will focus on over the coming weeks as recognizing your satisfaction levels is an important part of the Program. Another way to look at it is to ensure you are eating enough at each meal and snack, and not trying to eat less like you may have done on other diets.

5.   **I feel bloated and my clothes are tight, any tips?**

Feeling bloated can be normal as your body adjusts to the Food Plan and the changes that you are making. Follow the Program as designed and be as consistent as possible to help the body to adapt as quickly as possible. It is also normal to feel bloated when your weight is about to drop, and can be a sign of detox. If you feel that there may be something more going on, be sure to check in with your healthcare provider.

6.   **How important is the timing between my meals?**

The order you are eating your meals and snacks is important, but the timing between meals and snacks can change day to day. The time between all meals and snacks is ideally anywhere from 30 minutes to no longer than 3.5 hours apart.

7.   **Is there an alternate option for leafy greens?**

While there is no alternative to leafy greens, there are some vegetables that count as leafy greens. Vegetables like Brussels sprouts, bok choy and cabbage all count towards the vegetable and leafy greens component of your meals.

8.   **At what time should I finish drinking my water for the day?**

This will vary from person to person. It is a great idea to start drinking your water as early as possible in your day and avoid having it late into the evening, if it affects your sleep. The timing is something you can play around with based on your individual needs.

9.   **What if I have a question about supplements?**

For questions regarding supplements and your individual health needs, it's best to reach out to your pharmacist or healthcare provider.

Please take the time to head over to the Facebook Group or the Livy Method App and watch the quick video that accompanies this post.

LET'S TALK KEEPING A JOURNAL/USING THE LIVY METHOD APP

Why it can be a great idea to be tracking your progress along the way.

BENEFITS OF JOURNALING

A journal can be a great tool to help give you insight into how your body is responding to the process. It can help you pick up on patterns of behavior and responses and give you a better idea of what weight loss looks like and feels like, specifically to you.

It can also help you pick up on any food sensitivities, especially if you have digestive issues, track bowel movements if you struggle in that department and track your body's response to the supplements, or anything new you are adding in or taking out.

It is also beneficial for tracking your mood, which can motivate you to show up for yourself every day, take the time to think about how you are managing your emotions, and how you are feeling day to day.

THINGS TO TRACK

- Weight in the morning
- How you are feeling physically
- How you are feeling mentally
- Energy day to day
- Sleep
- Food
- Water
- Movement
- Bowel movements
- Notable responses from food
- Medications
- Supplements
- Non-scale victories

You can use good old pen and paper or the Livy Method App. Do what works best for you. As we progress, your journal can be a very helpful tool to give you insight and make the most of the time that you have while following the Program.

The more tools the better!

Please take the time to head over to the Facebook Group or the Livy Method App and watch the quick video that accompanies this post.

5 PRO TIPS TO BE MORE PROACTIVE WITH THIS PROCESS

It is important to be an advocate for yourself during this process. Down below, you will find some tips for being proactive and getting the most out of the Program.

Proactive - adjective

pro·ac·tive (proh-ak-tiv)

"Definition of proactive 1 [pro- entry 2 + reactive]: acting in anticipation of future problems, needs, or changes"

1. **Be sure to watch the Check In Video daily**

    In it, Gina not only guides you through the Program and gives you a heads up on what you need to focus on each day, she also goes over frequently asked questions that can give you insight on where we are at in the process.

2. **Be sure to read the posts a few times, even if you have done the Program before**

    Posts can resonate differently, depending on where you are at in your weight loss journey.

    There is quite a bit of information. It is a good idea to review it a few times and even make notes. Having a clear understanding of the process makes it so much easier to follow, which makes it so much more effective in the end.

3. **Make sure you are watching the videos that go along with the posts**

    The videos go more in-depth and may also touch on other elements not listed in the written content.

4. **It is progress over perfection, so keep moving forward**

    The changes you make week to week become the jumping off point for the following week. You want to avoid going back and repeating steps.

    The goal is to be all in and keep things moving forward.

    If ever you go off plan, simply pick up where you left off.

5. **Set your intentions and end of day reflections**

    Using the Livy Method App or Check In Video in the group, is a great way to keep this process at the forefront of your mind by setting your intentions each day. It can help remind you of the things that you need to focus on while working towards your goals.

    Taking some time to reflect at the end of your day is helpful in keeping you accountable and aware of the things that you are doing well and should be proud of, and help you focus on any areas that could use more attention.

    Setting intentions and end of day reflections can help with self-sabotage throughout the process, as it brings awareness to where you are at and what you are working through.

A BONUS TIP: Keep a journal and/or use the Livy Method App for tracking how your body is responding to the changes you are making. Journalling can help with any problem solving should it be needed along the way, and give you great insight into how to make the most out of this process.

LET'S TALK MAXIMIZING YOUR EFFORTS CHECKLIST

Maximizing refers to all of the other things you can do besides following the Food Plan, drinking the water and taking any supplements to be as proactive as possible.

Even though it is still too early in the Program to be concerned about the scale, as you move forward you may find yourself wondering if you are doing everything right, or if there is anything more you can do to help the process.

Below is a list of 20 questions and a checklist that you can use to highlight areas of opportunity and things you can focus on to make the most of your efforts while following the Program. Refer back to it daily, weekly, or whenever you are feeling like or wondering if there is more you can be doing. Utilize the blank spaces to add your own unique points you are hitting the mark on.

Please note, some posts listed in the checklist will be coming out in the coming weeks. As you move through the Program week to week, you may want to revisit this checklist to see if there is any area that you can level up!

20 QUESTIONS TO ASK YOURSELF:

1. **Are you following the Program to the best of your ability day in and day out?**

    The more consistently you do all of the things you need to do to follow the Program, the more successful you will be.

    ☐ Have you watched the six key videos that break down the rhyme and reason behind the order of the meals/snacks:

    - ☐ The Livy Method
    - ☐ The Food Plan
    - ☐ Let's Talk Detox
    - ☐ Let's Talk The Scale
    - ☐ Let's Talk Weight Loss
    - ☐ Let's Talk About Hunger

    ☐ Are you eating all meals and snacks?

    ☐ Are you having token amounts of meals/snacks when you're not hungry?

    ☐ Are you following the order of the Food Plan?

    ☐ Are you eating your meals/snacks 30 mins - 3.5 hours apart?

    ☐ Are you checking into the Livy Method App or Facebook Support Group daily?

    ☐ Are you using the Livy Method App, the tracking sheets or a journal to track your progress?

- [ ] Are you reviewing the information repeatedly until you are super clear on it?
- [ ] If you are a returning member, are you asking yourself the 4 Mindfulness Questions before each meal/snack? If you are new to the Program, the 4 Mindfulness Questions are introduced in Week 3.
- [ ] Are you open to your hunger levels changing day in and day out and adjusting portions accordingly?
- [ ] Are you weighing yourself and recording your weight every day to track your body's natural fluctuations and patterns?
- [ ] _____
- [ ] _____
- [ ] _____

2. **Has your body had time to make change and focus on fat loss?**

It is important to be real about the time your body needs to make change, and the time your body has had to focus on fat loss. Coming off of a super restrictive diet, being hit or miss with following the Food Plan, taking days off or having some off days or weekends, along with being sick or stressed can all affect the progress you are making while following the Program.

- [ ] Are you consistently following the Program Guidelines day to day, week to week?
- [ ] Are you consistently following the Food Plan?
- [ ] Are you consistently hitting all meals and snacks?
- [ ] Are you making sure to have the "stars" at each meal/snack?
- [ ] Are you having token amounts when you're not hungry?
- [ ] Are you consistently drinking enough water to meet your body's needs?
- [ ] Are you consistently taking your supplements (if you have added them in)?
- [ ] Are you setting intentions in the morning?
- [ ] Are you checking in mid-day?
- [ ] Are you reflecting at night?
- [ ] _____
- [ ] _____
- [ ] _____

3. **Have you had the flu or a cold or any other sickness that your body is dealing with, or had to focus on?**

It is all about priorities when it comes to your body focusing on fat loss. Being sick won't stop you from reaching your goal, but it can slow you down for a moment. Helping your body focus on healing is the quickest way to get the scale moving.

- ☐ Have you reviewed the Let's Talk Sickness post?
- ☐ Are you following the sickness protocol and helping the body heal so it can better focus on fat loss when the time comes?
- ☐ Are you forcing the Food Plan rather than giving your body time to recover?
- ☐ Are you getting enough rest to allow your body the time it needs to recover?
- ☐ Are you on antibiotics or any medications that might mess with digestion/make you dehydrated?
- ☐ Have you adjusted your water intake to help your body detox out the virus/process any medications you may be on?
- ☐ If you are sick, are you taking into consideration that the scale may be up simply because you are sick?
- ☐ Are you working hand in hand with your healthcare provider?
- ☐ _____
- ☐ _____
- ☐ _____

4.   Are you managing your stress levels?

Stress can play a major role in preventing the body from focusing on fat loss. Managing your stress can go a long way in getting the scale to move. Are you doing all you can do to help the body manage your stress?

- ☐ Have you revisited the Let's Talk Stress and Sleep post?
- ☐ Have you revisited the Meditation and Stress Management Share page?
- ☐ Are you being consistent with the basics of the Program?
- ☐ Are you allocating time for breath work?
- ☐ Are you stretching?
- ☐ Have you added in movement?
- ☐ Are you communing with nature?
- ☐ Are you having Epsom salt baths?
- ☐ Have you added in meditation?
- ☐ Are you taking the time to journal to process and work through all the feels/associations that may come up during this process?

☐ Are you eating as early into the evening as possible?

☐ Have you added in the suggested supplements that can help aid in stress relief?

☐ Are you redirecting your thoughts?

☐ Are you looking for things that bring you joy?

☐ Have you considered therapy?

☐ Are you keeping up with health issues and seeing healthcare providers?

☐ _____

☐ _____

☐ _____

5. Are you getting quality deep and REM sleep?

Getting quality sleep is a major factor when it comes to losing weight. When you sleep, your body repairs, rebuilds, regenerates, and rejuvenates in order to make change. Getting enough is integral to the detox process. Are you helping your body get the best sleep possible?

☐ Have you visited the Let's Talk Stress and Sleep post?

☐ Are you fostering good sleep hygiene habits?

☐ Are you avoiding blue light at night?

☐ Are you staying off screens/getting off them earlier?

☐ Are you avoiding stimulants like the TV and phone?

☐ Are you dimming/adjusting your lighting in the evening?

☐ Do you have a nighttime routine?

☐ Are you helping your body prepare for sleep by eating earlier in the evening?

☐ Are you making an effort to go to bed earlier?

☐ Are you taking naps when needed?

☐ Are you taking an Epsom salt bath in the evening?

☐ If you are having sleep issues (i.e., snoring, gasping) have you reached out to a sleep specialist?

☐ Are you reducing your caffeine intake if it is affecting your sleep?

☐ Have you added in the suggested supplements that can help aid in sleep?

☐ Are you keeping a journal beside your bed?

☐ _____

☐ _____

☐ _____

6. Are you drinking enough water?

Because we are piggybacking the body's natural detox response, drinking enough water is very important when it comes to fat loss. It's more than just setting an amount, it's about being consistent and adjusting to ensure you are meeting your body's daily needs.

- ☐ Have you reviewed the Let's Talk Water post?
- ☐ Have you reviewed the Let's Talk Low Sodium post?
- ☐ Are you starting your day with your morning lemon/ACV water?
- ☐ Are you consistently hitting your water goal day in and day out?
- ☐ Is the majority of your fluid intake flat water?
- ☐ Are you setting/hitting your water target daily and adjusting as needed?
- ☐ Are you adjusting your water intake according to your body's needs?
- ☐ Are you focusing on hydration early in the day?
- ☐ Are you spreading your water intake out, sipping and avoiding guzzling?
- ☐ Do you have a good water bottle or cup you are drinking out of?
- ☐ Have you measured the cup or vessel that you drink your water from to be sure of your intake?
- ☐ Are you setting timers/reminders?
- ☐ Are you adding in trace minerals/good quality salts to your water to avoid low sodium levels?
- ☐ Are you drinking the minimum amounts of water required for basic body functioning (2.7-3.5 L) and adjusting according to your body's needs?
- ☐ Are you aware of your body's signs that you have reached your optimal amount (You are no longer thirsty, lips/mouth no longer dry, bathroom trips have decreased)?
- ☐ Are you tracking your water?
- ☐ If your water is not appealing, are you adding in fresh fruit or lemon/lime juice?
- ☐ If drinking alcohol, are you adding in one extra cup of water per drink?
- ☐ _____
- ☐ _____
- ☐ _____

7. Are you making your meals and snacks as nutrient rich as possible?

It is important that your body is getting the nutrients it needs to address its needs and make change. Ensuring that your food choices are nutrient rich will also help with feeling more satisfied when it comes to your portions.

- ☐ Have you reviewed the Let's Talk Nutrient Rich Meals post?
- ☐ Have you reviewed the Let's Talk Proteins Carbs and Fats post?
- ☐ Are you adding in healthy fats to your meals and snacks?
- ☐ Are you consistent with making sure you are getting each component of each meal/snack?
- ☐ Are you going for foods that are more bang for your buck and avoiding grabbing what is convenient?
- ☐ Are you having protein-rich breakfast?
- ☐ Are you switching up your proteins?
- ☐ Are you adding in a good variety of healthy fats?
- ☐ Are you being mindful of your sugar intake?
- ☐ Are you avoiding artificial flavours/colours/sweeteners?
- ☐ Are you avoiding low fat/no fat dairy products?
- ☐ Are you avoiding processed foods?
- ☐ _____
- ☐ _____
- ☐ _____

8.   Are you moving your body enough?

Although you don't have to exercise in order to lose weight, your body is meant to move. Being active has its benefits and making sure to move your body as much as possible can make all the difference when it comes to getting the scale to move.

- ☐ Have you visited the Let's Talk About Exercise post?
- ☐ Are you being mindful to move?
- ☐ Are you being as active as possible?
- ☐ Are you getting your heart rate up?
- ☐ Are you getting your heart rate up as high as you can for as long as you can even just for a few minutes to evoke your fight or flight response?
- ☐ Are you taking the stairs instead of the elevator/escalator?
- ☐ Are you parking further away when buying groceries?
- ☐ Are you going for walks?
- ☐ Are you doing light movements throughout the day?
- ☐ Are you walking away from exercise feeling good and energized, not tired, taxed or drained?

- ☐ Are you choosing exercises that you enjoy and have a positive association towards?
- ☐ If you are lifting weights, are you lifting lighter and using higher repetitions?
- ☐ Are you giving your body adequate time to rest to repair and rebuild?
- ☐ _____
- ☐ _____
- ☐ _____

9. Are you helping the body while in detox?

Although the body naturally detoxes on its own, supporting the body and its needs can make all the difference when it comes to helping it specifically focus on fat loss, and following through with releasing fat.

- ☐ Have you visited the Let's Talk Detox post?
- ☐ Have you visited the Let's Talk Supporting the Body in Detox post?
- ☐ Are you consistent with your supplements?
- ☐ Are you consistent with eating all meals and snacks?
- ☐ Are you eating token amounts if not hungry?
- ☐ Are you mindful of portions to help the body stay focused on detox?
- ☐ Are you choosing easier to digest proteins while in detox?
- ☐ Are you keeping your heavier grains on the lighter side while in detox?
- ☐ Are you keeping leafy greens on the heavier side while in detox?
- ☐ Are you going to bed earlier while in detox?
- ☐ Are you taking Epsom salt baths while in detox?
- ☐ Are you getting in extra water while in detox?
- ☐ Are you moving your body while in detox?
- ☐ If you are menstruating, have you increased your Calm Magnesium?
- ☐ _____
- ☐ _____
- ☐ _____

10. Are you taking medications or have health issues that need to be factored in?

It is important to note, you can lose weight regardless of any health issues you may have. Because the Program is based on helping the body be as healthy as possible and carrying extra weight can be detrimental to your health, it is more than happy to release it. Doing everything you can to address your body's needs to maximize your efforts will make all the difference when it comes to reaching your goals.

- ☐ Have you visited the Let's Talk 4 Main Reasons Why Your Weight Might Be Slower To Move post?

- ☐ Do you think there are underlying issues that are affecting your health? And if so, have you addressed them or sought out help for them?

- ☐ Are you working hand in hand with your healthcare provider(s) when it comes to your specific medical conditions/medications?

- ☐ Have you seen a naturopath?

- ☐ Have you seen a chiropractor?

- ☐ Have you seen a physiotherapist?

- ☐ Have you seen an acupuncturist?

- ☐ Have you gotten your blood work done?

- ☐ Have you sought out a specialist/expert to address any health issues above and beyond what we are doing on the Program?

- ☐ Have you considered therapy to address mental health issues?

- ☐ Are you being patient in factoring in your health issues?

- ☐ Are you recognizing any limitations you may have?

- ☐ Have you looked into other ways you can help your body heal or deal with your health issues?

- ☐ Have you adjusted your water intake to accommodate for any medications/health issues?

- ☐ Have you introduced any supplements that may help?

- ☐ _____

- ☐ _____

- ☐ _____

11. Are you missing any organs?

Your body is amazing in how it can continue to function even when missing organs (kidney, spleen, gallbladder, reproductive organs, colon, etc.). Besides following the basics of the Program, there are things you can do above and beyond to help the body compensate and function at more optimal levels.

- ☐ Are you factoring in the need to compensate for any missing organs?

- ☐ Are you working hand in hand with your doctor, pharmacist, or healthcare practitioner when it comes to your specific medical conditions/medications?

- ☐ Are you going the extra mile to help your body manage any deficiencies?

- ☐ Are you helping the body compensate for missing organs by adding in supplements that may help? (Example: Bile salts/digestive bitters if you are missing your gallbladder)
- ☐ Are you supporting your body by getting quality sleep?
- ☐ Are you getting adequate hydration?
- ☐ Are you managing your stress?
- ☐ _____
- ☐ _____
- ☐ _____

12. Do you have hormone issues you need to address or that need to be factored in?

Dealing with hormonal issues will not stop you from reaching your goal. However, going the extra mile to address them can make all the difference in how you feel and how your body functions. It can also make a difference when it comes to movement on the scale.

- ☐ Have you visited the Let's Talk 4 Main Reasons Why Your Weight Might Be Slower To Move post?
- ☐ Have you looked into addressing hormonal issues you may be dealing with?
- ☐ Have you sought out a specialist/expert to address any health issues above and beyond what we are doing on the Program?
- ☐ Are you moving your body?
- ☐ Are you managing your stress?
- ☐ Are you getting good quality sleep?
- ☐ Are your meals truly nutrient rich?
- ☐ Have you added in breakfast?
- ☐ Is your breakfast truly protein rich?
- ☐ Have you considered decreasing or eliminating your consumption of alcohol?
- ☐ Are you adding in supplements that can help?
- ☐ Are you factoring in and giving the body the time that it needs to address any hormonal issues?
- ☐ Are you being consistent with the Food Plan and Guidelines?
- ☐ _____
- ☐ _____
- ☐ _____

13. Have you had your blood work done?

Getting your blood work done is one of the most important things you can do to help with leveling up your health and wellness. Knowing what is going on in all areas of health in regards to your body can give you great insight to all the things you can do to maximize your efforts when it comes to weight loss.

- ☐ Have you checked in with your healthcare provider recently?
- ☐ Have you had a physical done recently?
- ☐ Have you asked your healthcare provider for further blood work testing?
- ☐ Are you working with your healthcare provider to interpret your results?
- ☐ Do you have any deficiencies that could be affecting your body's ability to function properly?
- ☐ Have you added in any supplements that address deficiencies?
- ☐ _____
- ☐ _____
- ☐ _____

14. Are you taking any supplements and taking them consistently?

Supplements are designed to help supplement and address any deficiencies your body may have, to ensure your body is able to work at the most optimal level. This is especially important to this process as having deficiencies can affect your body's ability to focus on fat loss.

- ☐ Have you reviewed the Let's Talk Supplements post?
- ☐ Have you reviewed the Let's Talk Secondary Supplements post?
- ☐ Have you considered all the suggested supplements and added them in?
- ☐ Are you consistently taking them day in and day out?
- ☐ Are you setting reminders or have a plan for remembering to take them?
- ☐ Have you created a supplements schedule personalized to you?
- ☐ Are you considering your environment and the demands it has on your body (ie. lack of sunlight, working a high-stress job, living in a warmer climate)?
- ☐ Have you given your body enough time to adjust to and adapt to the supplements you have added in?
- ☐ Have you booked a consultation with your pharmacist to discuss the suggested supplements?
- ☐ Are you working hand in hand with your healthcare provider?

☐ _____

☐ _____

☐ _____

15. Has your body been focusing on repairing, rebuilding and making change? Are you noticing and tracking non-scale victories?

Paying attention to what your body is focused on and when, like physical changes that can't be seen on the scale, your body changing shape and size and various other non-scale victories can be another sign that your efforts are adding up. Focusing on these and not just on the scale can give you the motivation you need to keep working towards your goals.

☐ Are you recognizing the non-scale victories you are experiencing?

☐ Are you tracking your NSVs in the Livy Method App or in a journal?

☐ Have you been taking photos each week to track your physical changes?

☐ Do you recognize your body making change when the scale is not moving?

☐ Are your clothes fitting better?

☐ Do you have increased energy?

☐ Are your measurements changing?

☐ Are your rings looser?

☐ Has your complexion improved?

☐ Are you leaning into your non-scale victories for motivation?

☐ _____

☐ _____

☐ _____

16. Are you getting a good variety of protein in your diet to meet your body's needs?

Although The Livy Method is not a high protein diet, making sure you are eating enough and the right kind of quality protein will ensure the body gets what it needs, to make the changes that it needs to make. Protein also feeds into your satiety hormones helping you to feel more satisfied, which plays a role in adjusting portions.

☐ Have you reviewed the Let's Talk Groceries post for a breakdown on the variety of protein on plan?

☐ Have you reviewed the Let's Talk Proteins Carbs and Fats post?

☐ Have you reviewed the Vegan Meal Ideas Share page?

☐ Are you maximizing your food choices?

- ☐ Are you having a good balance of plant-based proteins and animal-based protein?
- ☐ Are you mindful to limit the amount of red meat you are consuming each week?
- ☐ Are you making an effort in adding fish and seafood into your diet?
- ☐ Are you being in tune and adjusting your proteins when you are in active detox (keeping harder to digest proteins to a minimum)?
- ☐ Are you choosing the best options, or are you stuck on eating what you like and love?
- ☐ _____
- ☐ _____
- ☐ _____

17. Do you have any digestive issues that you need to factor in or address?

Digestion is important for weight loss because if your body is unable to process food properly and get the nutrients it needs, it can affect your body's ability to function at more optimal levels and focus on fat loss. Although having digestive issues won't stop you from reaching your goals, factoring them in along the way and addressing your body's needs can make all the difference.

- ☐ Have you reviewed the Let's Talk Supplements post?
- ☐ Have you reviewed the Let's Talk Bowel Movements post?
- ☐ Have you reviewed the Let's Talk 4 Main Reasons Why Your Weight Might Be Slower To Move post?
- ☐ Have you seen your healthcare provider regarding your digestive issues?
- ☐ Have you seen a naturopathic doctor?
- ☐ Have you added in the suggested supplements that help aid in digestion?
- ☐ Are you taking a daily fiber supplement if needed?
- ☐ Are you maximizing your food choices to help your body better digest and process your food?
- ☐ Are you consistently adding in leafy greens?
- ☐ Are you journaling to track, and isolate any potential food allergies/sensitivities?
- ☐ Are you eating things you are sensitive to like dairy or gluten?
- ☐ _____
- ☐ _____
- ☐ _____

18. Do you have issues with bowel movements and if so, what are you doing to address them?

Bowel movements are the number one way the body detoxes. Given that we are piggybacking the body's natural detox response, focusing on regulating bowel movements can make all the difference when it comes to maximizing your efforts with this process.

- ☐ Have you visited the Let's Talk Bowel Movements post?
- ☐ Have you seen your doctor regarding your bowel movement issues?
- ☐ Are you being consistent with the Food Plan and water and allowing your body the time to adjust and adapt to the changes you have made?
- ☐ Have you followed up with a naturopathic doctor?
- ☐ Have you seen a hormone specialist if needed?
- ☐ Have you added in the suggested supplements that help aid in constipation/loose bowel movements?
- ☐ Are you consistent with your water intake and adjusting it according to your body's needs?
- ☐ Are you making your food choices as nutrient rich as possible?
- ☐ Are you consistently adding in leafy greens to your meals?
- ☐ Are you being mindful to add in fiber rich foods?
- ☐ Are you taking a daily fiber supplement if needed?
- ☐ Are you moving your body?
- ☐ Have you been journaling your foods to track and isolate potential sensitives or triggers?
- ☐ _____
- ☐ _____
- ☐ _____

19. Are you sabotaging yourself?

Dealing with self-sabotage can be part of the process. However, undermining your success can easily get in the way of you reaching your goal. Bringing awareness to how your actions are affecting your progress plays a major role when it comes to helping you work through it.

- ☐ Have you reviewed the Self-Sabotage posts?
- ☐ Are you continually getting in your own way of reaching your goals?
- ☐ Are you making choices that take you further away, not closer to, your goals?
- ☐ Have you identified your WHY?

- ☐ Are you setting realistic goals?
- ☐ Are you indulging in your frustration and festering in your funk?
- ☐ Are you having real conversations with yourself?
- ☐ Are you making a list of positive affirmations/self-talk and revisit them often?
- ☐ Have you made a list of all the things that can help you cope besides food?
- ☐ Have you identified your triggers/what you're afraid of?
- ☐ Are you journaling?
- ☐ Have you made a list of non-negotiables?
- ☐ Are you taking responsibility?
- ☐ Are you avoiding accountability?
- ☐ Are you comparing your journey to someone else's?
- ☐ Are you future tripping (anxious for what the future holds)?
- ☐ Are you committed to making life changing change, or looking for a quick fix?
- ☐ Are you being patient with the process?
- ☐ Are you trying to rush results?
- ☐ _____
- ☐ _____
- ☐ _____

20. Do you genuinely believe you have what it takes to follow through and finish?

When it comes to Finally & Forever it's about losing weight in a way that is not only healthy for your body, but equally healthy for your mind. It means having faith in yourself, working through issues and associations, creating new habits and beliefs, and doing all the things you can do to maximize your efforts. Most importantly, it is about following through, finishing and reaching your goal and not giving up until you get there.

- ☐ Do you have faith that you can lose your weight Finally & Forever?
- ☐ Do you trust yourself?
- ☐ Have you established and solidified your WHY?
- ☐ Have you reassessed your WHY to ensure it still resonates?
- ☐ Have you considered what is motivating you to keep showing up and following through till the end?
- ☐ Are you setting your intentions every day?
- ☐ Do you check in on yourself mid day?

☐ Are you reflecting at the end of each day?

☐ Have you visualized yourself at your Finally & Forever?

☐ Have you asked yourself what Finally & Forever will look and feel like to you?

☐ Have you asked yourself what losing your weight will truly mean to you?

☐ Do you truly see yourself still here at the end?

☐ Do you believe it without a shadow of a doubt?

☐ _____

☐ _____

☐ _____

Visit this post often as these questions are designed to help you self reflect and account for all of the things that you can do to level up your efforts when it comes to losing weight with The Livy Method. They can help highlight areas of opportunities and things you can work on to keep yourself organized throughout this process to maximize your efforts.

If after going through this there are still boxes left unchecked that you need to revisit, get excited as this means that there are more things you can be doing to be proactive with this process.

As you move forward, you can use this post as a daily checklist or if ever you find yourself wondering what more you can do to get and keep the scale moving to the best of your ability, be sure to refer back to this post as needed.

MAXIMIZING YOUR FOOD CHOICES

In the first few weeks of the Program, the focus was on settling into the routine. Now it is time to maximize your efforts when it comes to following the Food Plan, including leveling up your food choices.

Here are some questions to ask yourself that might highlight some small changes that can make a difference when it comes to getting and keeping the scale moving.

1.   **Are you still eating bread?**

     The Food Plan is designed to help decrease the amount of insulin your body is used to using. Bread, pasta, flour and crackers in general, require more insulin than whole foods when the body breaks them down, regardless of the type or source. While trying to lose weight, you want to decrease and balance out blood sugar levels, so adding them in can be counterproductive.

2.   **Are you eating popcorn or snacking at night?**

     It can take time to make the changes you need to make to address cravings, and no doubt some of you are still working on that. Popcorn was added in the beginning to help with that transition. Since then, we have talked about hunger and how to address it. Be sure to review the Let's Talk About Hunger post if you haven't already. We have also talked about how the body doesn't need food after dark and how eating and snacking can mess with your sleep and prevent your body from doing the work it needs to do during sleep. So now that you understand that, it's time to cut out the popcorn or any night time snacking.

3.   **Are you still having heavier carbs at dinner?**

     You may love your potatoes and rice at dinner, but the body does not necessarily need heavier carbs at night. Unless you are working out or playing sports in the evening, you might want to consider minimizing heavier carbs at dinner. Instead, a better option is to add them to your lunch, if and when you feel you need them.

4.   **Are you eating breakfast?**

     Although it is fine to skip it, having a protein-packed breakfast is absolutely beneficial to the weight loss process. You might want to be more consistent about adding it in, even if it is just as simple as an egg or a few spoonfuls of yogurt with hemp hearts.

5.   **Is your breakfast truly protein rich?**

     When eating oatmeal, cereals, or yogurt with added sugar and/or fruit for breakfast, are you making sure that protein is the star of the show? The more sugar and carbs in your breakfast, the more protein and fat you need to counteract that. Be sure you are bumping up the protein as much as you can.

6. **How's Your Sugar Adding Up?**

Although we do say that it's perfectly fine to have sugar in coffee or tea, with oatmeal or in yogurt, it quickly adds up. Be mindful of how much you are having in total and look for ways you can minimize any added sugar.

LET'S TALK ABOUT PRE-PACKAGED AND PROCESSED FOODS

Eating pre-packaged and processed food on occasion is nothing to worry about and can be a great convenience when needed. Minimally processed foods are totally fine to have. For example, canned beans, tuna, salad mixes in a bag, frozen vegetables etc. However, not all processed foods are created equal.

Here are some things to keep in mind when checking the ingredients:

- Avoid artificial colours, flavours or sweeteners, as well as partially/hydrogenated oil or trans fats.

- Be mindful of added sugar. There are over 50 different names for sugar on food labels. Some examples are: glucose, sucrose, dextrose, maltose, maltodextrin and anything ending in the word syrup or sugar such as brown rice syrup and beet sugar.

- Keep in mind that the first ingredient is the largest quantity ingredient and descends from there, with the last ingredient being the smallest. It is a good idea to look at the first 3 ingredients, as they make up the largest part of what you are eating. It is best to choose a product with the least number of ingredients.

- Just because you can't pronounce it, doesn't mean it's something to avoid. Some hard to pronounce ingredients are actually harmless. One example is Xanthan Gum, which you might see as an ingredient in salad dressings or sauces that is added as a thickener.

- When you are not sure about an ingredient, search it on your phone in the store or take a picture of the list, and look it up when you get home if you want to learn more.

This information is here to highlight some of the things you can do to further maximize your efforts when it comes to the Food Plan. Some people might want to be hard core, while others prefer a more relaxed approach. Everyone is different. As long as you keep showing up, you can't mess it up. It's important to make choices that make you feel good and you are comfortable with along the way.

LET'S TALK SUPPLEMENTS

The following are basic supplements that can be helpful to aid in deficiencies in the body that may affect its ability to focus on fat loss. They can also help support your efforts with this process by addressing the body's needs and have it function at more optimal levels.

Please note: You do not need to add in any supplements, they are only suggested. It is up to you to decide if you want to add them in.

Before we get started:

- Although the supplements suggested here are all beneficial to the human body and basic health in general, before you run out and buy any for the sake of weight loss, you want to understand why they are a benefit and assess if they are right for you.

- With regards to particular brands, there are a lot of great products to choose from. Get to know the knowledgeable staff at your local pharmacy and/or health store to help make the best choice for you.

If you have questions or concerns about adding in any supplements in regards to health issues you have or medications you take, be sure to check in with your healthcare provider.

BASIC SUPPLEMENT LIST:

- Vitamin D
- Omega 3
- Calm Magnesium
- Probiotic
- Prebiotic
- Digestive Bitters
- Collagen

LET'S BREAK THEM DOWN:

VITAMIN D, D3:

Vitamin D is essential in supporting the body's metabolism. Low levels of vitamin D are often found in people who have weight to lose. When someone is lacking vitamin D, the hypothalamus (the very small part of your brain that regulates hormonal functions, amongst other things) senses the lower levels and responds by increasing body weight.

- Vit D comes in drops or pills.

- Vit D2 is the vegan form.
- Vit D3 is the most effective for raising levels as it is more easily absorbed.

DOSE

600-2000 IU/day is the recommended dose range. Follow package directions for dose.

WHEN TO TAKE

It is best taken with a meal that contains fat for better absorption, ideally breakfast or lunch because adding it in too late in the day can interrupt the body's production of melatonin and mess with your sleep.

ALTERNATE SOURCES FOR VITAMIN D:

Very few foods contain significant amounts of vitamin D, so sun exposure is the best source if you are not supplementing.

- Your skin produces more vitamin D from the sun during mid-day, when the sun is at its highest point.
- The more skin that is exposed the more vitamin D the body will make.
- Darker skin tones require more sun exposure to absorb vitamin D.

OMEGA 3:

One way you can support the fat loss process is to add in more good fat. Without enough good fat in your diet, the body will be reluctant to let go of stored fat.

30% of your diet should come from fat, and ideally 10% of that should come from Omega 3. A primary source of Omega 3 is fish, and unless you are eating it at least two to three times a week, it can be difficult for the body to get enough.

- Omega 3 comes in pill or liquid (oil). Both are equally good.
- If you do not like fish oil or are allergic, you can use vegan alternatives.

DOSE

500-3000 mg per day is the recommended dose range. Follow the directions on the product label and adjust as needed.

WHEN TO TAKE

Best taken with food and added fat for best absorption. Because it can be hard to digest, you can divide the dose and take it at breakfast and lunch. Avoid taking before bed or before exercise as the increased activity can cause heartburn or reflux.

PLEASE NOTE: If you are on prescribed blood thinners or have any other health issues, consult with your healthcare provider before adding in.

OMEGA 3 FOOD SOURCES

- Best fish Sources:
- Mackerel
- Salmon
- Seabass
- Oysters
- Sardines
- Shrimp
- Trout

Other Omega 3 Food Sources

- Seaweed and algae
- Chia seeds (ground or soaked for better absorption)
- Hemp Seeds
- Flax seeds (ground is best for absorption)
- Walnuts
- Edamame
- Kidney Beans

CALM MAGNESIUM (MAGNESIUM CITRATE):

There are many forms of magnesium. Calm Magnesium is specifically suggested because it is easily absorbed by the body and supports the detox process. Although magnesium is responsible for over 300 actions in the body, it is specifically important while losing weight because it not only helps to convert your foods into usable energy, it also helps calm the nerves and address cortisol levels (caused by stress). This will help your body to relax, which can help with getting deep and REM sleep. Deep sleep is important because that is the kind of sleep you need for the body to best repair, rebuild, and detoxify.

- The most effective Calm Magnesium is in powdered form. The pill form does not have the same effect.

- You can purchase plain or flavoured.

- When using the powder, dissolving in warm to hot water activates the ingredients.

DOSE

1-2 tsp per day is generally recommended on the product label. Start with the recommended dose and adjust as needed.

WHEN TO TAKE

Beneficial before bed, but can also be taken during the day.

PLEASE NOTE: When it comes to magnesium, there are other types than the one suggested here. However, for the purpose of weight loss, the magnesium citrate powder works best. Natural Calm Mag is a good brand, but there are other magnesium citrate powders available on the market. **CALM Mag. is NOT the same as CAL Mag. (calcium magnesium).**

MAGNESIUM FOOD SOURCES:

- Dark Leafy Greens - spinach, kale, collard greens, Swiss chard
- Pumpkin Seeds
- Nuts - especially almonds, cashews and Brazil nuts
- Tuna
- Avocados
- Bananas
- Legumes
- Whole grains

PROBIOTICS

Probiotics are good bacteria added to your digestive system that promote a healthy immune system and can help with weight loss by improving digestion.

- Probiotics come in pill, powdered, or liquid form.
- They come in a variety of different potencies and strains.

Look for a probiotic with a variety of strains. Some common beneficial ones include:

- L. acidophilus (Lactobacillus acidophilus)
- B. Longum (Bifidobacterium longum)
- B. bifidum (Bifidobacterium bifidum)
- L. rhamnosus (Lactobacillus rhamnosus)
- L. fermentum (Limosilactobacillus fermentum)

DOSE

5-10 billion CFUs is an average potency. Follow the recommended dosage on your product's label.

WHEN TO TAKE

Ideally taken on an empty stomach or with breakfast. You can also take it before going to bed. Whichever time you choose, try to be consistent with it.

PLEASE NOTE: If you're following SIBO or the FODMAP diet while also following the plan, you might be advised NOT to add in a probiotic. If unsure, always check in with your healthcare provider.

PROBIOTIC FOOD SOURCES

- Yogurt
- Kefir
- Buttermilk
- Some cheeses such as Gouda, Cheddar, Parmesan and Swiss
- Sauerkraut
- Kimchi
- Pickles that are naturally fermented. (If they contain vinegar they are not naturally fermented.)
- Tempeh
- Miso
- Kombucha - be mindful of sugar content

PREBIOTIC WITH ADDED CLEAR FIBER:

Prebiotic helps to feed the good bacteria in your gut which can be beneficial in addressing inflammation, digestive issues and helps to promote healthy bowel movements.

- It is being used more and more in gut therapy to address things like high histamine levels, inflammation, insulin resistance, Crohns, and Colitis.

DOSE

Follow directions on the product label.

WHEN TO TAKE

Prebiotic can be taken any time of day.

PREBIOTIC FOOD SOURCES

- Garlic (raw)
- Onions (raw or lightly cooked)
- Leeks
- Asparagus
- Radishes
- Bananas
- Apples
- Flaxseeds
- Cabbage
- Dandelion greens and root
- Shiitake mushrooms
- Oats, Bran, Barley
- Hemp seeds
- Unpasteurized apple cider vinegar

DIGESTIVE BITTERS:

If you have known digestive issues, are missing your gallbladder, or simply feel bloated after eating raw vegetables or nuts and seeds, you may want to add in some digestive bitters.

- Digestive bitters are drops that are added to water.
- Digestive bitters stimulate digestion and help to produce enzymes that aid in processing and getting the nutrients you need from your food.
- Best to look for Canadian bitters which is specifically a digestive aid, as opposed to Swedish bitters which contain an added laxative (senna), which is not necessarily needed when following the Program.

DOSE

1-2 ml up to 3 times per day as directed on the label.

WHEN TO TAKE

Take between meals or 15 mins before meals.

COLLAGEN:

Collagen can help with tissue repair, improving the quality of hair and nails, but more importantly skin, which is important when it comes to weight loss.

- It is a non-essential protein naturally found in the body that starts to deplete after the age of 21.

- Collagen can help with internal tissue repair as well as maintaining muscle mass.

- Most commonly sold in powder form and can be mixed into coffee, tea, water, oatmeal, yogurt etc.

- Collagen comes in either bovine sourced or marine sourced. Marine is better for skin and bovine is better for maintaining muscle mass, but both are effective. Speak to someone at your local pharmacy or health food store to see which source is best for you.

DOSE

5-10g is the average dose recommendation. Follow the directions on your product's label.

WHEN TO TAKE

Collagen can be taken any time of day.

FINAL NOTE ON SUPPLEMENTS:

When it comes to these suggested supplements, there is no rush to add them in or start taking them all at once. You can pick and choose what you add in, take your time adding them in, and can add them in at any time during your weight loss journey.

Everyone has different needs. It's best to grab a pen and paper and make some notes on what times work best, given your individual situation. Check in with your pharmacist or healthcare provider if you have any questions or to inquire about any medications that could have any interactions or affect the timing of supplements.

FREQUENTLY ASKED QUESTIONS

1. **Where can these supplements be purchased?**

   Your local health food store or pharmacies are great if you want to talk to someone for recommendations. Here are a few good online shopping options as well:

   - Well.ca (Canada)

   - Vitamart.ca (Canada)

   - COSTCO (Canada & US)

   - Amazon.ca and .com (Canada & US)

- Bedrugsmart.ca (Canada & US)
- Vitaminshoppe.com (US)
- Thrivemarket.com (US)

2. **Can I continue to take any other supplements that I am already taking?**

You can continue to take any supplements that you are already taking or have been recommended by your healthcare provider. If you have any questions, be sure to check in with them.

3. **Can a multivitamin be taken instead?**

A multivitamin generally does not contain the recommended dose of each individual supplement suggested.

4. **Can supplements be taken in gummy form?**

Gummies are not as effective. They also contain artificial colour and sweeteners.

5. **What if I am having acid reflux when taking omega 3?**

Be sure to check the quality and expiry date.

Try taking it just before a meal instead of after.

Switch brands or try the oil if using capsules.

Try putting the capsules in the fridge or freezer.

6. **Can magnesium citrate pills be used instead of the powder?**

If the powder is not available you can take capsules. Keep in mind the powder tends to be more effective.

7. **Can Calm Magnesium be added in while also taking another type of magnesium supplement?**

You can continue using other types of magnesium supplements and add in the Calm Magnesium. There are many different magnesium supplements out there used to address various issues. The Calm Magnesium (or magnesium citrate powder) is suggested specifically to complement this Program. Be sure to speak with your pharmacist or healthcare provider if you have any concerns.

8. **If taking a probiotic in the morning, should it be taken before or after lemon water or ACV?**

You can take it before or after. It is best to wait about 10 minutes in between.

9. **Can you mix the collagen and Calm Magnesium and take them together?**

You can mix these together and take at the same time. Be sure to activate the Calm separately in hot water and once it stops fizzing you can add the collagen, mix together and take.

10. **Can collagen count as protein for breakfast?**

The non-essential protein in collagen is not a good source of dietary protein, so you do not want to use it as a source of protein at meals.

11. **Is there a vegan form of collagen?**

Collagen is animal-based, however, there are vegan collagen boosters that help your body make more of its own. Check your local health food store as they would be able to guide you best.

Please take the time to head over to the Facebook Group or the Livy Method App and watch the quick video that accompanies this post.

LET'S TALK NON-SCALE VICTORIES (NSVS) — ANOTHER MEASURE OF SUCCESS!

Non-Scale Victories (NSVs) are measures of success that do not show up on the scale. They can be lost inches, having more energy, feeling more in-tune to your body's needs and being more proud of yourself, to name a few. Some will present themselves early and easily and some you may have to look to find and work towards.

In the pursuit of weight loss, we have been conditioned to be hyper focused on the number on the scale and only feel we are moving in the right direction to our Finally & Forever if the scale is moving in the perceived right direction. While doing The Livy Method, we want you to look beyond the scale, open your mind and expectations, and measure your success with NSVs.

Here is a list of some of the NSVs that you can experience while following the Program. You will notice that some can be seen, and others have to be felt. We encourage you to make your own list or add to this one.

EXAMPLES OF NSVS:

- Increased energy
- Changes in your body
- Lost inches when measuring
- Clothing fitting looser
- Tightening belt loops
- Tightening watch straps
- Wedding rings fitting again
- Seeing/feeling your hips, cheeks, and collarbones
- Improved complexion
- Towels feel bigger when wrapped around
- More regular bowel movements
- Less uncomfortable and strained bowel movements
- Sleeping better
- Not needing an afternoon nap
- No longer snoring
- Easier time getting up in the morning
- Symptom management of chronic illness
- Decreased chronic pain
- Decreased medications – blood pressure, cholesterol, blood sugar meds, antacids, etc.

- Menopause and PMS symptoms improved
- Migraines diminishing or less frequent
- No more heartburn
- Less gas and less bloating
- Improved overall digestion
- Less Inflammation
- Improved Mobility
- Being comfortable with doing simple activities
- Not being out of breath doing chores/daily activities
- Ability to be on the floor playing with your kids/grandkids
- Crossing your legs comfortably
- Having coffee because you like it, not because you need it
- Wanting to drink water
- Moved your car seat closer to the steering wheel
- Fitting in chairs, seats that you were previously uncomfortable in
- Friends/family commenting that they are noticing positive change
- Inspiring kids/family/friends to change their own poor diet habits
- New friends/relationships
- More in-tune with your body's needs
- Improved relationship with food
- Being hydrated
- Less brain fog
- More focus and concentration during the day
- Increased libido
- Diminished cravings and snacking urges
- Trying new foods and not being afraid of delicious food and fat
- Changing and enhanced taste buds
- Appreciating how food smells
- Learning how to fuel your body
- Learning new information, understanding how your body works
- _____
- _____

- _____
- _____
- _____

We like to level up around here so let's take it one step further and talk about NSVs that have nothing to do with your body or a physical feeling. These are the ones that come from trusting yourself and your mind-body connection.

Intuition: "having the ability to understand or know something without any direct evidence or reasoning process" and "using or based on what one feels to be true even without conscious reasoning; instinctive."

NSVS THAT ARE MORE INTUITIVE:

- Making yourself a priority
- More positive mood and attitude
- More focus
- Feeling confident
- Happier
- More patience
- Pride for being open to learning and doing this
- Pride of sticking to something
- Hope, not fear, that you can succeed
- Not wanting to quit when one day doesn't go your way
- Calmer about your choices knowing you will be ok
- Calm about grocery shopping, buying real food and not diet food
- Recognizing stress and not running from it but understanding it
- Less anxiety around food and feeling deprived
- Being in-tune with how certain foods make you feel
- Knowing what you actually want to eat instead of just eating
- Developing positive eating habits and associations
- Not missing the types of food you thought you would because you don't feel deprived
- Realizing that you want to exercise, not feel like you HAVE to exercise
- Not feeling shame and guilt and having food freedom
- Trusting you can do new things

- _____
- _____
- _____
- _____
- _____

Here is a collection of NSVs that have been personally experienced and shared by members of our community:

- My best NSV is getting my mind and body to realize they're on the same team.
- I am putting myself first instead of everyone else and taking the time to know I deserve this.
- I am acknowledging and managing my stress much better.
- My best NSV is not wanting to snack at night anymore.
- I am living each day with renewed energy.
- I am learning to love my body.
- My NSV is last Saturday at the gym I noticed when doing a spin class that my knees and my stomach were no longer connecting.
- I am scared but I am trusting the process and putting myself first!
- I am able to do up buttons as my arthritis is better.
- I am eating the right amount of food for me, not what a tracker says or just because it's on my plate.
- Today I had to move my car seat up. Suddenly I couldn't reach the pedals – sure sign my bum is getting smaller!
- After many years on my anxiety meds, I have finally been able to start dropping doses to get off them. This is such a huge non-scale victory for me. My numbers on the scale may not always drop day to day, but my negative thoughts about myself do.
- What a wonderful non-scale victory! Recognizing when I have eaten to satisfaction, so I don't have that feeling of having eaten too much and feel uncomfortable.
- Last week, a colleague said to me "you look really good these days" to which I replied, "Thanks, I feel really good." And in that moment, I realized that I meant it. I had been so focused on the scale that hadn't been moving that I wasn't paying attention to how all over awesome I have been feeling lately and all the little victories that have been piling up. Lesson learned - this Program is also a wellness journey, not just a weight loss one.

Recognizing and embracing your non-scale victories can be just as important, if not more so, than the goal you are trying to reach number-wise. Writing them down, reviewing and appreciating them can keep you more motivated along the way than what is happening on the scale each day.

IS IT A FRUIT OR VEG?

This question gets asked a lot, especially in relation to tomatoes and avocados. Because they are technically fruits, we get asked if they can be eaten at fruit snack, but on this Program, we classify tomatoes as a vegetable and avocado as a healthy fat.

DID YOU KNOW….

A fruit develops from a flower and produces seeds or a pit. Like tomatoes and cucumbers and many other fruits we think of as vegetables in this Program.

The word "vegetable" is only a culinary term. In the botanical world, the word "vegetable" doesn't even exist. What we call vegetables they refer to as leaves, stems, roots, flower buds etc. Like celery is a stem and radishes are roots.

Watermelon is both a fruit and a vegetable, but we use it as a fruit on plan and rhubarb is actually a vegetable as per the stem example that was used with the celery above.

There are many foods on plan that are technically fruits, but we use them as vegetables. And then there are some fruits that we categorize as healthy fats.

Are you confused yet?!

LET'S BREAK IT DOWN…

FOODS THAT ARE TECHNICALLY FRUITS, BUT ARE USED AS VEGETABLES ON PLAN:

- Tomatoes
- Cucumbers
- Peppers
- Peas
- Green beans
- Eggplant
- Okra
- Corn
- Zucchini
- Pumpkin
- Squash

FOODS THAT ARE TECHNICALLY FRUITS, BUT ARE USED AS HEALTHY FATS ON PLAN:

- Avocado

- Nuts

- Olives

- Coconut (technically a fruit, a nut, and a seed!) But we use it as a healthy fat on plan.

Don't overthink it! We could go down a scientific rabbit hole with this subject but just wanted to provide some clarity as well as some fun facts! When in doubt, refer to the Let's Talk Groceries post for clarification.

WEEK 3 GUIDELINES: MINDFULNESS

The goal this week is to follow the Program as consistently as possible to allow the body to calm down and adjust to the changes you have made. This is also where you start to address issues and associations when it comes to food and work to be more in tune with your portions by introducing 4 Mindfulness Questions.

LET'S TALK CONSISTENCY

During Prep Week, we introduced the basic Food Plan and the changes you were to implement. Week 1 was about fine tuning and adjusting those changes, as well as introducing Bonus Snacks if needed.

Week 2 had you working on consistency and maximizing your efforts, along with introducing Supplements.

Consistency continues to be a major focus as we are still in the phase of making the body feel confident that it no longer needs the stored fat it has been hanging onto for whatever reason; high stress, lack of sleep, long periods of time without eating, years of restrictive dieting, just to name a few.

Moving into Week 3 you are continuing to follow the basic Food Plan and being as consistent as possible to allow the body time to calm down and adjust from the changes you have made in the past few weeks so it can focus less on digestion and inflammation and more on making changes.

This part of the process is also where you start to address your associations to food. For example, if you use food for anything other than nutritional requirements, like eating out of boredom, distraction, stress, reward and so on. So this is a great week for helping you get more in tune with your body's needs over your wants.

This week also allows the body time to adjust its hunger levels, which can naturally have you feeling more satisfied on smaller portions.

It's important to note, when being so consistent for so long you might start to feel bored with the routine or the foods you are eating. Rest assured; this is normal for where we are in the process. Rather than looking for alternatives or swapping recipes to make things more exciting, I want you to indulge in the boredom.

If you are not bored, that is OK too, as some people enjoy the routine.

Now for the main focus this week, which is Mindfulness. Although it is not the most exciting week, it is a very important one. Being mindful of how your body is responding to the changes you are making as well as being in-tune to your body's needs is essential to building a strong mind body connection.

LET'S TALK MINDFULNESS

Mindfulness is how we start to address portion sizes with The Livy Method.

Because we do not count, weigh, or measure, before you start adjusting portions, the first step is to pay attention to how the body is responding before, during, and after you eat.

As you move forward in the Program, you are going to transition into more of a natural way of eating. But first, you need to make sure you are completely in tune with where you are at now.

INTRODUCING THE 4 MINDFULNESS QUESTIONS:

ASK YOURSELF THESE 4 SETS OF QUESTIONS:

1. **Before you eat, ask yourself:**
   - Am I hungry?
   - How is this portion for me?
   - Is this enough?
   - Is this too much?
   - How would I feel if I ate all of it?

2. **While eating your food, pay attention to how you feel and ask yourself:**
   - Is my choice of food satisfying?
   - Do I feel any physical effects of eating?
   - Am I starting to feel satisfied?
   - How would I feel if I took a few more bites?
   - How would I feel if I stop eating now?

3. **When you are done eating, ask yourself:**
   - How do I feel?
   - How do I know when I have eaten enough?
   - Do I feel satisfied and if so, what is my definition of satisfaction?
   - How do I feel physically?

4. **15 minutes after you are done eating, ask yourself:**
   - How do I feel?
   - Do I still feel satisfied?
   - Could I have eaten more?
   - Could I have eaten less?

The goal here is to bring awareness to your changing hunger levels. You may not get a really strong response or any answer from your body at first, but trust that the more consistently you ask, the more your body will start to talk back.

While following the Program, you may notice that your portions will naturally decrease on their own. However, your hunger levels may change day to day so keep in mind that when it comes to portions, they are always what they feel like and not what they look like, so each day might look different, portion size wise.

Please note: While you may feel inclined to start cutting and decreasing portions thinking it's going to get you ahead, rest assured, it won't. It will only lead to confusion down the road if you miss this very important step. This week is the set up for Week 4 where we mindfully start to adjust portion sizes, so it is very important that you work on understanding what satisfaction means to you.

FREQUENTLY ASKED QUESTIONS

1. **I am struggling to overcome the habit of eating all of the food on my plate, even after I am satisfied. Any tips?**

   You could be dealing with food waste issues if throwing out the uneaten portion feels uncomfortable for you. Save the remaining portion for another meal, or another day. Over time, these new habits will become wired in your brain, especially as you start to feel better about yourself and more in tune with your body's hunger and satiety signals.

   When serving your portions ensure you are asking yourself the 4 Mindfulness Questions, especially "How is this portion for me?". It is a good way to start thinking about what the portion feels like, as opposed to what it looks like.

2. **Any other tips to strengthen the mind-body connection?**

   Asking yourself the 4 Mindfulness Questions with every meal and snack will really help you to develop this connection. Practice, repetition and consistency will help to strengthen this connection. Over time you will find the more you get in tune with your body the clearer your body will communicate its needs.

What makes The Livy Method different from all the other diets out there, is that apart from the Food Plan, another main focus is on developing a mind-body connection. Keep following the Food Plan as many of these strategies are built into the weekly tweaks as we progress through the Program.

3.   **Is it ok to graze while eating your meals?**

It is totally fine to take your time while eating your meals. Just be sure to ask yourself the 4 Mindfulness Questions with every meal and snack and keep in mind that your hunger levels will change day to day. Once you have finished your meal or snack, allow at least 30 min and up to 3.5 hours before you have the next one.

4.   **How do I know the difference between my hunger and migrating motor complex?**

Hunger is just another way the body communicates its needs. It is the body letting you know where it is at, and what it needs throughout the day. Once you have eaten to satisfaction the hunger feeling should subside.

The migrating motor complex (MMC) is an important mechanism of digestion, signified by the "grumblings" and "churning" of the stomach. This takes place after the body processes and digests food. Because we are eating so often during the day, the body is doing most of this work at night. As we move through the Program and phase you into more natural patterns of eating, this will also include the downtime your body needs in between meals to self regulate.

5.   **I eat until I am satisfied but am hungry not long after, any tips?**

If you find you are still hungry after eating to satisfaction, be sure you are making your meals nutrient rich and adding in good fats to help with sustaining energy. If you find you need, add some starchy vegetables or grains to your meals.

If your hunger cues are based on your stomach grumbling, this can be due to your migrating motor complex as opposed to real hunger. If you are still hungry 10-15 min after eating, you can always go back for more or wait until your next meal and snack.

6.   **Should I be reducing my portion sizes?**

It is very important to not be decreasing portions intentionally at this point. You want to be eating to satisfaction while asking the 4 Mindfulness Questions. As you continue to focus on your hunger levels and how you are feeling at each meal and snack, you may notice that your portions will naturally start to decrease. We will be addressing portions more as we move forward in the Program.

7. **I do not understand the purpose of why I'm asking the 4 Mindfulness Questions. Any tips?**

The practice of asking the 4 Mindfulness Questions is to bring awareness to how your body is responding to the food choices that you are making and the portions that you are eating. It is also important to understand what satisfaction feels like to you. This will play an important role when it comes time to start decreasing portions and adapting to the changes we will be making to the Food Plan week to week.

8. **When meal prepping, should I pack extra and eat to satisfaction, or pack exactly what I think I'll need?**

Hunger levels will vary from day to day and from meal to meal and you want to ensure that you are eating enough to feel satisfied. Being prepared by packing more than you need can help if you find yourself feeling extra hungry.

Please take the time to head over to the Facebook Group or the Livy Method App and watch the quick video that accompanies this post.

LET'S TALK BEING IN TUNE TO YOUR BODY'S CUES

Your body should tell you when to eat, what to eat and how much to eat. However, over the years we learn to tune out our body's cues; not drinking when thirsty, sleeping when tired, or eating when hungry.

Growing up and being taught not to waste food and finish everything on the plate and sometimes not being allowed to leave the table until everything was finished leaves a lasting impression.

This idea that you must clean your plate, goes back in history tied to food shortages beginning in World War 1. It has become normal for parents to urge their kids to finish everything on their plates, regardless of how they feel. As a result, we start learning to disconnect from our body's cues at a young age.

Disconnecting is also reinforced through years of dieting. With most diets, the goal is to purposely ignore your body's cues and not eat when hungry to help force the body to burn fat. The Livy Method is about doing the exact opposite, which is why mindfulness is key.

This brings us to why this week is so important. We need to take the time to unlearn all of that training and start to feel and understand what our bodies are trying to tell us.

THESE ARE SOME THINGS THAT YOU CAN BRING AWARENESS TO AND FOCUS ON:

- Set your intentions at the beginning of each day
- Check in on yourself throughout the day
- Reflect on your intentions at the end of the day
- Pay attention to how your body is responding to the changes that you are making
- Be in tune to how you feel when you wake up
- Be aware of your mood and energy levels
- Pay attention to when you are tired
- Pay attention to when you are thirsty
- Pay attention to when you are hungry/not hungry
- Pay attention to your internal dialogue
- Be mindful of the energy that you are bringing to this process
- Be aware of your environment and set yourself up for success
- Learn to listen to your gut and trust your instinct

Learning to listen to your body's cues is especially important when it comes to portion sizes and figuring out what satisfaction means to you.

TIPS FOR BEING MORE MINDFUL WHEN EATING:

CONSISTENTLY ASK THE 4 MINDFULNESS QUESTIONS AT EACH MEAL AND SNACK

The more you ask, the more in-tune you will become. Asking the 4 Questions makes you more aware of your body's cues before, during, and after you eat. Eventually, it will become second nature and you will no longer need to ask, as your body will tell you when to eat, what to eat and how much to eat.

TRY NOT TO EAT WHILE DISTRACTED

Watching television, being on your phone, driving, etc. can take the focus away from connecting with your body's cues. Try to eat in a calm state where you can slow down and pay attention. If you have to eat while distracted, be extra diligent about checking in with yourself.

EAT WHAT'S MOST APPEALING ON YOUR PLATE

You still want to prepare your meals using the guidelines of more vegetables at lunch and more protein at dinner, but do not put too much focus on that while eating and being mindful. Instead, eat what is most appealing to you in the moment, eat to satisfaction and do not worry if you end up having more protein at lunch or less at dinner because you are leaving food on your plate.

WHEN ASKING THE 4 QUESTIONS, MAKE THEM RESONATE WITH YOU

Eating to satisfaction can be a hard concept to grasp at first, so try rewording the questions. For example, are you still hungry, is your body wanting more or does it just taste really good so you want to keep eating? Feel free to come up with your own questions to make it easier for you to connect with them.

AVOID TRYING TO CONTROL YOUR HUNGER LEVELS OUT OF FEAR

It is normal to feel anxious about being hungry after you eat because you think you did not eat enough. Keep in mind, you cannot eat more food and have it last longer. As long as you are making your food choices nutrient rich and eating to satisfaction in the moment, trust you are eating enough. If you feel hungry in between meals, remember the next meal or snack is right around the corner and you can always add in Bonus Snacks if you need them.

SAVE YOUR LEFTOVERS

If you find yourself struggling with food waste issues, remember when you do not finish what is on your plate you can always save it for later. Save your leftovers and incorporate them into your next day's meals and snacks.

Being in tune with your body's needs takes practice. Be patient and consistent. In time, the more you ask the 4 Mindfulness Questions and the more self aware you are, the stronger your mind body connection will become. Losing weight Finally & Forever is more than just what you are eating and when. It's being mindful, in tune and understanding your body's needs.

THE 4 MINDFULNESS QUESTIONS

Asking yourself the 4 Sets of Mindfulness Questions is an important aspect of learning to become in tune with your body and its needs. Since we don't count, weigh or measure our food, asking these questions is what we use when it comes to addressing portion sizes.

Let's do a quick review of the 4 Sets of Mindfulness Questions:

1. **Before you eat, ask yourself:**
   - Am I hungry?
   - How is this portion for me?
   - Is this enough?
   - Is this too much?
   - How would I feel if I ate all of it?

2. **While eating your food, pay attention to how you feel and ask yourself:**
   - Is my choice of food satisfying?
   - Do I feel any physical effects of eating?
   - Am I starting to feel satisfied?
   - How would I feel if I took a few more bites?
   - How would I feel if I stop eating now?

3. **When you are done eating, ask yourself:**
   - How do I feel?
   - How do I know when I have eaten enough?
   - Do I feel satisfied and if so, what is my definition of satisfaction?
   - How do I feel physically?

4. **15 minutes after you are done eating, ask yourself:**
   - How do I feel?
   - Do I still feel satisfied?
   - Could I have eaten more?
   - Could I have eaten less?

Though these questions may seem very simple, the thinking involved when asking them is more complex. They are meant to strengthen your mind-body connection, have you more in tune with your portions and recognize your body's needs over your wants.

PAY ATTENTION TO PHYSICAL CUES TO KNOW WHEN YOU HAVE HAD ENOUGH

Sometimes your body may give you a particular cue, sign, or tell you that you have finished your meal. Some of those cues may be:

- Burping
- Sighing
- Change in your breathing patterns
- Sitting back in your seat
- Moving food around on your plate
- Moving away from your food
- Pushing your plate away

It may take many tries to slowly figure out how you know you are done and satisfied. Make progress over perfection your focus in this process. It is okay to not get it right every single time, but it is also important to keep trying. At some point, it will become second nature that you will no longer have to formally ask the questions, and you will intuitively know what to do in portioning and preparing your food, and in knowing when you are satisfied with your meal and snack choices.

Asking the 4 Mindfulness Questions is an important aspect of this Program to lose weight, and for continued success in maintenance, Finally & Forever.

Check out the video in the Livy Method App or Facebook Support Group to watch Rebecca, who has lost over 110 lbs using The Livy Method, share how she uses the 4 Mindfulness Questions.

LET'S TALK STRESS AND SLEEP

Managing your stress and getting enough sleep can make all the difference when it comes to getting and keeping the scale moving.

Although following the Program helps with both stress and sleep in general, there are quite a few things above and beyond the basics that you can focus on to help with this process.

When it comes to stress, keep in mind the goal isn't to make it completely go away, it is more about recognizing it, and managing it better so you can capitalize on it.

TIPS FOR MANAGING STRESS:

- Be consistent with the basics of the Program; the food, water and any supplements.
- Be in tune with and recognize your stress levels.
- Move your body more.
- Find activities you enjoy doing like sports and other leisure activities.
- Get outside and commune with nature.
- Practice deep breathing exercises.
- Have a warm Epsom salt bath before bed.
- Keep up with health issues. Seeing a naturopathic doctor, chiropractor, acupuncturist, massage therapist and other healthcare providers can be helpful.
- Add in helpful supplements like Omega 3, and add good fats to your meals along with being consistent with magnesium.
- Look for things that bring you joy. Look to have fun with this process. Don't underestimate the power of having a good conversation and laughs with a friend or spending quality time with a loved one.

Stress is challenging to the body. If you are consistently supporting the body and its needs, it will work hard to make you stronger and healthier, putting a greater focus on fat loss.

Focusing on improving your sleep can also help with managing stress. The body needs deep and REM sleep to repair, rebuild and detox. Here are a few things you can do to improve the quality of sleep you are getting.

TIPS FOR IMPROVING SLEEP QUALITY:

- Eat as early in the evening as possible.
- Set up your sleep environment for success.
- Establish a good evening and bedtime routine.

- Take Calm Magnesium before bed.

- Keep a journal beside your bed to organize your thoughts.

- Turn lights down low in the evening.

- Stay off of screens or get off them earlier.

- Use blue light glasses.

- Take naps when you feel the need. In general, naps are not advised when trying to improve sleep patterns, but when it comes to this process, the body is working hard to make change. So when you are tired, be sure to rest.

Making small improvements to manage your stress and improve your sleep quality can make a huge difference when it comes to getting and keeping the scale moving. For some, focusing on these two things can be just as important as following the Food Plan when it comes to losing weight Finally & Forever.

Please take the time to head over to the Facebook Group or the Livy Method App and watch the quick video that accompanies this post.

WHAT PROGRESS IS REALLY LIKE

(An excerpt from the book Atomic Habits written by James Clear, I think will be sure to resonate)

"Imagine that you have an ice cube sitting on the table in front of you. The room is cold and you can see your breath. It is currently twenty-five degrees. Ever so slowly, the room begins to heat up.

Twenty-six degrees.

Twenty-seven.

Twenty-eight.

The ice cube is still on the table in front of you.

Twenty-nine degrees.

Thirty.

Thirty-one.

Still, nothing has happened.

Then, thirty-two degrees. The ice begins to melt. A one-degree shift, seemingly no different from the temperature increases before it, has unlocked a huge change.

Breakthrough moments are often the result of many previous actions, which build up the potential required to unleash a major change. This pattern shows up everywhere.

Cancer spends 80 percent of its life undetectable, then takes over the body in months.

Bamboo can barely be seen for the first five years as it builds extensive root systems underground before exploding ninety feet into the air within six weeks.

Similarly, habits often appear to make no difference until you cross a critical threshold and unlock a new level of performance. In the early and middle stages of any quest, there is often a valley of disappointment.

You expect to make progress in a linear fashion and it's frustrating how ineffective changes can seem during the first days, weeks, and even months. It doesn't feel like you are going anywhere. It's a hallmark of any compounding process: the most powerful outcomes are delayed.

This is one of the core reasons why it is so hard to build habits that last. People make a few small changes, fail to see a tangible result and decide to stop. You think, "I've been running every day for a month, so why can't I see any change in my body?" Once this kind of thinking takes over, it's easy to let good habits fall by the wayside. But in order to make a meaningful difference, habits need to persist long enough to break through this plateau - what I call the plateau of latent potential.

If you find yourself struggling to build a good habit or break a bad one, it is not because you have lost your ability to improve. It is often because you have not yet crossed the Plateau of Latent Potential.

Complaining about not achieving success despite working hard is like complaining about an ice cube not melting when you heated it from twenty-five to thirty-one degrees. Your work was not wasted; it is just being stored. All the action happens at thirty-two degrees.

When you finally break through the Plateau of Latent Potential, people will call it an overnight success. The outside world only sees the most dramatic event rather than all that preceded it. But you know that it's work you did long ago when it seemed that you weren't making any progress, that makes the jump today possible."

You can see how this relates to what we are doing here, and as frustrating as it can be. Keep going and you will get there.

LET'S TALK CELEBRATORY WEEKENDS

Life is going to happen. It is all about progress over perfection.

Because The Program covers a span of three months, chances are you are going to encounter those moments that are made for indulging. However, they are nothing to worry about because The Program takes them into account.

Here are some tips to navigate them:

1. **Take some time to set your intentions before the weekend. Are you going to focus on following the Food Plan, choose to indulge, or take each day as it comes?**

   There is no right or wrong answer to this, it's all about how you want to feel when it's time to get back at it. Regardless, make a plan so you are prepared.

2. **Make a point of eating normally the day of any big event, or in anticipation of a big/festive meal.**

   Follow the Food Plan leading up to your event as consistently as possible. This will help keep your digestive system stimulated so you are able to digest your meal better and feel less bloated after eating a bigger meal and prevent you from overindulging.

3. **Start your day higher in protein and fat and minimize carbs. For example, choose eggs over oatmeal. This will get your body working harder from the get-go and give you more sustaining energy.**

   Also, if you start your day higher in carbs like cereal, oatmeal or bread, you run the risk of setting yourself up to crave more carbs and sugar the rest of the day. If there is a lot of food around, you may be more tempted by it.

4. **Stay on top of your water and start drinking earlier in the day.**

   Staying hydrated helps keep your energy up and your cravings down which will help you continue to make choices that make you feel good, even when off routine. If you are on the road or out and about, make a plan and get it in when you can.

5. **Get right back at it the day after indulging.**

   Trying not to eat or punishing yourself for overeating only makes the situation worse. The more consistent you are with getting back to following the Food Plan, the better you will feel and the quicker you will be back to working towards your weight loss goals.

At the end of the weekend, there is nothing you can do that can't be undone by getting right back at it. The Program is designed to keep you moving forward, so all you need to do is pick up exactly where you left off. Keep in mind, what you learn by not following the plan can be just as insightful and as much of a value as following it perfectly. It's all part of the process.

That being said, the more consistent you are in following the Program, and the more you can minimize any indulgences along the way, will help to maximize your efforts and get you closer to reaching your goals.

Please take the time to head over to the Facebook Group or the Livy Method App and watch the quick video that accompanies this post.

WEEK 4 GUIDELINES: DOWNSIZING

Week 4 is where you start to adjust portions, which is less about how much food you are eating and more about the issues and associations that you may have created around food over the years, especially when it comes to trying to lose weight.

You have spent the past three weeks addressing your body's needs by following the Food Plan and eating to satisfaction. You have worked hard to lay a strong foundation. Moving forward, the focus is on getting and keeping the scale moving.

This week brings us to DOWNSIZING

After bringing awareness to portions in Week 3, downsizing is the next step in addressing them without counting, weighing or measuring. This is also where food waste issues and feelings associated with any past dieting can pop up, as this is the one week that most resembles a typical weight loss diet.

The goal this week is to continue to ask yourself the 4 Mindfulness Questions before, during, and after eating and aim to eat to feel **SLIGHTLY** unsatisfied, while being as consistent as possible with the Food Plan and Maximizing your efforts day to day.

In downsizing, you will eat a few bites less than when you were eating to satisfaction, to decrease the amount of food that you are used to eating and therefore, the amount of insulin your body produces as a result. The body's response to getting less than it is used to, to sustain its current set point, will be to release fat and adjust to the amount of food coming in. Because you have spent the last few weeks eating to the point of satisfaction, even the slightest decrease in portion size will be noticed by the body.

Rest assured, you will still be eating enough to meet your body's needs by following the Food Plan and eating nutrient rich foods. In decreasing your portions by even a few bites less, the body will take notice and ask for more, which means you will feel hungry.

The key is to SLIGHTLY decrease portions, so the body feels SLIGHTLY unsatisfied.

The only thing that you are changing is the amount of food you are eating. You do this by simply decreasing your portion sizes by a few bites less than when you were eating to satisfaction in the previous weeks.

The Food Plan remains the same:

- Higher protein breakfast
- Fruit snack
- Lunch
- Vegetable snack
- Nuts/seeds snack
- Dinner

The kinds of foods you have been eating and the components of your meals and snacks, along with your water intake and any added supplements stay the same. You can continue to add in Bonus Snacks if you need them.

HERE IS HOW IT WORKS:

1. You are going to decrease portions for each meal and snack by a few bites less than you were eating to feel satisfied. You can do this by leaving a few bites left on your plate, or by portioning out less food to begin with.

2. Ask the 4 Mindfulness Questions, and rather than eating just enough to feel satisfied, leave yourself feeling slightly unsatisfied.

3. The body will feel unsatisfied at the end of the day for a few days, this is normal and to be expected, so you may find yourself hungry when going to bed.

4. After a few days, when you don't give the body what it needs, it will start to drop fat or make changes to adjust the amount of food you are giving it.

5. You are going to downsize for Week 4, and then for Week 5 you will be back to eating to satisfaction. Then you are going to repeat the process.

You may feel like your portions are already small enough, but keep in mind you have been eating to the point of satisfaction for the size of body you are now.

Please note: You do not want to decrease your portions too quickly or by too much. More is not more and will NOT get you ahead. It will only slow you down. The key is to SLIGHTLY decrease portions, so the body feels SLIGHTLY unsatisfied.

FREQUENTLY ASKED QUESTIONS

1. **Do we downsize every day and for every meal and snack and for how long?**

   Yes, you are to downsize every meal and snack every day for the week and then we will be back to eating to satisfaction in Week 5.

2. **What if my breakfast is already small?**

   Although it is a benefit, breakfast is not necessary to eat because when you wake up you are already full of energy and any food you eat will take hours to break down before it is of any use. You can't feel unsatisfied from food your body doesn't need so if your breakfast is already small, do not worry about downsizing. However, if you wake up hungry and have room to downsize, then you should downsize.

3. **Do we still use Bonus Snacks?**

   If you have been using Bonus Snacks, you can still keep them in and downsize them as well. If you have not been utilizing Bonus Snacks up to this point it is best not to add them in.

4. **What if I am feeling hungry at the end of the day?**

   The whole point is to feel unsatisfied, especially at the end of the day. You are decreasing the amount of food the body is used to getting.

   Remind yourself this is just one phase of the Program and not how it is going to be forever. You will be eating enough nutrient rich foods during the day, that even with downsizing you do not need to be worried about not eating enough, even if you are feeling hungry before bed.

   Try switching up your routine or having some tea which can help.

5. **Will I burn fat and ruin my metabolism by doing this?**

   NO.

   You have spent the past few weeks giving your body what it needs, so it no longer feels the need to store fat. By following the Food Plan, you are eating nutrient rich foods every few hours so your body will be getting what it needs, just not as much as it is used to.

6. **Should I prepare a smaller portion or prepare my usual portion size and leave a few bites on my plate?**

   Either way works, so do what is best for you. You can prepare a smaller portion, and if you need more you can add more later or, you can prepare your normal portion and leave a few bites on your plate. Keep in mind that hunger levels can change day to day and throughout the day, so when packing your meals and snacks it can be a good idea to be prepared to make sure you have enough. If you have leftovers, you can always save it for the next day.

7. **How do I downsize my fruit snack if I am eating a whole fruit such as an apple or a banana?**

You still will want to downsize your fruit, regardless of the size. Purchasing smaller sized fruits or slicing them can help when gauging your hunger level in the moment. Some days you may only need half of a fruit to feel slightly unsatisfied, other days you may require more. Be sure to ask the 4 Mindfulness Questions and leave enough behind to feel slightly unsatisfied.

8. **My portions for snacks and meals are inconsistent. How do I figure out what a few bites less means for me?**

It is normal to feel a bit unclear about what downsizing may look like for you. The fact that you are identifying that your portions for your meals and snacks are inconsistent shows that you are identifying that your hunger levels change day to day. During downsizing, be sure to ask the 4 Mindfulness Questions.

9. **I have not been feeling hungry, how do I downsize?**

If you are not hungry and only having token amounts then you wouldn't have to downsize your 4-5 token bites. As our portions naturally begin to adjust to the changes we are making, you may perceive your portions to be smaller than when you started. You will find with each new tweak, your hunger levels will change. For example, downsizing your meals may make you hungrier for your snacks.

Please take the time to head over to the Facebook Group or the Livy Method App and watch the quick video that accompanies this post.

LET'S TALK FAT

We talk a lot about fat in the Program but always in very general terms; like helping the body release fat or focusing on fat loss. But we don't really talk about the different kinds of fat and what fat is used for.

Did you know there are actually three different types of fat cells in the body: white, brown, and beige. They can be stored as essential, subcutaneous, or visceral fat.

Each type of fat serves a different role. Some promote healthy metabolism and hormone levels, while others contribute to health issues.

LET'S TALK WHITE FAT:

White fat is what makes up most of the fat in your body and is also what makes you visibly fat.

It's made up of large, white, cells that are stored under the skin or around the organs in the belly, arms, buttocks, and thighs. These fat cells are the body's way of storing energy for later use. White fat cells contain large lipid droplets and are involved with the body's endocrine system:

- Metabolism
- Growth and development
- Emotions and mood
- Fertility and sexual function
- Sleep
- Blood pressure

White fat cells are found just beneath the skin (called subcutaneous fat). It's the type of fat that makes you look fat and tends to accumulate around the hips, butt, thighs, and arms and is attributed to cellulite.

Contrary to popular belief, this is not the fat that is linked to health issues. That title belongs to visceral white fat.

WHAT IS VISCERAL WHITE FAT?

Visceral fat is the fat that accumulates around the belly, located in the abdominal cavity, and intertwined around your organs. It's this kind of fat that can increase your risk for a number of diseases.

Now, believe it or not, there is a third kind of white fat; this fat is called ectopic fat.

WHAT IS ECTOPIC FAT?

Ectopic fat refers to the fat that the body stores when it runs out of places to store it. Usually found in locations not normally associated with fat storage, like your liver (Fatty liver for example). It can interfere with cellular function in the body, which, in turn, can affect organ function. Some of you may know it well, as it's also associated with insulin resistance.

Although the body needs some white fat to function, too much white fat can have detrimental effects, and can put you at risk for health issues like type 2 diabetes, heart disease, high blood pressure, stroke, hormone imbalances, pregnancy complications, kidney disease, liver disease & cancer.

LET'S TALK BROWN FAT:

Brown fat is found in smaller quantities in the body than white fat. It gets its brown colour from iron, is denser than white fat and helps to regulate body temperature. This process is called thermogenesis. During this process, the brown fat also burns calories.

Brown fat tends to be stored around organs like your heart, liver, kidneys, and pancreas, as well as your shoulder blades and spinal cord. Babies, for example, are born with a lot of brown fat to help regulate body temp.

This type of fat burns fatty acids to keep you warm. This is also why when following a program like The Livy Method, you may find ketones in your blood while losing weight.

This is not indicative of the body being in ketosis like people tend to believe, but more so of the body naturally burning fat as it's designed to do for purposes other than weight loss.

LET'S TALK BEIGE FAT:

Ok, so here's where things get a bit weird.

Beige fat is basically white fat that has been coerced by the body to act more like brown fat.

Beige fat (also known as brite fat), is relatively new in terms of research. It's believed that certain hormones and enzymes get released when the body is stressed like when you are cold or even when you exercise. This can cause the body to convert white fat into acting more like brown fat. These beige fat cells can do the job of white and brown fat cells. Similar to brown fat, beige cells can help burn fat rather than store it.

The question now of course would be, how do we increase brown or beige fat cells in the body and decrease white fat cells?

The Program itself addresses the white fat cells so you already have that covered!

In terms of increasing brown fat cells, more and more research is being done on the effects of cooling your body temperature, as exposing your body to cold temperatures may help recruit more brown fat cells. For example, taking a cold shower or having an ice bath. Turning the thermostat down or going outside in cold weather are other ways to cool your body and possibly create more brown fat. Just keep in mind before you start purposely freezing your butt off, that the research on this is still fairly new!

Other methods suggested for increasing brown fat cells include eating more often (being sure to eat enough) and exercising to help increase metabolism, which of course we also cover on plan.

Now that we have talked about the different kinds of fat...Let's talk about the three different ways the body stores fat.

1. **Essential Fat:**

    Essential fat is necessary for a healthy, normal functioning body. This fat is found in your brain, bone marrow, nerves and membranes that protect your organs. It plays a major role in hormone regulation, including the hormones that control fertility, vitamin and nutrient absorption, and regulating body temperature.

2. **Subcutaneous Fat:**

    Subcutaneous fat refers to the fat stored under the skin. It's a combination of white, brown and beige fat cells. Most of your body fat is subcutaneous. It's the fat that you can grab and pinch. It's the fat that makes you look fat. Most notably, subcutaneous fat is the body's method of storing energy for later use.

3. **Visceral Fat:**

    Visceral fat, also known as belly fat, is the white fat that's stored in your abdomen and around all of your major organs, such as the liver, kidneys, pancreas, intestines, and heart. Too much visceral fat can increase your risk for health issues like diabetes, heart disease, stroke, artery and even some cancers.

LET'S TALK BENEFITS OF FAT:

Because as much as fat gets a bad rap, it does have its uses and benefits, such as:

- Regulating body temp
- Helps to balance hormones
- Key for reproductive health
- Ensures vitamin storage
- Important for brain health & neurological function
- Essential for healthy metabolism
- Helps to balance blood sugar

NOW LET'S TALK RISKS ASSOCIATED WITH FAT:

Having too much white fat, particularly white visceral fat, can be detrimental to your health and can increase your risk for the following health conditions:

- Heart disease
- Stroke
- Coronary artery disease
- Atherosclerosis
- Pregnancy complications
- Type 2 diabetes
- Hormone imbalances
- Some cancers

LASTLY, LET'S TALK WHAT HAPPENS WHEN YOU GAIN AND LOSE WEIGHT:

Contrary to popular belief, the total number of fat cells you have remains the same when you gain and lose weight. When you gain weight, fat cells expand and then shrink when you lose.

You cannot get rid of fat cells unless you have them surgically removed for example, by way of liposuction. Key to note here, when you have liposuction and gain weight back, it will come back in the places where you still have fat cells, which can make for a very odd appearance.

Like all cells, fat cells do die off but are replaced with new ones every year. Once you become an adult (age of 20) the number of fat cells you have essentially stays the same.

Keep in mind this info doesn't really affect your weight loss journey and there is nothing that needs to be done with it. It is more of an FYI in the hopes of helping you have a deeper level of understanding when it comes to the complexities of fat and fat loss.

LET'S TALK SUPPORTING THE BODY IN DETOX

Detoxing is something the body does every day on its own. By supporting the body and its needs while following the Program, we piggyback this natural process to help the body specifically focus on fat loss.

You will hear me talk a lot about the importance of supporting the body in detox. This refers to the things you can do to better capitalize on this natural process when it comes to the body releasing fat.

While following the Program, we generalize a lot when using the term detox, as it can refer to a variety of things relevant to your weight loss journey. For example, when your body is releasing fat, when you are menstruating, and when you are sick the body uses the same detox process.

Here are some ways that you can support your body in detox in order to get and keep that scale moving. You will notice they are all very similar, but with slightly different intentions:

WHEN IN DETOX AND THE SCALE IS MOVING:

The Food Plan and the changes that you are making week to week are designed to capitalize on the detox process. Your body releases fat when you poop, pee, breathe and sweat. When the scale is moving, you want to focus on:

- Increasing water intake as the body needs more when releasing fat.
- Being consistent with any supplements you have added in.
- Consistently following the Food Plan.
- Making sure your meals and snacks are nutrient rich.
- Eating even if you are not hungry, eat a token amount to stimulate the digestive system to keep things moving.
- Going lighter on the carbs and heavier on the leafy greens at lunch and dinner.
- Choosing easier to digest protein like fish as opposed to red meat.
- Eating as early as possible.
- Going to bed earlier to ensure a good night's sleep.
- Moving your body, sweating, and focusing on getting your heart rate up, avoiding taxing your muscles. Nothing too heavy that will cause damage and sidetrack the body into focusing on repairing and rebuilding instead of detoxing.

The intention: To keep the body focused on detox for as long as possible to capitalize on fat loss when the scale starts to move.

WHEN YOU ARE MENSTRUATING:

This is a great opportunity for you to capitalize on the body's natural detox process. Your period each month is a time where the body looks to reset. The goal is to focus on:

- Drinking extra water.

- Being consistent with supplements (increase the Calm Magnesium, if taking).

- Consistently following the Food Plan.

- Being extra in tune to portions and mindful not to overeat.

- Going lighter on the carbs and heavier on the leafy greens at lunch and dinner for increased roughage to help keep moving things in and out.

- Eating dinner as early as possible.

- Relaxing, like having an Epsom salt bath in the evening.

- Going to bed earlier to help the body get extra rest.

- Being mindful of intensity when it comes to moving your body. Doing what feels best.

The intention: To help the body stay focused on and support menstruation and capitalize on this natural detox process to also release fat.

WHEN YOU ARE SICK:

Most people associate being sick with weight loss, when in fact with this process, it's normal for your weight to go up when you are sick. This is simply due to the body retaining water and not real weight gain. The body automatically detoxes when you are sick, so there is no need to force the Food Plan to capitalize on it. To support the body when you are sick, focus on:

- Being mindful of increasing your liquids in addition to drinking extra water.

- Getting lots of rest.

- Be consistent with any supplements you are taking.

- Add in immune support and manage symptoms if needed.

- Be in the moment with meals and snacks, if you are not hungry, don't force yourself to eat.

- Avoid heavier carbs and harder to digest proteins and go for easy to digest foods like soup to help keep your energy up but not divert resources from healing.

- Go to bed earlier and take naps to help the body get the rest it needs to heal.

- Keep your activities nice and light. Maybe some light stretching or going for a walk to get some fresh air.

The intention: To help your body recover as quickly as possible and to give it what it needs to capitalize on the natural detox process that comes with sickness.

As you can see, the process is similar in each situation but the intention is slightly different.

Keep it simple, check in on where your body is at and what it is focused on, and be sure to support the body in detox when needed. Don't overthink it, show up day to day and assess where you are at and what your body needs in the moment to help get and keep the scale moving.

Please take the time to head over to the Facebook Group or the Livy Method App and watch the quick video that accompanies this post.

LET'S TALK SKIN AND WEIGHT LOSS

When it comes to loose skin and weight loss, it's all about how you lose it.

When doing a traditional quick fix, burn the fat diet, you can lose weight fast. The downside is that the body takes fat from where it least needs it. This creates pockets or certain areas where you lose more fat than in other areas. Although it can look like you have lost a lot of weight in certain areas, it's not so great for the skin.

The key to minimizing loose skin is how you lose your weight. When you detox, releasing fat naturally by pooping, peeing, breathing, and sweating you release it in layers. This overall gradual loss, which we use with the Livy Method, makes it much easier for the body to regenerate your skin around your new sized body frame.

Top tips for helping the skin during and after weight loss:

1.   Dry brushing

It's like a loofah except you don't get it wet. Dry brushing is beneficial because it stimulates the nervous system, helps to increase overall circulation, and removes dead skin cells, which promotes regeneration and leaves the skin feeling invigorated.

Dry brushing is most beneficial in the morning, because of its energizing qualities. Start at your feet and brush upward toward the heart. Similarly, with your arms, begin at the hands and work upward. Use firm, small strokes upward or work in a circular motion. For the stomach, work in a clockwise direction.

Dry brushing or any kind of exfoliation should be gentle on the skin, so avoid being too harsh. Ideally, dry brushing is done 1-2 times a week.

2.   Collagen

Collagen is what keeps our skin from sagging, giving us that plump and youthful look. Collagen starts to decrease in the body as we age.

It can be beneficial to add in a collagen supplement. Adding in a collagen supplement helps to promote the production of proteins that help structure your skin, including elastin and fibrillin. (Review the Let's Talk Supplements post for more information on collagen supplements.)

You may also want to read the ingredients label, as some products may contain additional ingredients to support skin health, including silica, hyaluronic acid, or vitamin C.

Collagen is also found in the connective tissues of animals. Thus, foods like chicken skin, pork skin, beef, and fish are natural sources of collagen. Additionally, foods that contain gelatin, such as bone broth, also provide collagen.

Here is a list of some more food sources that either contain collagen or help promote collagen production by providing key building blocks.

- Fish
- Chicken
- Egg whites
- Citrus Fruits
- Berries
- Red and yellow vegetables
- Garlic
- White tea
- Leafy greens
- Cashews
- Tomatoes
- Bell peppers
- Beans
- Avocados
- Soy
- Also herbs high in collagen include: Chinese knotweed, horsetail, gynostemma
- Herbs that help to produce collagen include: Gotu kola, bala, and ashwagandha

Keep in mind that it can be hard to get what the body needs naturally, so adding in a supplement is your best bet when looking to increase collagen.

3.   Use natural oils and creams.

Because fat stores are full of toxins from the products you use, the foods you consume and also from the environment, you want to avoid adding in more toxins by using creams on your skin that contain perfumes, dyes and synthetic ingredients.

When a cream, lotion or oil is applied to the skin, the ingredients are absorbed into the bloodstream. From there, they have a direct effect on many of the body's processes. Meaning, if the ingredients are beneficial, they'll have beneficial effects. If they are a detriment, they'll have adverse effects on the body.

Some ingredients to avoid: parabens, sulfates, petrochemicals, synthetic dyes, propylene glycol, and triclosan.

Some natural oils to use on your body:

OLIVE OIL

The antioxidants in olive oil help to soothe the skin and repair damaged cells due to excessive dryness. It can also help in preventing age related wrinkles and fine lines.

GRAPESEED OIL

Because it contains high levels of vitamin E, this oil may contribute to better skin and reducing UV damage.

COCONUT OIL

Coconut oil is a powerful antioxidant that works to eliminate free radicals that can damage your skin. In addition, coconut oil hydrates and moisturizes your skin, which prevents sagging. Coconut oil can clog pores so best to use on the body and not the face.

ALMOND OIL

It's highly emollient, which means it helps to balance the absorption of moisture and water loss. Because it is also antibacterial and full of vitamin A, almond oil can be used to treat acne and some skin conditions. Its concentration of vitamin E can also help to heal sun damage, reduce the signs of aging, and fade scars.

Lastly, the things not mentioned here, are all the things you are doing while following the Program. Making nutrient rich food choices, adding in supplements, being hydrated, moving your body, managing your stress and getting quality sleep!

Right now you have your body focused on making change. A lot of the repairing of the skin happens after you have lost weight, when your body is working on stabilizing and maintaining your weight.

Just like when you cut your hand and your body repairs the skin, the same happens when you lose weight. Although it takes a while, your skin will regenerate around your new frame and anything you can do to help it along the way adds up and can make a difference.

Please take the time to head over to the Facebook Group or the Livy Method App and watch the quick video that accompanies this post.

WEEK 5 GUIDELINES: LEVELLING UP — MAXIMIZING AND EATING TO SATISFACTION

This week you are taking a break from Downsizing and instead, will focus on levelling up by Maximizing and being even more in tune with your portions while following the Food Plan and eating to satisfaction.

This means digging your heels in and relentlessly doing everything you can do to get the body to focus on releasing fat. Which means stepping up your game like never before, and taking everything you have learned and not just implementing it, but also building on it so you can take things to the next level.

Think of this week as taking everything you have learned up to this point and using it to level up and maximize your efforts and help the body focus on fat loss. Week 5 is a key week because it's a jumping off point for downsizing again one last time next week.

WHEN MAXIMIZING YOU ARE FOCUSING ON:

- Continuing to use the Let's Talk Maximizing Your Efforts Checklist post
- Consistently following the Food Plan
- Eating all of your meals and snacks
- Making your food choices as nutrient rich as possible
- Drinking enough water

- Consistently taking any supplements that you have added in
- Being super mindful about portions, continuing to ask the 4 Mindfulness Questions, and eating just enough, so you are feeling satisfied and not full 10 - 15 minutes later.

Please note: Eating to Satisfaction in Week 5 is with a different intention than in the first few weeks.

Portion wise, the goal is to not feel hungry or full. It is to feel like you have had just enough so that when you walk away 10 - 15 minutes later, and you ask yourself the fourth set of questions, you feel satisfied and not stuffed. Alternatively, if you feel hungry 10 - 15 minutes later, you can always go back for more. Pay attention and adjust your portions to see what works best for you.

For week 5, you are still asking the 4 Sets of Mindfulness Questions:

1. **Before you eat, ask yourself:**
   - Am I hungry?
   - How is this portion for me?
   - Is this enough?
   - Is this too much?
   - How would I feel if I ate all of it?

2. **While eating your food, pay attention to how you feel and ask yourself:**
   - Is my choice of food satisfying?
   - Do I feel any physical effects of eating?
   - Am I starting to feel satisfied?
   - How would I feel if I took a few more bites?
   - How would I feel if I stop eating now?

3. **When you are done eating, ask yourself:**
   - How do I feel?
   - How do I know when I have eaten enough?
   - Do I feel satisfied and if so, what is my definition of satisfaction?
   - How do I feel physically?

4. **15 minutes after you are done eating, ask yourself:**
   - How do I feel?
   - Do I still feel satisfied?
   - Could I have eaten more?
   - Could I have eaten less?

Each stage and phase or the Program is meant to get the body's attention and to get it to take action, and Week 5 is no different. There will be plateaus or stabilizing periods as they are a normal part of the process, but from this point moving forward, you should expect to see your body change or the scale drop, even when eating to satisfaction and regardless of the stage and phase you are in.

Sometimes, there is a delayed reaction before the numbers show on the scale, so stick with it and keep working. Think of the end game. Getting caught up on the day-to-day numbers can sidetrack you. When it comes to the scale, it is all about that downward trend and seeing how it all adds up at the end, based on all of the things you are doing to get and keep that scale moving.

FREQUENTLY ASKED QUESTIONS

1. **If I am maximizing, should I take out the heavier carbs even if my body wants them?**

   You are looking to continue to ask yourself those 4 Questions and be in tune with what your body is asking for. If you feel your body needs starchy carbs or grains then you can add them in. The best time to add them is to your lunch so that your body can use the energy from them throughout the day.

2. **If I did not maximize downsizing last week, should I redo it?**

   Recognizing that you could have done better is a great sign that you are becoming more in tune. It is not recommended to go back and redo weeks. If you have not been following at all or needed to take time off of the Program for any reason, it is best to pick up where you left off and keep things moving forward.

3. **What is the difference between being full and being satisfied?**

   Being full can leave you feeling bloated and uncomfortable with a feeling that you ate too much.

   Being satisfied is when you can walk away 10 - 15 min after your meal or snack and not feel the effects of eating.

   By following the Food Plan, asking the 4 Mindfulness Questions and becoming mindful of how you are feeling after eating will all help with learning the difference between full and what satisfaction feels like to you.

4. **I have still not lost any weight, is this normal?**

   For various reasons, it can be normal for some not to lose until later on in the Program. How quickly or how much you lose in the first few weeks is not an indication of how successful you will be in the end. If your weight is not moving, then you should be noticing your body changing in other ways and experiencing non-scale victories. Continue being consistent with your food, water and supplements and doing all the things to keep supporting your body referred to in the Let's Talk Maximizing Your Efforts Checklist post.

Many members have found that they've seen bigger drops on the scale in the latter half of the Program.

Please take the time to head over to the Facebook Group or the Livy Method App and watch the quick video that accompanies this post.

LET'S TALK ABOUT THE MESSY MIDDLE

Given we are half way through the Program, let's talk about what Finally & Forever weight loss is all about. How to achieve it and what you can expect on the road to reaching your goal.

There are 4 stages to Finally & Forever:

1. The first stage is losing your weight and reaching your goals. Which is why you are here, and following the Program is a very effective way to accomplish that.

2. The second stage is helping your body to solidify the weight you have lost. Meaning, giving your body time to make your new weight your new norm.

3. The third stage is where you start to test the waters.

4. The fourth stage is where you wake up, you look good, you feel good. You just go about living your life.

This isn't something you need to focus on or be concerned about yet. We will be breaking down next steps further as we move forward in the Program. This is just to give you an idea of the journey ahead.

Because when it comes to sustainable weight loss, there's more to it than eating less and exercising more like the diet industry would like you to believe.

It's about being in-tune with your body's needs, and the relationship you have with not only food, but with yourself.

It's about working through the issues and associations you have tied in and around food over the years.

It's also about working through old habits, while creating new ones and busting through beliefs that can keep you stuck in the past.

This is where working through the feels and the mental part of the process becomes just as important as what you are eating and when.

This is what makes The Livy Method different than other diets and why as long as you keep showing up, you can't mess it up.

LET'S TALK 4 MAIN REASONS WHY YOUR WEIGHT MIGHT BE SLOWER TO MOVE

Every extra pound of fat is hard on the body, so contrary to popular belief your body is not looking to store fat and carry excess weight.

However, the reality is that although weight loss will come easier for some, others will have to work a little harder and dig a little deeper because they have some underlying issues their body is dealing with.

If your weight is dropping and or your body is changing and you are noticing non-scale victories like increased energy, sleeping better, and even pooping better, then chances are you have nothing to be concerned about as your body is responding well to the process.

If your weight isn't dropping and your body isn't changing and you are not noticing any non-scale victories, then chances are you have some issues you need to address.

4 MAIN REASONS WHY YOUR WEIGHT MIGHT NOT BE MOVING:

1. Inflammation

Inflammation is an issue because weight gain is associated with increased inflammation in the body. It can lead to insulin resistance which is an issue when it comes to weight loss because it leads to higher blood sugar levels, as well as fatty liver.

It's key to note, there are different types of inflammation which can be caused by a variety of conditions, so it's best to check in with your healthcare provider as this is just a general overview.

Causes of inflammation:

- Hormonal issues like insulin resistance, Hashimotos and high cortisol levels
- Digestive issues including food sensitivities or allergies
- Autoimmune diseases like arthritis, lupus, psoriasis
- Medications
- Stress
- Lifestyle and environmental factors (ie. exposure to chemicals and irritants)

It is worth pointing out there are also foods that can cause or contribute to inflammation.

These include:

- Sugar
- Refined carbohydrates
- Alcohol
- Processed meats
- Trans fats

These are foods we try to minimize and things we address while following the Program. But if your body isn't responding in the way it should, then a visit to your healthcare provider to further investigate can be just what you need to get the scale moving.

2. Food Sensitivities

When it comes to food allergies, you generally know when you have them as they tend to be pretty noticeable and, in some cases, extreme. Symptoms often involve swelling, itching and wheezing and can require immediate medical attention and medication.

Food sensitivity, on the other hand, is usually GI-related. They can happen when the body has a hard time digesting certain foods and can affect the weight loss process simply because they make people feel unwell. They can also cause bloating and discomfort that may mimic weight gain, which doesn't help when it comes to staying motivated.

Food intolerance symptoms usually begin about half an hour after eating or drinking, but in some cases, you might not notice them for a few days after consuming.

Symptoms include:

- Nausea
- Stomach pain
- Gas, cramps or bloating
- Vomiting
- Heartburn
- Diarrhea
- Headaches
- Irritability or nervousness

As you progress through the Program, you will become very in tune to your body's needs. Using the Livy Method App or keeping a journal to track how your body is dealing with the foods you eat can help give you insight into any food sensitivities you might have.

3. Gut Dysbiosis

I'm hesitant to use this word because it seems to be the new buzzword of the year, so it's key to keep in mind this is a general term used to describe when the bacteria in your digestive system becomes unbalanced.

There can be many causes and a variety of symptoms, so if you feel there is something off with your digestion, be sure to consult with your healthcare provider.

Causes of Dysbiosis:

- Consuming processed foods, including sugar and artificial sweeteners like sucralose, food additives, preservatives and artificial ingredients
- Chemicals like pesticides on unwashed fruit and veg
- Environmental toxins, skin care products
- Alcohol
- Any new medications added in
- Use of antibiotics that affect your microbiome
- Parasites
- Poor oral hygiene
- High levels of stress or anxiety

Some symptoms can include:

- Nausea, upset stomach
- Constipation
- Diarrhea
- Bad breath
- Trouble urinating
- Vaginal or rectal itching
- Bloating
- Extreme fatigue
- Chest pain
- Rashes
- Trouble concentrating
- Anxiety

There are tests your healthcare provider can perform to diagnose. And there are medications and different types of treatment including changes in lifestyle (like following the Program) that can help.

4. Hormonal Health

When people think of hormones, they tend to think of sex hormones, when in reality there are over 50 different types of hormones that factors into your weight loss journey. These hormones control a number of functions in the body including; heart rate, appetite, sleep cycles, metabolism, mood, and of course sexual health to name a few.

Hormones are key to the weight loss conversation because your body storing fat and releasing it are regulated by certain hormones in the body. Hormones also influence your energy expenditure (or the number of calories your body burns on a daily basis, not that we care or talk about calories).

Hormones work like chemical messengers that can make or break your weight-loss efforts. While following the Program, we leverage the benefits of certain hormones while minimizing the downside of others. For example, following a balanced diet that feeds into your satiety hormone (Leptin) and minimizing the need for as much insulin as your body is used to using, which are things you are already doing by following the Food Plan.

Please note: I am NOT highlighting these four things to say that you can't lose weight if you are dealing with them. It's more so to highlight that if the scale isn't moving, there can be underlying issues the body needs to focus on more than others, in order to help it start focusing on weight loss.

If you suspect you are dealing with any of the issues below, have faith following the Program and maximizing your efforts will help to address them. But it is also worthwhile to work with your healthcare provider to address these issues, which can be a game changer when it comes to the scale.

LET'S REVISIT EXERCISE

Exercise is a great complement to the Program. It's great for heart health, bone density, stress release, as well as toning and shaping your changing body.

As great as exercise can be for your health and wellness, it's not the best weight loss tool, which is the reason why it's not a mandatory component of the Program. But given where we are at now, it's not unusual to start thinking about adding in more movement as your body gives you access to more energy.

Now that you're feeling more energetic, let's talk about how to implement exercise that will fall in line with your weight loss goals:

- If you are new to exercise, start by simply being more active. Things like taking the stairs and parking further away when getting groceries, going for walks or doing some push-ups or squats in your kitchen, can add up and have a big impact.

- It is best to start slow to minimize the stress on the body and build up to it.

- Choose activities that you enjoy so you make a positive association to exercise moving forward, and it becomes something you look forward to doing.

- You also want to walk away from any exercise feeling good and energized, not tired, taxed or drained.

LET'S TALK CARDIO AND GETTING YOUR HEART RATE UP:

Cardio exercise gets your heart rate up and is very effective for fat loss. When it comes to exercise and weight loss, it's all about the message you are sending to the body. Your physical brain that runs your body doesn't see what you are doing for exercise, it only interprets what you are doing based on your movements and heart rate.

This is where you can use the body's natural FIGHT or FLIGHT response by getting your heart rate up to maximize your results. If you repeatedly evoke the fight or flight response, your body will look to make you as strong and efficient as possible and will look to get rid of extra fat that could be slowing you down.

Cardio doesn't have to be running. It can be walking, skipping, swimming, dancing, lifting lighter weights with higher reps, sports activities, and anything else that helps get your heart rate up.

LET'S TALK LIFTING WEIGHTS:

When lifting weights, you are purposely creating damage to your muscles so your body repairs them and makes them stronger. This is great for increasing muscle mass, bone density, and toning and shaping your body.

With where you are at now in the process, adding some resistance training is a great complement to the Program with all the changes your body is already making due to all the nutrient rich food you have been focused on giving it.

With lifting heavier weight you need to make sure that you give your body adequate rest in between workouts. If you choose to exercise daily it can be a great idea to alternate muscle groups or lift a little lighter using higher repetitions to get your heart rate up and build muscle with minimal damage.

LET'S TALK REST:

If you are going to work out to the point of being sore, you need to make sure you are giving your body adequate time to repair and rebuild, or you will run the risk of over-training.

Overtraining happens when the body can't catch up to the damage that's been done, leaving your body feeling weak and in a deficit, which in turn can cause the body to feel the need to hold on to fat or store more fat for easy energy.

Be mindful of taking rest days, making sure to drink enough water, and getting good quality sleep to help the body recover.

It's always a great idea to speak to your healthcare provider before starting any new routine.

LET'S REVISIT WHY MY WEIGHT IS UP?

Fluctuations on the scale are going to happen and are something you need to be comfortable with. It's important to remember that throughout this Program, your weight will continue to naturally fluctuate, no matter what you do.

When following the Program, consistently eating all meals and snacks, making foods nutrient rich and eating to satisfaction you are not going to gain weight. Here is a reminder of all of the things that can have your weight up that don't amount to real weight gain.

REASONS YOUR WEIGHT CAN BE UP:

- Stress
- Lack of sleep
- Salty food
- Hard to digest food
- Dehydration
- Body fighting an illness
- Body sore from a workout
- Body reacting to change in routine
- Body reacting to change in food
- Body reacting to new medication or change in medications
- Body reacting to any new supplements or change in supplements
- Deficiencies like being low in iron
- Hormones fluctuating
- PMS
- Your scale needing new batteries

And the most important reason is that your body is detoxing and your weight is about to drop.

If you continue to show up, you are going to be successful and lose your weight regardless of the little ups along the way. The ups are normal and to be expected. Embrace the fluctuations on the scale and remember, it's all about the downward trend.

WEEK 6 GUIDELINES: DOWNSIZING ONE LAST TIME

This week you are repeating Downsizing One Last Time while Maximizing and being even more in tune to your body's needs while bringing awareness to how your body is responding both physically and mentally to the process.

BACK TO DOWNSIZING ONE LAST TIME

You may be wondering how you are going to downsize again if your portions are already small. Remember, when it comes to downsizing, you are only eating a few bites less from what you were eating to feel satisfied. It is about what the portions feel like, not what they look like.

It is important to keep in mind, the downsizing phase is just one of many techniques designed to get the body's attention to take action and focus on dropping fat. The real secret to the Program and to your success is showing up every day and being consistent with the changes you are making. For example, following the Food Plan, taking supplements, drinking your water, and Maximizing everything you can while making as many choices as possible that fall in line with your goals.

In the first round of downsizing, you were decreasing portions by a few bites. This was more of a practice round for you to get a sense of how it works, to test the waters, and start to address any issues and associations that start to pop up.

In Week 6, you are going to take things to the next level by being mindful with the portions, Maximizing everything you can to get and keep the scale moving and challenging yourself a little more now that you are starting to understand the process.

The idea is to get your body's attention and get it to focus on detox and dropping fat when normally fat loss is low on the list of the body's priorities day to day. In getting the body's attention, you may feel unsatisfied to the point where you will notice and may need to step outside your comfort zone.

Please note: The goal is to feel SLIGHTLY unsatisfied, not to feel hungry like you are starving and depriving your body. It is just enough of a decrease that will get the body's attention.

Also keep in mind that you will be dealing with fluctuating hunger levels that need to be factored in. There will be some days where the body will be naturally hungrier than others. Where one day you might be hungry every 30 minutes, and then the next day, 3 hours can go by and you won't be hungry at all. This is normal and to be expected. On the days you are not hungry, you still want to eat a token amount. You may find after a few bites, you will start to feel hungry, in which case, you still want to leave yourself feeling slightly unsatisfied.

It should also be noted that the point of downsizing is to see the scale move. Just because you eat less, it doesn't mean the scale will move right away. Depending on where your body is at, and what it is currently focused on, there can be a delayed reaction when it comes to the scale. What you do this week can reflect on the scale next week. Therefore, it is very important that you stay as consistent as possible, Maximize, and stay on top of everything you need to get and keep the scale moving.

ON A FINAL NOTE: Keep in mind that how you are eating now is only a means to an end. How and what you eat will change and evolve as we move forward in the weeks to come. Other stages in the Program will include eating more and more often and then eating more in tune with your body's needs as we progress through the Program.

This is the last week you will be purposely reducing portions as we will not be Downsizing again, so do your best to be all in! If you are unsure or need a refresher on Downsizing, be sure to review the Week 4 Guidelines.

FREQUENTLY ASKED QUESTIONS

1. **I am eating to slightly less than satisfaction but am really hungry shortly after. Any tips?**

    Keep in mind, in getting the body's attention with this tweak, chances are, you will feel hungrier than normal. Make sure the foods you are eating are nutrient rich and eat breakfast if that is something you tend to skip. Keep asking yourself the 4 Mindfulness Questions. If you are feeling like you are distractedly hungry after your meals or snacks, this may be a signal that you are downsizing too much, so you can always have more or you can hold off and have your next meal or snack earlier than expected.

2. **Do we downsize both meals and snacks this week?**

    When downsizing, you want to try and downsize all of your meals and snacks if possible.

Hunger levels will be different every day, so the amount you need each day will change. If you are not hungry and have only token bites, then you don't need to downsize those.

3.   **I get symptoms such as headaches during downsizing. Is this normal or a result of hunger?**

Headaches can be a side effect of detox. However, because we are eating nutrient rich food six times a day, you should not feel deprived and get headaches as a result of eating a few bites less. Side effects from the Program should never be severe, so if you're concerned, be sure to check in with your healthcare provider.

4.   **I am going on vacation and will not be able to downsize, should I eat to satisfaction instead this week?**

Vacations can do wonders for weight loss. Change of environment, less stress, abundance of good fresh foods and some decent sleep can be exactly what the body needs to get the scale moving. If you find you are unable to follow the week while away, then try to maintain regular eating habits as much as possible. Once you are back you can pick up from where you left off and follow through with the week of Downsizing.

Please take the time to head over to the Facebook Group or the Livy Method App and watch the quick video that accompanies this post.

LET'S TALK SECONDARY SUPPLEMENTS

The following are suggested supplements that can help level up your health and wellness and support the body with the fat loss process.

This list is for those of you who may be interested in taking things to the next level when it comes to your health and wellness. If you have not yet added in the basic supplements, you should consider those first.

After spending the past few weeks laying a strong foundation and addressing the body's basic needs, these supplements can help take things to the next level and may even help to speed up the process. With that said, they are not a mandatory part of the Program or make or break when it comes to reaching your goals. More important than any supplement that you can take is all the work you are putting into this process day to day.

Read over the information and decide if you think any of the listed supplements could be a benefit to you and always remember that if you have any questions or concerns when considering adding in any supplements, be sure to talk to your healthcare provider.

MCT OIL

MCT oil is a medium-chain triglyceride (MCT). Unlike other fat sources that need to be broken down, digested, and stored before it is used by the body, MCT oil is sent directly to your liver where it has a thermogenic effect and the ability to support your metabolism (the rate at which your body functions and burns calories).

Because MCT oil is instantly utilized for fuel instead of being stored as fat, it can help to calm the mind (since your brain is floating in cholesterol, it needs good fat for energy to function) and keep the body revved up and working extra hard.

Look for MCT oil derived from 100% coconut oil, NOT coconut oil itself.

It comes in oil or powder form. You can take it straight, add it to beverages, or use as a dressing on salads.

DOSE

Start with 1 teaspoon and work your way up to a tablespoon per serving or as directed on the product's label. Take up to 3 times a day.

WHEN TO TAKE

Ideally taken in the morning. It can also be added later in the day, around 3-4 pm, and after dinner. Side effects can include digestive upset if you use too much too soon, so start with less instead of more and work your way up.

This does not replace your omega 3 supplements, as MCT oil is not an essential fatty acid.

ADAPTOGENS

Adaptogens are supplements derived from plants that can help support the body's ability to cope with stress by decreasing sensitivity to stressors, and can help it return to a balanced state when experiencing stressful situations. This can help to decrease your body's cortisol levels. This is important to weight loss because when you are stressed, your adrenals produce and control cortisol.

Cortisol is known as the stress hormone because of the body's stress response. When you are stressed, your adrenals can produce too much or not enough which can signal the need to store fat in the body. Most of the cells in your body have cortisol receptors that use it for a variety of functions including: regulating blood sugar, reducing inflammation, regulating metabolism, and memory function.

COMMON EXAMPLES OF ADAPTOGENS:

- Ashwaganda
- Ginseng
- Reishi
- Rhodiola
- Schisandra
- Holy Basil

SOME SIGNS YOU CAN BENEFIT FROM ADAPTOGENS:

- Feeling tired; struggling to wake up in the morning
- Trouble falling asleep
- Anxiety, or feeling on edge
- Mood swings
- Depression
- Weight gain
- Autoimmune issues
- Brain fog
- Body aches
- Hair loss
- Lightheaded

These symptoms are pretty general, which is one of the challenges because there are many variables that affect how your body functions.

DOSE

Follow the directions on your product's label for dosage.

WHEN TO TAKE

Take as directed and be sure to check with your healthcare provider, especially if you are taking medications as there can be interactions.

B COMPLEX

Vitamin B Complex is a group of water-soluble vitamins, which play a very important role in maintaining the growth and the metabolism of cells in the body. When it comes to weight loss, B12 is especially important because it helps the body convert fats and proteins into energy. It is mainly found in red meat, chicken, fish, dairy and eggs.

A B Complex can help the body maintain sufficient levels of a variety of B vitamins so that it can efficiently utilize carbohydrates, fats, and proteins and help the body maintain energy, stamina, and control appetite.

B vitamins are water-soluble, meaning they are not stored in the body. Though they don't stick around long, B vitamins are vital for supporting a variety of bodily functions. Each B vitamin supports different bodily functions, so your healthcare provider will be able to pinpoint the supplements you need and help you decide between B12 vs. B complex.

- B1 (thiamine): Helps convert nutrients into energy, making it essential to your metabolic system. It strengthens the immune system and supports nerve function. Naturally found in pork, sunflower seeds and wheat germ.

- B2 (riboflavin): Riboflavin works with thiamine to convert food to energy, while also serving as an antioxidant. Naturally found in organ meats, beef, and mushrooms.

- B3 (niacin): Niacin helps your cells communicate and plays a role in metabolism and DNA production. Naturally found in chicken, tuna, and lentils.

- B5 (pantothenic acid): Converts food to energy, supports hormone and cholesterol production. Naturally found in liver, fish, yogurt, and avocado.

- B6 (pyridoxine): Facilitates energy production, regulates hormone activity, blood glucose levels, hemoglobin production, and aids in the creation of neurotransmitters. Found naturally in chickpeas, salmon, and potatoes.

- B7 (biotin): Biotin specifically helps metabolize carbohydrates and fats. Can be found naturally in yeast, eggs, salmon, cheese, and liver.

- B9 (folate): Folate metabolizes amino acids, assists in the formation of blood cells, and helps your cells develop and divide properly. Found naturally in leafy greens, liver, and beans.

- B12 (cobalamin): Involved in neurological function, DNA production, and red blood cell development. Found naturally in animal sources like meat, eggs, seafood, and dairy.

Typically, it is B1, B6 and B12 deficiencies that are an issue. Your healthcare provider can order a blood or a urine test to assess and provide recommendations.

DOSE

Range varies depending on the B vitamin. Follow directions on your product's label.

WHEN TO TAKE

B vitamins can boost energy and can be hard to process, so it is best to take them earlier in your day and with a meal.

COQ10

CoQ10 is an antioxidant that also plays a fundamental role in the production of energy by the cells. A deficiency can contribute to lower energy levels and a slower metabolism. It is believed that CoQ10 production decreases with age, which may help explain one of the reasons why it can be harder to lose weight as you get older.

CoQ10 can enhance healthy weight loss because it helps to support increased metabolic function. In addition, it can work to decrease body fat while boosting energy levels by maximizing your body's ability to convert food to fuel.

It's also great for skin. Lack of CoQ10 results in decreased production of collagen and elastin. Collagen is important because it makes your skin firm, while elastin gives your skin flexibility. The loss of collagen and elastin can cause your skin to wrinkle and sag.

DOSE

Follow the directions on your product's label. 90–200 mg of CoQ10 per day is usually recommended, though some conditions may require higher doses of 300–600 mg.

WHEN TO TAKE

CoQ10 is fat soluble, so it should be taken with a meal containing fat so your body can better absorb it. Check with your healthcare provider before adding this in, especially if you are taking medications as there can be interactions.

L-THEANINE

L-theanine is an amino acid found in green and black tea leaves as well as mushrooms. It is thought to be effective in decreasing brain chemicals that contribute to stress and anxiety while increasing brain chemicals that encourage a sense of calm.

L-theanine elevates levels of GABA, as well as serotonin and dopamine. These chemicals are known as neurotransmitters, and they work in the brain to regulate emotions, mood, concentration, alertness, and sleep, as well as appetite, energy, and other cognitive skills. Increasing levels of these calming brain chemicals promotes relaxation and can help with sleep and stress. Some research also suggests that L-theanine may improve the function of the body's immune system and help to improve inflammation in the intestinal system.

DOSE

Dose ranges from 100-400mg. Start with a smaller dose and work up.

WHEN TO TAKE

Follow the directions on your product's label.

Due to its calming effects, L-theanine may also help lower blood pressure so you may want to keep that in mind and consult with your healthcare provider if you have low blood pressure.

Women who are pregnant or breastfeeding should consult their healthcare practitioner before adding L-theanine or supplementing with green or black tea.

TURMERIC

The primary antioxidant in turmeric the spice is curcumin, which is an anti-inflammatory. While increasing your intake of turmeric isn't a lone strategy for weight loss, it may help you address inflammation and help with metabolism.

Curcumin, which is an antioxidant in turmeric, suppresses the inflammatory messaging in many cells, including pancreatic, fat and muscle cells. This can help curb insulin resistance, high blood sugar, high cholesterol levels, and other metabolic conditions resulting from excess fat.

Turmeric is a readily available spice, and adding it to your diet has no side effects unless you have an allergy, so it can easily be added to foods. However, in order to get the amount of curcumin necessary to aid in weight loss you would have to use a lot of it. Therefore, if you want to experience the full effects, you would need to take a supplement that contains significant amounts of curcumin.

WHAT TO LOOK FOR

The best curcumin supplements contain piperine, which substantially increases the absorption and therefore effectiveness.

DOSE

Follow the directions on your product's label for dosage.

WHEN TO TAKE

Follow the directions on your product's label. Check with your healthcare provider before adding this in, especially if you are taking medications as there can be interactions.

TRACE MINERALS

Minerals are needed for important metabolic functions in the body. Even though trace minerals are only required in small amounts, they are indeed essential. Not only for good health, but also weight loss.

There are two classes of minerals:

1. Major
2. Trace

Major minerals include: calcium, potassium, chloride, phosphorus, magnesium, sodium, and selenium.

Trace minerals include: chromium, germanium, manganese, rubidium, vanadium, cobalt, iron, molybdenum, zinc, copper, lithium, nickel, and silica.

Adding in trace minerals that include sodium are beneficial in preventing low sodium levels caused from changes in your diet, taking medications, excessive sweating, and electrolyte loss.

DOSE

Follow recommendations on your product's label.

WHEN TO TAKE

Add to your water following directions on your product's label.

Check with your healthcare provider before adding any new supplement to your daily routine.

Please take the time to head over to the Facebook Group or the Livy Method App and watch the quick video that accompanies this post.

LET'S REVISIT WATER

Let's revisit how much you need and why, relevant to where you are now in this process.

KEY TAKEAWAYS WHEN IT COMES TO WATER:

- Everyone is different and every day is different. Consider your body's needs and adjust day to day to find the right amount. Your needs can change throughout the Program.

- When the scale is bouncing up and down the same few pounds this is usually a sign the body is trying to detox but needs more water. Try increasing by a few cups.

- When you crave carbs and sugar specifically, this is usually a sign you are dehydrated and the body is trying to get you to eat high water content foods like fruit. So, when craving sugar, bump up your water intake.

- It's normal to be extra hungry and extra thirsty heading into the evening right before your weight is about to drop. Drink more water to help support detox.

- When you are drinking lots of water but your lips are dry and or you are thirsty, this is a sign your body is asking for even more water. You can trust your body so drink more.

- If the scale is moving and you find the water hard to drink or particularly unappealing, this can be a sign you are in active detox, so support the body and the scale dropping by increasing it slightly.

- If you drop weight and the next day the scale is the same or even up, this can be a sign the body is retaining water to continue to drop, so support the body's needs and continue to stay on top of your water to keep the scale moving.

- If the more water you drink, the more you have to pee. That can be a sign you are still dehydrated. Once properly hydrated, you will be able to go longer periods of time without having to go to the bathroom as often. Try drinking earlier in the day and spreading it out, sipping rather than guzzling so it won't go right through you.

WHY WATER IS KEY:

- The Livy Method utilizes the body's natural detox process. Because the body releases fat when you poop, pee, breathe and sweat, drinking enough water continues to be key.

HOW MUCH DO YOU NEED?

- Everyone requires different amounts, so you will have to play around with it to see what works for you. Your water intake can also change from day to day depending on a variety of factors.

- The average person needs at least 2.7 - 3.5 litres of water for basic body functions like digestion, pumping blood through your veins, sweating, bowel movements etc. (Refer to the original post, Let's Talk Water, in the Livy Method App or Facebook Support Group for source.)

- When following the Food Plan and to help the body get into detox mode (focus on fat loss), you need to drink above and beyond what it needs for basic body functions.

- Since your goal here is weight loss, aim for 3.5 litres. You can adjust from there depending on your height, weight and other factors listed below.

WHEN TO DRINK MORE THAN 3.5 LITRES:

- You are taller than average (over 5'5" for women, 5'9" for men).

- You have more weight to lose.

- Your body is releasing fat.

- When the scale is bouncing between the same 2 numbers.

- You are fighting an illness.

- You have your period.

- You take medication that causes weight gain or dehydration.

- You work or live in a dry environment.

- You exercise or are active enough to sweat.

- You drink alcohol.

- You eat salty food.

HOW DO YOU KNOW YOU ARE DRINKING ENOUGH?

- You no longer feel thirsty.

- You no longer have a dry mouth or lips.

- Your trips to the bathroom have decreased (they will increase until you are properly hydrated).

- Your sugar cravings are decreasing.

HOW MUCH IS TOO MUCH?

Overhydration and water intoxication happen when you drink more water than your kidneys can get rid of through urine. You have a greater risk of developing water intoxication if you drink a lot of water in a short period of time. When you drink too much too fast, your kidneys can't get rid of the excess water.

Therefore, to avoid hyponatremia (low salt in blood) or overhydration from excess water, you should not drink more than 1 L of water per hour, and be mindful to include salt in your diet or add in trace minerals. If you have any concerns, speak with your healthcare provider.

WHEN INCREASING WATER INTAKE:

- Increase slowly.
- Start early and spread your water drinking throughout the day.
- Sip and don't chug a large amount at once.

TIPS FOR GETTING IT IN:

- Make it fun! Make it a challenge!
- Start drinking early in your day. Most people find it easier to get the majority in the first half of the day.
- Sip, don't guzzle or it will go right through you.
- Get a good water bottle.
- Track your water (and other fluids such as coffee, tea, bone broth) intake by using the Livy Method App.
- Set reminders to drink.
- Add fresh or frozen fruit, cucumber slices, and/or fresh herbs or ginger.
- Slow down your water intake in the evening, if it messes with your sleep.

When it comes to water, it's not about drinking more and more. It's about drinking enough. Do what's right for you and always consult with your healthcare provider if you have any concerns.

Once you have lost the weight and are in maintenance, you can adjust and scale back on the amount you are drinking to maintain hydration without having to drink more for the sake of weight loss.

WEEK 7 GUIDELINES: MAXIMIZING & FEEDING THE METABOLISM

This week has you consistently following the Food Plan and Maximizing your efforts to help the body focus on fat loss. Mid-week, we will be introducing the Feeding the Metabolism tweak.

As we move into Week 7, we are going to move on from Downsizing. For the first 1-3 days of the week, you are to eat to satisfaction while maximizing. For the last 4-7 days, you will be shifting gears and Feeding the Metabolism.

DAYS 1-3 YOU ARE MAXIMIZING AND EATING TO SATISFACTION

With Maximizing and eating to satisfaction, you are doing everything you can to get and keep the scale moving while supporting your body and its needs.

WHEN MAXIMIZING, YOU ARE FOCUSING ON:

- Drinking enough water
- Being consistent with any supplements you are taking
- Eating all of your meals and snacks
- Making your food choices as nutrient rich as possible
- Being super mindful about portions
- Asking the 4 Mindfulness Questions
- Make sure you eating just enough so when you walk away 10 - 15 minutes later, you are feeling satisfied and not overly full

- Avoiding eating too late in the evening as it will mess with sleep and the detox process
- Managing stress levels and getting quality sleep
- Being more active, and moving your body

DAYS 4 - 7 YOU ARE GOING TO INTRODUCE FEEDING THE METABOLISM

With Feeding the Metabolism you are going to split up your meals and snacks. This is designed to feed into your increasing metabolism and get you even more in tune to your portion sizes. You are going to continue to be super consistent with the Food Plan, water, and any supplements you take.

You are to split your meals into 2 portions. After eating your first portion, you will eat the second portion 20 - 30 minutes later, while still asking the 4 Mindfulness Questions for both.

You can do this with one meal or all of your meals. You can also do this with your snacks.

FOR EXAMPLE: For lunch, prepare a portion that you have been eating to satisfaction and then divide it in two. Eat one portion, continuing to be mindful of how you feel, while asking the 4 Mindfulness Questions. 20 - 30 minutes later, you will have the second portion.

If you are hungry for the second portion, you will ask the 4 Mindfulness Questions again, and eat just enough, so when you walk away you are feeling satisfied and not stuffed 10 - 15 minutes later. Alternatively, if you are not hungry for the second portion, make sure you still have a token amount (4 - 5 bites).

Keep in mind there is no hard and fast rule for this. You can split up all of your meals and snacks, some of your meals and snacks, or even just one. The goal is to eat more often than what your body is used to. So, it can be once more a day to six more times a day, and that can change from day to day.

TO TAKE IT ONE STEP FURTHER: When dividing meals and snacks, separate your protein from your carbohydrates. As an example, for lunch eat your protein first, and then eat your vegetables and any added heavier carbs in your second portion.

Healthy fats and leafy greens can be eaten with either portion, or both.

Protein decreases your hunger hormones (ghrelin) and stimulates your satiety hormones (leptin) that help you feel more satisfied. Eating your protein first will help with getting you even more in tune with the foods that you are eating and the portions you are having. You may find with eating more often; you are either not as hungry or hungrier. Both are beneficial responses from the body.

When it comes to soups, stews, chili etc., where it's harder to separate the protein, just separate the portion into 2 servings and do not worry about separating the protein.

Please note: If you're concerned that you will not be able to split up as many meals and snacks as you would like, keep in mind at this point your body wants your fat gone just as much as you do, so it will be looking to get rid of it. If you just follow the Food Plan and Maximize your efforts, you should still expect the scale to move.

TO RECAP:

Days 1-3 you are eating to satisfaction and Maximizing.

Days 4-7 you will implement Feeding the Metabolism.

Remember you can split up all or some of your meals and snacks. Do the best you can. This is only for a few days. For more information, review the Let's Talk Feeding the Metabolism post.

FREQUENTLY ASKED QUESTIONS

1. **Do I have to wait until mid-week to start the splitting process? Or can I start at the beginning of the week?**

   To maximize your efforts, it's important to follow the Program as designed. Feeding the Metabolism works best off the heels of Maximizing and eating to satisfaction. To recap, days 1-3 you are eating to satisfaction and Maximizing. Days 4-7 you will implement Feeding The Metabolism. It is not recommended to switch up the order. Everything is for a rhyme and a reason, and if you do switch up the order of this tweak, it won't have the same effect.

2. **I work full time and struggle to split my meals and snacks throughout the day. Any tips?**

   Some members find that setting timers or alarms as reminders to eat really helps with this process. Keep in mind, you don't need to split all your meals and snacks for the tweak to be effective. Do the best you can while at work and split other meals and snacks if, and when you can.

3. **Do I eat 20 - 30 minutes after starting or finishing my last portion?**

   It is 20 - 30 minutes after your last bite of your last meal or snack.

4. **Do I have to split the same meals each day?**

   The great thing about this tweak is that there is no hard and fast rule. You can split all of your meals and snacks, or even just one of them in a day for this tweak to be effective. This can change day to day.

5. **If I normally skip breakfast do I start with splitting my morning fruit snack?**

   As always, breakfast is beneficial to have. However, if you do choose to skip it, start with splitting your morning fruit snack.

6. **What if I am not hungry for the second half of my meal or snack?**

   If after 20 - 30 minutes you find you are not hungry for the second portion, you still want to eat a token amount (4-5 bites).

7.   **If I am already eating token bites for most of my snacks, how do I split them?**

If you are not hungry for a meal or snack and are having only token bites, then you would not need to split those meals or snacks.

Please take the time to head over to the Facebook Group or the Livy Method App and watch the quick video that accompanies this post.

LET'S REVISIT THE 4 MINDFULNESS QUESTIONS

For the past few weeks you have been working hard to strengthen your mind-body connection. The 4 Mindfulness Questions that we introduced in Week 3 are a great tool for that, especially when it comes to your portions.

You want to continue to ask the 4 Questions until they become second nature, where your body lets you know WHEN to eat, WHAT to eat, and HOW MUCH to eat and you don't need to ask them anymore. As we move forward, we are going to transition into a more natural way of eating, so being in tune with how your body responds to these questions will be key.

THE 4 SETS OF MINDFULNESS QUESTIONS:

1. **Before you eat, ask yourself:**
   - Am I hungry?
   - How is this portion for me?
   - Is this enough?
   - Is this too much?
   - How would I feel if I ate all of it?

This is to bring awareness to your hunger levels and your portion sizes.

2. **While eating your food, pay attention to how you feel and ask yourself:**
   - Is my choice of food satisfying?
   - Do I feel any physical effects of eating?
   - Am I starting to feel satisfied?
   - How would I feel if I took a few more bites?
   - How would I feel if I stop eating now?

This is to bring awareness to how you are feeling while you are eating, and your body's cues when it comes to eating to satisfaction.

3. **When you are done eating, ask yourself:**
   - How do I feel?
   - How do I know when I have eaten enough?
   - Do I feel satisfied and if so, what is my definition of satisfaction?
   - How do I feel physically?

This is to bring awareness to how you are feeling when you are done eating, and if you are satisfied or need to eat more.

4. **15 minutes after you are done eating, ask yourself:**

- How do I feel?

- Do I still feel satisfied?

- Could I have eaten more?

- Could I have eaten less?

This is to bring awareness to how you are feeling after your body processes and digests your food, which can give you more insight to whether you have had enough or too much.

Following these steps for the past weeks you may have noticed that your portions have naturally decreased. At this point in the Program you are becoming even more in tune with your body's needs. Continue to work on that internal dialogue to fine tune your portions and maximize your efforts each day.

LET'S REVISIT NUTRIENT RICH MEALS

With where we are in the Program, it can be easy to fall into old habits and start choosing foods that you like and love, or are easy and convenient instead of choosing foods that will maximize your efforts.

Using salad as the example below, you want to add in as many nutrient rich elements as possible, as opposed to having just lettuce with some chicken on it. Keep in mind this can be applied to any meal, prepared in any way.

- Spring Mix/Greens = leafy greens + roughage + vitamins + minerals + protein
- Variety of Vegetables = energy + fiber + vitamins
- Avocado = energy + healthy fat + potassium + fiber
- Chicken = protein
- Feta cheese = energy + healthy fat + protein
- Nuts and Seeds = energy + healthy fat + protein
- An all-natural vinaigrette or dressing = healthy fat when made with good quality oils

EASY THINGS TO HAVE ON HAND THAT QUICKLY BUMP UP YOUR MEALS:

- Nuts and seeds
- Nut Butters
- Olives
- Pickled and marinated vegetables like artichoke hearts, pickled beets, roasted red peppers, etc.
- Hemp Hearts
- Natural oils, dressings and dips
- Cheese or other dairy such as yogurt or cream
- Coconut milk
- Salsa
- Avocados
- Hummus
- Nutritional Yeast
- Condiments and spices
- Protein Powder

As your portions are naturally becoming smaller, bumping up the nutrient value is not only a great way to give the body what it needs, it can also help give you more sustaining energy which can lead to feeling more satisfied. Even if you can add in one or two extra things like a drizzle of olive oil, an extra veg, or a few nuts... it can make all the difference.

LET'S TALK FEEDING THE METABOLISM

The tweak for Week 7:

- **Day 1-3 has you eating to satisfaction and Maximizing.**
- **Day 4-7 you are going to introduce Feeding the Metabolism.**

Feeding the Metabolism is meant to be used as another way to stimulate and utilize your digestive system to help feed into your increasing metabolism, and have you even more in tune to your portions.

In Feeding the Metabolism, you are going to continue to follow the Food Plan, and be consistent with the water and any supplements you take. The only thing that changes is you are going to split your meals and snacks into smaller portions and eat as often as possible.

- You can split your breakfast into 2 portions, your lunch into 2 portions, and dinner into 2 portions.
- You can also split each of your snacks into 2 portions.

After eating the first portion, you are going to wait 20 - 30 minutes and then consume the second portion. If you are hungry for the second portion, ask the 4 Mindfulness Questions and eat just enough so that when you walk away 10 - 15 min later, you are feeling satisfied and not stuffed. If you are not hungry for the second portion, you still want to eat a token amount.

You may find with eating more often, you are either not as hungry or hungrier. Both are normal and beneficial responses from the body.

Keep in mind there is no hard and fast rule for this. You can split up all of your meals or some of your meals or just one of your meals, and the same rules apply with the snacks. The goal is to eat more often than what you are used to eating. This can be 1 more time a day or 5 more times a day, and that can change day to day.

To take it one step further when dividing meals, separate your protein from your carbs.

As an example, for lunch, eat your protein first and then eat your vegetables 20 - 30 minutes later. Healthy fats and greens can be eaten with either portion or both.

For something like soup, stews, or chili where it's harder to separate the protein, just separate the portion into 2 servings.

With vegetable protein you can do the same. With chickpeas for example, which are a protein but have carbohydrates in them, there is still a benefit to separating them from the extra vegetables and any added carbs.

If you're concerned that you will not be able to split up as many meals and snacks as you would like, keep in mind that at this point, your body wants your fat gone just as much as you do, so it will be looking to get rid of it. If you just follow the Food Plan and Maximize your efforts, you should still expect the scale to move.

Please take the time to head over to the Facebook Group or the Livy Method App and watch the quick video that accompanies this post.

LET'S REVISIT PROTEINS CARBS AND FATS

As we begin Feeding the Metabolism, it is the perfect time to revisit the protein, carbs and fats list.

Remember, it's not an exhaustive list and keep in mind you don't need to worry about serving sizes or percentages. This is just to give you examples of what foods fall under each category.

SOURCES OF CARBOHYDRATES (Foods that break down into energy)

- Fruits
- Vegetables
- Starchy vegetables like potatoes, squash, cassava, plantain
- Naturally occurring sugar, found in things like beans, lentils and chickpeas
- Rice and grains like black rice, quinoa, barley and buckwheat
- Oatmeal and cereals
- High fiber crackers and dark, dense, or sprouted grain breads

SOURCES OF PROTEIN (Feeds the muscles helping to repair and rebuild along with maintaining and building muscle mass)

- Meat (Any kind, including organ meat)
- Eggs
- Fish
- Seafood
- Beans, lentils, legumes
- Nuts (all)
- Seeds (all, including hemp hearts and chia seeds)
- Dairy - cheese, yogurt, milk products (not to be used as a main source)
- Tofu

PLANT BASED PROTEIN (AS YOU CAN SEE BELOW, THERE IS PROTEIN FOUND IN LOTS OF THINGS BESIDES ANIMAL SOURCES)

- Broccoli - 2.6g per 1 cup
- Asparagus - 2.4g per 1 cup
- Peas - 9g per 1 cup
- Cauliflower - 2g per 1 cup
- Brussels - 3g per 1 cup
- Bok choy-1g per 1 cup
- Spinach, collard greens - 1g per 1 cup

- Mung bean sprouts - 2.5g per 1 cup
- Beans (kidney, pinto, black beans, chickpeas etc.) - 7.5g per 1/2 cup
- Lentils - 9g per 1/2 cup
- Quinoa - 4g per 1/2 cup
- Tempeh - 11g per 1/2 cup
- Tofu - 7g per 1/2 cup
- Buckwheat - 6g per 1 cup
- Soybeans/Edamame - 10g per 1/2 cup
- Rice - 7g per 1 cup
- Hemp seeds - 10g per 3 tbsp
- Pumpkin seeds - 5g per oz
- Chia - 4g per 2 tbsp
- Nut butter -15g per 2 tbsp
- Hummus - 7g per 2 tbsp
- Spirulina - 4g per 1 tbsp

Keep in mind you still do not need to worry about these measurements. They are for reference only and to point out the fact that some proteins have carbs in them, some vegetables have protein in them, and that protein adds up.

SOURCES OF FATS (ESSENTIAL FOR CELLULAR FUNCTION, PROVIDING ALTERNATIVE ENERGY AND BRAIN FUEL)

- Fish/Fish oil
- Omega 3 and or 369
- Oils like olive oil, coconut oil, avocado oil, grape seed oil, flax and hemp oil
- Salad dressings made with good quality oils
- Olives
- Avocado
- Nuts (all)
- Seeds (all, including hemp hearts and chia seeds)
- Dairy

This is not a complete list, this is just to remind you of the kinds of foods suggested when talking about incorporating proteins, carbs, and fats to your meals.

FOOD FACTS - ANTI-INFLAMMATORY FOODS

WHAT IS INFLAMMATION?

Inflammation is the body's normal reaction to injuries and infection. Short term bouts of inflammation is called acute inflammation and is your body's way of protecting yourself.

In contrast, too much inflammation for a long period of time leads to chronic inflammation, where the body thinks it's under constant attack, so the immune system continually fights back. It is linked to many diseases like arthritis, diabetes, heart disease, cancer and bowel diseases like Crohn's disease.

CAN CERTAIN FOODS HELP REDUCE INFLAMMATION?

A diet rich in anti-inflammatory foods isn't a magic cure when dealing with chronic inflammation. Medication and other treatments are important so be sure to be working with your healthcare provider. However, the combination of treatment and changes in diet can have a noticeable impact on low-grade inflammation.

FOODS THAT CAN HELP LOWER INFLAMMATION

The good news is anti-inflammatory foods tend to be the same foods that help keep you healthy in other ways as well. So even if you don't suffer from inflammation, it's a great idea to incorporate more of these nutrient rich foods into your diet.

- **Plant-based proteins** - Bump up those beans and lentils
- **Fresh fruit** - Intense colours are a sign that fruits are high in antioxidants. Look for dark blues & purples, like blackberries, plums and grapes. Bright reds, oranges and yellows like pomegranate, apples, raspberries, strawberries, papaya, mango and pineapple
- **Vegetables** - Especially broccoli, Brussels sprouts, cauliflower, and bok choy
- **Fatty fish** - Salmon, sardines, albacore tuna, herring, lake trout, and mackerel
- **Leafy greens** - Kale, spinach, and romaine lettuce, the darker the better
- **Foods with healthy fats** - Olive oil, avocados, nuts, and seeds (especially walnuts, almonds, hemp, flax, and chia seeds)
- **Whole grains** - Oatmeal, dark rices, barley, wheat kernels, etc.
- **Other foods/beverages high in antioxidants** - Ginger, turmeric, green tea, coffee and red wine (in moderation)

WHAT FOODS MAKE INFLAMMATION WORSE?

- Refined carbohydrates, such as white bread, pastries, and sweets
- Foods and drinks that are high in sugar, including excessive alcohol, soda and other sugary beverages
- Processed meat, such as hot dogs and sausages
- Fried foods
- Artificial food additives often found in highly processed foods and fast food
- Any foods that you may have a sensitivity to
- Too much saturated fat

BOTTOM LINE IS...

- Eat more plants
- Focus on antioxidants
- Consume Omega 3s
- Cut out highly processed and sugary foods
- Be mindful of having too much saturated fat

If you are following the Program, you have likely added in lots of great anti-inflammatory foods already. This is just another way to get you thinking about how you could level up your efforts. Whether you suffer from inflammation or not, adding in anti-inflammatory foods increases your health in general and can help prevent any inflammation from getting out of control.

LET'S REVISIT ALCOHOL

At this point in the Program, with your body working more efficiently and after weight loss, you may notice that your tolerance to alcohol has changed, and you are unable to consume as much as you did before.

When it comes to losing weight, the issue with alcohol is less about the kind you are drinking and more about the food you are eating with it. If you are following the Food Plan this is a non-issue. Here are a couple of things to keep in mind if you find yourself drinking and indulging:

- Drinking alcohol slows down the metabolism & your digestive system. If you are snacking it's best to choose protein, fats (like cheese and nuts) and veggies, leaving out any heavy carbs.

- Keep in mind alcohol can affect weight loss in other ways. For example, interrupting your sleep, messing with estrogen levels, and causing dehydration.

- Alcohol increases the production of galanin, a neuropeptide in the brain, which causes you to crave greasy food. Pair that with the effects of dehydration that causes you to crave sugar and you are ready to eat your face off the next day!

- Bumping up good fats like oils, nuts, seeds, and avocados, increasing your water along with having a banana, which is high in potassium, first thing the next day will help the body metabolize the alcohol and reduce the galanin.

- Drinking can also affect the good bacteria in your digestive system, so if your stomach always feels off the next day, try adding in or doubling up on your probiotic.

If you like to enjoy an alcoholic beverage every now and then, let's revisit your drink of choice and the impact it may have:

WINE

- There are benefits to choosing red wine over white. Although both are fine, red has more antioxidants and is slightly better for you. That isn't a reason to give up your white if that's what you prefer.

ROSE & CHAMPAGNES

- A little higher in sugar so don't be surprised if you wake up with a headache but also totally fine to have.

BEER/CIDERS

- Darker beers like Guinness are higher in nutrient value but any of your regular, all-natural ales, lagers, pilsners etc. are totally fine.

- When it comes to Ciders the same rules apply. Be mindful of added sugars and artificial ingredients.

- Be mindful of added ingredients and preservatives when drinking "light" or "low-cal" beer. Some are better quality than others.

- When it comes to non-alcoholic beverages, be mindful of artificial ingredients and added sugar.

HARD LIQUOR

- When it comes to the hard stuff, be mindful about what you are using as a mix. Try to avoid pop/soda, including diet versions and artificially flavoured juice.

- If you enjoy something like rye and coke or gin and tonic once every now and then, it's no big deal.

- When it comes to coolers and premixed drinks, look for quality ingredients and avoid anything artificial.

The best thing you can do to offset any negative effects of alcohol consumption is to add in that extra water of one cup per drink. Besides that, enjoy your beverages!

WEEK 8 GUIDELINES: MAXIMIZING & FEEDING THE METABOLISM ONE LAST TIME

Week 8 is a repeat of Week 7. You will be Maximizing and mindfully eating to satisfaction for the first THREE days of the week followed by Feeding the Metabolism One Last Time for the last FOUR days.

If you feel like you didn't have the chance to work Week 7 to the best of your ability, then this is your second chance. For a refresher, please review the Week 7 Guidelines and check out the Let's Talk Feeding the Metabolism post.

OVERVIEW:

DAYS 1-3 MAXIMIZING AND EATING TO SATISFACTION:

- Follow the Food Plan.

- Eat all meals and snacks.

- Make your food choices nutrient rich.

- Ask yourself the 4 Mindfulness Questions.

- Eat to satisfaction with an emphasis on portions, eating just enough so 10 - 15 minutes later you feel satisfied and not full.

- Continue to Maximize using the Let's Talk Maximizing Your Efforts Checklist post.

DAYS 4-7 FEEDING THE METABOLISM:

- Continue to Maximize your efforts.

- Continue to ask the 4 Mindfulness Questions.

- Split meals and snacks into 2 portions.

- Take it one step further, separate your protein from carbs (healthy fats and leafy greens can be included with either portion).

- Eat the first half, then wait 20 - 30 min before you eat the second half.

- If you are hungry for the second portion, ask the 4 Mindfulness Questions again and eat just enough so that 10 - 15 minutes later you feel satisfied and not full.

- If you are not hungry for the second portion, eat a token amount (4 - 5 bites).

- Be super mindful of portions and adjusting to hunger levels day to day.

This will be the last week we will be following the basic Food Plan. Moving forward, we will be changing things up to adapt to the changes your body is making. We have a lot of time left to get and keep that scale moving. Your focus moving forward should be following through and finishing just as strong, if not stronger than when you started. Your body is on your side, continue to be all in to Maximize your efforts in the time frame we have left.

FREQUENTLY ASKED QUESTIONS

1. **Is it normal to be hungry during the Feeding The Metabolism tweak?**

   It is totally normal to feel hungry during the Feeding The Metabolism tweak. You may find with eating more often, you are either not as hungry as usual or feel hungrier. Both are normal and beneficial responses from the body.

2. **I am not hungry for the second portion, should I still eat it?**

   It is normal to not feel hungry for the second portion after waiting 20 - 30 minutes. However, you will still want to eat a token amount.

3. **Can I eat the second portion later than 30 minutes, or should I skip it?**

   If you know you will not be able to eat the second portion within 20 - 30 minutes, then it is best not to split the portion at all. If for whatever reason, you split the portion and you are unable to eat the second half 20 - 30 minutes later, it is best to wait for your next meal or snack.

Please take the time to head over to the Facebook Group or the Livy Method App and watch the quick video that accompanies this post.

SELF-SABOTAGE PART 2

At this point in the Program, self-sabotage can start to pop up once again, though reasons can be a bit different than earlier on in the process.

Let's highlight a few different ways you may find yourself dealing with self-sabotage. These are just a few examples with some suggestions on how you can start to address them.

1. Rewarding yourself for reaching a milestone

It's common practice to use food as a reward which can be problematic while you are trying to lose weight. Make a list of things other than food that you can reward yourself with. Here are some ideas to get you started:

- A new book or magazine.
- A new skin care product or something for the bath.
- Treat yourself to time with a friend or loved one.
- Schedule yourself some 'me' time, whatever that looks like for you.

2. Being bored

Boredom can sometimes feel like a lack of motivation, tempting you to quit. Regardless, you are going to have to keep doing what you have to do, for as long as you need to do it to reach your goals, even if it's not all that exciting.

- Embrace being bored and recognize routine and consistency is exactly what your body needs to focus on fat loss.
- Lean into the changes that you are making week to week and try to have fun with them. Be open to what you can learn as you progress through the Program and the process.
- Step out of your comfort zone. Try a new fruit or vegetable or find a new recipe to try. Or just try something new in general like a new hobby, a new exercise routine, take a class, or learn something new.

3. Being tired of constantly focusing on yourself and doing all of the things

Prioritizing yourself and being mindful of making the most of this process can be exhausting. The time it takes to reach your goals can sometimes impact your enthusiasm, ambition to lose weight, and follow through on your journey.

- Take a moment to think back to when you started and why. Make a list to remind yourself and reflect back often to help keep you motivated along the way.
- Watch or listen to some of the Facebook Lives or guest segments for some motivation and inspiration.

- Try simplifying or pre-prepping your meals and snacks as much as possible so there isn't as much thinking involved.

- Set timers and reminders on the Livy Method App to help keep you on track.

4.   Thinking of quitting and starting fresh in the next group

Perhaps you feel you didn't do as well as you could, or there is not enough time left to reach your goal. So you may be thinking, why bother when you can just start fresh in the next group.

- Recognize that this could be a habit for you if you always start and stop a diet in the hopes of starting fresh each time. Following through is the only way to break that habit.

- Remember you still have time. Time is going to go by anyway, you might as well make the most of it.

- It's not really a fresh start, your weight loss journey is a continuation until you reach your goal. You will still need to put the same amount of time and effort in, regardless of how many times you start and stop.

- There is a lot of time between now and the next group to still lose more weight. Finishing this one will only set you up for success when it comes time to start the next Program.

- It's progress over perfection that adds up and makes a difference. Keep going and you will be one step closer to reaching your goals.

5.   Getting frustrated with lack of movement on the scale, or because you feel it is taking too long

Weight loss can be frustrating and more often than not, it takes longer than you think. Keep in mind, the goal is to lose your weight Finally & Forever, and that takes time and effort.

- Ask yourself, if you give up now, what will you do next? Try another burn the fat diet, lose some weight, and then gain it all back plus more?

- Remember, even if you haven't lost any weight yet or as much as you'd like, you are making your body healthier as you work towards reaching your goal.

- Dig deep and Maximize your efforts. Refer back to the Let's Talk Maximizing Your Efforts Checklist post as often as you need.

- Make a list of non-scale victories and focus on all of the amazing things that are happening, which can be more motivating and rewarding than the numbers on the scale.

- If you feel there is an underlying issue or that there is something else going on, be sure to check in with your healthcare provider.

6.   Future-tripping

Maybe you are worried about what lies ahead. Thinking, how will you keep the weight off or what life will look like after weight loss. Or perhaps you don't trust that you can follow through and reach your goals, or are concerned you might go back to old habits.

- Work on staying in the moment. Focus on what you need to do day to day.

- Practice gratitude for all you have accomplished and trust yourself to be able to handle whatever the future holds.

- Practice a more positive internal dialogue by saying kind things to yourself and being your own cheerleader.

- Visualize yourself at the end and what that will look like and feel like, and what it will mean to you.

Self-sabotage often goes unnoticed if you don't take the time to stop and self-reflect. Bringing awareness to it is the first step in addressing it. Remember, it's all about progress over perfection and even when it comes to self-sabotage, it's all part of the process on the road to Finally & Forever.

LET'S REVISIT THE SCALE

Over the past few months, no doubt that you have experienced ups, downs and plateaus on the scale. Remember the scale is not a measure of success, it is a tool to use while you are losing weight and you should be using it as such.

Your weight loss journey will **NOT** be a straight line down. When it comes to the scale, it is all about the downward trend.

THINGS TO KEEP IN MIND:

- When it comes to the scale using The Livy Method, a drop is always a drop. When the scale moves down you can count on it being because of actual fat loss, and that is your true weight.

- When the scale goes up, it's not real weight gain. When following the Program, increases on the scale are always superficial based on what you did or didn't eat or drink the day before. (Check out the Wondering Why Your Weight Is Up? post for a list of other reasons why the scale can be up.)

- It's normal when your body releases fat to see your weight go down, and then see the scale go back up again as it retains water because it is in detox mode and looking to drop even more, so be sure to stay on top of drinking your water.

- It's normal to wake up feeling like you have lost weight, only to have the scale showing the same number as the day before or in some cases, it might even be up. This is usually a sign you are about to drop.

- It's normal to feel bloated and gross and have your weight be up the day before you see a drop on the scale. This is just the body retaining water as it prepares to release fat.

- If your weight is bouncing up and down the same few pounds, that usually means your body needs more water to support it in detox and focus on releasing fat.

- You are going to have plateaus. Plateaus are part of the process. They are your body's way of adjusting to your new lower weight, so your new weight becomes your new norm.

- You need and want plateaus as they are necessary to help the body adjust and solidify the weight you have lost, which will factor in to making your weight loss easier to maintain.

Although plateaus are a normal part of the process, while you are on one, you still want to Maximize your efforts and show up like you are expecting the scale to move. Refer to the Let's Talk Maximizing Your Efforts Checklist post to make sure you are doing everything you can to get the scale moving again.

LET'S REVISIT 4 MAIN REASONS WHY YOUR WEIGHT MIGHT BE SLOWER TO MOVE

If your weight is dropping, your body is changing, or you are noticing non-scale victories like better sleep, increased energy, or even better bowel movements, chances are you are doing great and your body is responding well to the process.

If you are finding or feel that your body is not responding in the way you think it should, here is a recap of the **4 Main Reasons Why Your Weight Might Not Be Moving.** For some expanded information on how these things can affect your weight loss efforts please visit the **Let's Talk 4 Main Reasons Why Your Weight Might Be Slower To Move** post in Week 5.

1. **Inflammation:**

This can be an issue because increased inflammation in the body can lead to insulin resistance. It's important to note that different types of inflammation can be caused by a variety of conditions so it's best to check in with your healthcare provider, to further work with them if you suspect that inflammation may be contributing to your weight being slower to move.

2. **Food Sensitivities:**

Food sensitivity is usually GI-related. They can happen when the body has a hard time digesting certain foods, and can affect the weight loss process because they can make people feel unwell and cause bloating and discomfort which may mimic weight gain.

3. **Gut Dysbiosis:**

Gut Dysbiosis is a general term used to describe when the bacteria in your digestive system becomes unbalanced. There are a variety of causes and symptoms, so if you feel there is something off with your digestion be sure to consult with your healthcare provider. There are tests that they can perform to diagnose, and treatments they may suggest that can help.

4. **Hormonal Health:**

There are 50 different types of hormones that factor into your weight loss journey. These hormones control a number of functions in the body including; heart rate, appetite, sleep cycles, metabolism, mood and sexual health to name a few. Hormones are key to the weight loss conversation because your body storing fat and releasing it are regulated by certain hormones in the body.

As you continue to follow the Program, have faith in your body and the work you are doing and continue to maximize your efforts. If you suspect you may be dealing with any of these issues listed, it is worthwhile to check in and discuss with your healthcare provider.

SPRING/SUMMER WEIGHT LOSS

As the temperature continues to rise and we head into the summer, here are a few things you need to know.

LET'S TALK WEIGHT LOSS AND THE HEAT:

In the last few months, your body has been busy transitioning from working like a heater in the winter months where you crave grains and starchy vegetables, fatty meats and foods that create heat when you eat them, to working more like an air conditioner in the warmer months.

This transition has your body giving you more energy, increasing your metabolism and naturally looking to drop any fat it would have stored over the winter months to help keep you warm. Which is a benefit when it comes to weight loss.

So let's talk about adjustments you can make so you can capitalize on the warmer weather rather than be set back by it.

LET'S TALK HUNGER IN THE HEAT:

When it's hot your body works hard to keep you cool. This can affect your energy and your appetite. It is normal to not be hungry in the heat. Which can make following the Food Plan tricky. This is where switching up some of your food choices can help:

- Increasing your fruit intake by way of adding fruit to meals in lieu of heavier carbs. So ditch the potatoes, rice and other grains and increase fruit. Try adding berries to a salad at lunch or some grilled pineapple at dinner.

- Increasing fruit and decreasing the heavier carbs will ensure the body still gets the energy foods it needs without having to work so hard. Potatoes for example can take 90 mins to process into energy, while fruit can take less than 30 mins.

- When it comes to main meals you will find that less is more, fresh vegetables and salad will seem more appealing than soups and stews.

- When it comes to salads, be sure to load them up and make them nutrient rich. Just keep in mind you are still looking to lose, so even with salads you need to be mindful of portions.

LET'S TALK CRAVING SUGAR IN THE HEAT:

Craving sugar in the cooler months is usually a sign you need more water. But in the warmer months, craving sugar can mean more sugar due to a drop in your energy levels.

If you are feeling your energy drain from being out in the heat, you may find you need to add small amounts of juice/frozen lemonade or natural popsicles will help to get your energy back up quickly.

By staying on top of drinking your water and eating meals and snacks, this drop in energy shouldn't happen often, so we are not talking about drinking juice every day. But when the heat is extreme or you are over-taxing your body in the heat, you will want to be mindful of how to manage that.

Because you are much more in tune at this point, your body will let you know when this happens. Making sure to hit all meals and snacks and adjusting your food choices can help minimize any drop in energy levels due to heat or over exhaustion.

When it comes to meal planning in the summer, consider adding in easier-to-digest proteins like fish and seafood as well as including more plant protein in lieu of harder-to-digest meats.

LET'S TALK CRAVING SALT:

When you are craving salt that can mean your body is looking for good fat. Because your body associates salty food with higher fat foods, you tend to crave salt when your body is in need of fat.

However in the summer, craving salt can mean your body is looking for salt. In the heat, your body needs salt to retain water and electrolytes. So, it's important to make sure that you are adding it in and getting enough in your diet.

LET'S TALK HYDRATION IN THE HEAT:

Drinking enough water is key when trying to lose weight, but in the summer it can be more of a challenge.

- Make sure you get started on it early.
- Be sure to spread it out during the day.
- Be sure to sip and not guzzle to help with hydration.

There will be days when it will be so hot you won't be able to drink enough. Adding in some fruit or vegetable slices can help to keep you hydrated.

Eating healthy can sometimes result in less sodium intake. That combined with drinking more water and sweating can put you at risk for low sodium levels. Be sure to get enough salt in your diet and/or add in some trace minerals.

You can also try adding some coconut water to the mix on those days. It helps to get you hydrated quickly and is loaded with electrolytes.

The warmer months can be a great time to focus on fat loss, with a few slight tweaks here and there, you can help your body adapt and capitalize on the change of seasons.

LET'S REVISIT SLEEP AND STRESS

Some of you may be noticing changes in your sleep and how you manage stress just from the changes you have made so far by following the Program and maximizing your efforts.

Although following the basics of the Program can help with both stress and sleep in general, there are quite a few things you can do to help with this process.

TIPS FOR MANAGING STRESS:

- Be consistent with the basics of the Program; the food, water and any supplements.

- Be in tune with and recognize your stress levels.

- Move your body more.

- Find activities you enjoy doing like sports and other leisure activities.

- Get outside and commune with nature.

- Practice deep breathing exercises.

- Have a warm Epsom salt bath before bed.

- Keep up with health issues. Seeing a naturopathic doctor, chiropractor, acupuncturist, massage therapist and other healthcare providers can be helpful.

- Add in helpful supplements like Omega 3 and add good fats to your meals along with being consistent with magnesium.

- Look for things that bring you joy. Look to have fun with this process. Don't underestimate the power of having a good conversation and laughs with a friend or spending quality time with a loved one.

TIPS FOR IMPROVING SLEEP QUALITY:

- Eat as early in the evening as possible.

- Set up your sleep environment for success.

- Establish a good evening and bedtime routine.

- Take Calm Magnesium before bed.

- Keep a journal beside your bed to organize your thoughts.

- Turn lights down low in the evening.

- Stay off of screens or get off them earlier.

- Use blue light glasses.

- Take naps when you feel the need. In general, naps are not advised when trying to improve sleep patterns, but when it comes to this process, the body is working hard to make change. So when you are tired, be sure to rest.

When it comes to stress, remember the goal isn't to make it completely go away, it is more about recognizing it, and managing it better so you can capitalize on it. And when it comes to sleep, you may not be able to get more sleep but you can work to improve the quality of the sleep you do get.

Focusing on improving your sleep quality and stress management can make a huge difference when it comes to getting and keeping the scale moving.

LET'S REVISIT KEEPING A JOURNAL

It's not too late to start tracking your progress.

Earlier on in the Program, we talked about the benefits of keeping a journal or using our Livy Method App to track your progress. With where we are now in the process, it can be even more important to help you capitalize on the time you have left …which by the way, is still a lot of time left to lose weight.

BENEFITS OF JOURNALING:

- Journalling can be a great tool to help give you insight into how your body is responding to the process.

- It can help you pick up on patterns of behavior and responses, and give you a better idea of what weight loss looks like and feels like, specifically to you.

- It can help you pick up on any food sensitivities, especially if you have digestive issues.

- It can help you keep track of bowel movements if you struggle in that department.

- It can help you track your body's response to the supplements you have been taking, and/or anything new you are adding in or taking out.

- Tracking your mood can be beneficial to help keep you motivated to show up for yourself every day. Take the time to think about how you are managing your emotions and how you are feeling day to day.

THINGS TO TRACK:

- Weight in the morning
- How you are feeling physically
- How you are feeling mentally
- Energy day to day
- Sleep
- Food
- Water
- Movement
- Bowel movements
- Notable responses from food
- Medications
- Supplements
- Non-scale Victories

You can use good old pen and paper, or the Livy Method App. Do what works best for you!

We are at the point in this process where keeping a journal can be a very helpful tool to problem solve and make the most of your efforts. It is one more way to maximize and level up!

FOOD FACTS - CRUCIFEROUS VEGETABLES

Did you know that the word "cruciferous" originates from the Latin word for "cross bearing"? That's because the flower petals resemble a cross.

Cruciferous - [KROO] + [SIF] - [UH] - [RHUS]

Not sure what cruciferous vegetables are? Here's a list of the most common ones:

- Arugula
- Bok choy
- Broccoli
- Brussels sprouts
- Cabbage
- Cauliflower
- Collard greens
- Kale
- Radish
- Turnips

These tasty veggies are packed with folate, vitamins C, E, and K and also loaded with fiber. Fiber helps to make these vegetables filling.

Cruciferous vegetables can help to support many areas of our health, like detoxification, antioxidant protection, and provide anti-inflammatory benefits. They help neutralize and eliminate toxins, providing more energy, improved health, and may aid in the prevention of some serious illnesses like cancers, autoimmunity, and neurodegenerative disorders.

They contain a sulfur rich substance called sulforaphane which is a powerful antioxidant. Sulforaphane is only activated when these vegetables are chopped or chewed, mixing the enzymes together with other components.

Sulforaphane cannot be formed after cooking, so if you want to get the most out of your cruciferous veggies you can chop and let them rest for 40 minutes. This allows time for the enzymes to mix and the sulforaphane to be formed before cooking. Once it's there, it won't be destroyed by cooking.

Cruciferous vegetables are super versatile. They can all be enjoyed raw or cooked, added to salads, soups, stir frys, stews, roasted, steamed, sauteed, and pureed.

Here are some ideas of how to easily incorporate more of these amazing veggies into your diet!

ARUGULA

It's zesty and peppery and can be enjoyed cooked or raw. Perfect as a leafy green side dish, simply drizzled with olive oil or your favourite dressing. Toss it in soup or stir fry to add some extra leafy greens to your meal.

Did you know that arugula is one of the easiest leafy greens to grow yourself? Just toss some seeds in a planter or your garden and watch them grow. They will continue to reproduce as you cut them so they can last all season long.

BROCCOLI AND CAULIFLOWER

These versatile veggies are delicious and prepared in so many different ways. You can steam, roast, and grate into a "rice". Try pureeing a combination of both together for a tasty mashed potato substitute. Pick up some broccoli sprouts to add to salads for an even bigger boost of the powerful sulforaphane.

BRUSSELS SPROUTS

Brussels sprouts are versatile. You can roast them which helps to bring out the sweetness or add some parmesan cheese on top. You can also steam, or pan fry them. Brussels sprouts are just as good raw and make a great coleslaw or addition to any salad. Just slice them thinly or run them through a food processor and add your favourite coleslaw dressing.

CABBAGE, COLLARD GREENS AND KALE

All of the above are equally good cooked or raw. Cabbage is perfect for coleslaw of course, and also great cut into "steaks" brushed with olive oil and roasted in the oven. Collard greens make a great wrap instead of using bread, but they are also delicious chopped and fried with some oil and garlic. Kale will not wilt for days so is perfect for make-ahead salads. Remove the tough stems, slice into ribbons and toss with a dressing. Bok choy is a great addition to stir frys, soups and stews.

TURNIP AND RADISH

Thinly sliced radish is a welcome peppery addition to any salad but did you know they are also delicious roasted? Roasting them releases the sweetness and mellows out the peppery bite. Turnips are versatile and can be enjoyed raw or cooked. Boil or steam and mash as a potato substitute. Grate them raw into salads and soups or roast them on their own or with a mixture of roasted veggies to bring out their sweetness.

WEEK 9 GUIDELINES: FOOD PLAN REVAMP

This week is about supporting the body working at a more optimal level by feeding into your satiety hormones, making it easier for the body to get the nutrients it needs and working to be even more in tune with your portions.

Off the heels of Feeding the Metabolism and making the body work extra hard for its food, this week we are going to slightly revamp the Food Plan and make it easier for the body to get the nutrients it needs.

We are going to do that by scaling back on the number of times you eat each day, along with giving you more flexibility when it comes to snacks. You will also be switching up the star of the meal for lunch and dinner while bumping up your protein and fat which will feed into your satiety hormones to give you more sustaining energy.

This is where you start to phase off the basic Food Plan moving forward to eat more in tune to your body's needs, while still very much following the guidelines.

It is important to continue to ask the 4 Mindfulness Questions with every meal and snack, as the slight change in routine can affect your portion sizes and hunger levels.

Portion wise, the goal is still to eat just enough, so that 10 - 15 mins later you don't feel full or stuffed, while still following all of the guidelines and Maximizing your efforts.

LET'S BREAK DOWN THIS WEEK'S TWEAK:

1. You are going to drop your 2 afternoon snacks down to 1. For example;
   - **Breakfast**
   - **Morning Snack**
   - **Lunch**
   - **Afternoon Snack (only one)**
   - **Dinner**

2. You are going to decrease your starchy vegetables and grains (if you have been adding them in), while still incorporating nutrient rich carbs, such as vegetables and fruit.

3. You are going to increase your protein and fat by way of adding a protein and fat source to your snacks.

4. Maximizing your high protein breakfast.

5. Switch the focus of the meals making protein the main component at lunch and vegetables the main component at dinner.

6. Continue to ask the 4 Mindfulness Questions as you may notice this slight change can affect your hunger levels.

7. Continue to Maximize your efforts using the Let's Talk Maximizing Your Efforts Checklist post.

MEAL AND SNACK IDEAS:

BREAKFAST:

Protein is still the focus, however, you want to maximize your choices, ideally taking out any carbs like bread, crackers, oatmeals (if you have been having), along with minimizing any fruits, using vegetables instead. This is also where you can start adding in protein shakes.

- Eggs and egg whites (can add sautéed vegetables and/or greens)
- Yogurt or cottage cheese with hemp hearts, nuts/seeds (can also add protein powder)
- Beans or lentils with sauteed vegetables and avocado
- Meat, Fish, or plant protein (can add sautéed vegetables and/or leafy greens)
- Protein shakes (make sure to use natural protein powders). If adding fruit, keep it to a minimum and add in good fat by way of oils, avocados, nut butter, nuts, seeds, unsweetened coconut, coconut milk etc.

MORNING SNACK:

This can still be fruit but you will want to add protein and fat to it. You also have the option of switching it up altogether and have just protein and fat.

- Fruit with nuts, seeds, nut butter, cheese or avocado
- Nuts and/or seeds on their own
- Yogurt or cottage cheese (if you didn't have it for breakfast)
- Boiled egg
- Protein shake (If you didn't have it for breakfast) make sure to use natural protein powders. If adding fruit, keep it to a minimum and add in good fat by way of oils, avocados, coconut etc.

LUNCH:

Protein is now the star of the meal with vegetables, leafy greens, and healthy fats. Although the goal is to minimize any starchy carbs. If you feel you still need them, just be sure to keep the portion on the smaller side.

- Eliminate or minimize any starchy vegetables like potatoes, and heavier carbs like white rice and grains (if you have been adding).
- This protein focused meal can be in any combination of soup, salad, stew, stir fry or however you would like.

AFTERNOON SNACK:

There is now only one afternoon snack. The easiest thing to do is to combine the vegetable snack with the nuts/seeds snack, or you can now choose from the other ideas/options listed below.

- Raw veg with nuts and/or seeds
- Nuts, seeds, or cheese
- Yogurt or cottage cheese (if you didn't have it in the AM)
- Vegetables with natural dips, guacamole, hummus, or nut butter
- Fruit and protein (like nuts, cheese, boiled eggs, yogurt)

DINNER:

Vegetables are now the star of the meal with added protein, leafy greens and healthy fats. Please note, the added carbs by way of the vegetables at dinner will help balance out the day of eating higher protein.

- Protein, leafy greens and healthy fats (protein should now be the smaller portion and vegetables are now the star of the meal).
- You can choose from the same types of meals you have been having all along, just be sure

to make vegetables the focus. Check out the individual meal and snack posts for meal ideas and the Recipe section of the Livy Method App for more ideas.

These are just a few options to get you started and to give you an idea of the kinds of food that you can incorporate at each meal and snack, but feel free to come up with your own. Below you will find a sample list (not exhaustive) of protein and fat sources you can choose from when preparing your meals and snacks.

PROTEIN SOURCES:

- Fish
- Meat (Any Meat)
- Eggs
- Seafood
- Beans, lentils, legumes
- Nuts and Seeds
- Dairy - cheese, yogurt, milk products
- Tofu, Tempeh
- Nut butter
- Hummus
- All-natural protein powder
- ...and don't forget about the protein in the vegetable/grains you are eating!

FAT SOURCES:

- Olives
- Avocado
- Nuts
- Seeds
- Hemp hearts
- Dairy...like yogurt, cheese, butter, sour cream etc.
- Olive oil, coconut oil, avocado oil, grape seed oil, flax and hemp oil
- Salad dressings made with good quality oils
- Omega 3 and 369
- Plus, any others you might think of

It's a few simple tweaks, so try not to overthink it. Make sure to continue to eat to satisfaction (just enough) and still be mindful of portions and your changing hunger levels day to day. You may find portions may be smaller or larger this week. Both are normal responses from the body and as always, portions are always what they feel like and not what they look like.

Continue to follow the basic guidelines of the Program, like eating all of your meals and snacks, making them nutrient rich, asking the 4 Mindfulness Questions, eating dinner as early as possible, being consistent with any supplements you are taking, staying hydrated and maximizing your efforts all around.

FREQUENTLY ASKED QUESTIONS

1. **What vegan/vegetarian protein sources are on Plan?**

   There are lots of plant-based protein options available that you can have. For example, you can have tofu, beans, lentils, dairy-free yogurts, protein shakes with dairy-free "milk" etc. Be sure to check out Let's Talk Groceries for more plant-based options.

2. **What protein powders/shakes are on Plan?**

   To maximize your efforts, it's best to have your protein shake either at breakfast or at morning snack (if you didn't have it at breakfast). You'll want to look for protein powders that are all natural with no artificial colours, flavours, and sweeteners. Make sure to add in good fat which will balance out any carbs (fruits or vegetables) you add in. Be mindful about the amount of fruit you are using. Like all meals and snacks, be in tune with the portion size of your shake. With liquid nutrients it can be harder to gauge satisfaction levels. Finally, keep in mind you do not need to add in protein shakes. You can get everything you need to be successful with this week's tweak without adding them in.

3. **Can we still only have fruit for our first snack?**

   You can, however, it is best to add some protein and fat to your fruit if you are still having it for your morning snack. You can also skip the fruit and just have protein and fat.

4. **I am confused about the afternoon snack, can you clarify what this should look like?**

   Since you are removing one of the afternoon snacks, the easiest option would be to combine your veg snack with your nuts and seeds snack. There are also other options you can now choose from. For example, fruit with added protein, or yogurt or cottage cheese if you didn't have it in the morning. Or any of the other options listed in the Week 9 Guidelines.

5. **Should I be increasing my protein amount this week?**

   The goal is to increase your protein intake slightly by adding it to your snacks, while also minimizing any heavier/starchy carbs.

6. **Are carbs completely eliminated from this tweak?**

   Ideally, you are to take out or minimize any heavier carbs like bread, crackers, oatmeals, white rice and grains, along with starchy vegetables like potatoes from your meals (if you have been adding). You will still be incorporating nutrient rich carbs by way of vegetables and fruits.

7. **Do I continue to add healthy fats to my lunches and dinners?**

    Yes. Healthy fats are an important component of the Program. Our bodies need good fats. You will want to continue to add them in with your meals and snacks.

8. **Are we still keeping our nuts to the same amount per day?**

    The amount of nuts you eat for your snack can change day to day depending on your hunger level. Ask yourself the 4 Mindfulness Questions and determine in the moment how many you will need to feel satisfied.

9. **If I was incorporating Bonus Snacks can I continue to do so?**

    If you have been utilizing the Bonus Snacks, you can continue to do so. With that said, be sure you are eating breakfast, making your meals nutrient rich, and only add them in if you need them.

10. **I've been skipping breakfast most days. Is it a good idea to eat breakfast this week to get extra protein?**

    Although breakfast is optional when following the Food Plan, it can be greatly beneficial to have a high protein breakfast, especially if you are looking to maximize your efforts this week.

Please take the time to head over to the Facebook Group or the Livy Method App and watch the quick video that accompanies this post.

LET'S TALK PROTEIN SHAKES

Although convenient to have, consuming protein shakes for meals and snacks can make it diffi-cult to be in tune to portion sizes. Which is why up to this point, you have been advised to leave them out, or at the very least, keep them to a minimum.

With where we are at in the process now, and with you being more in tune to your portion sizes and what it feels like to be satisfied, this is where you can start to add them in if you wish.

If you are thinking of adding in a protein shake, here are some things to keep in mind:

1. There are a variety of protein powder options out there, find one that works best for you.

2. Check the ingredients, make sure you are buying natural protein powder and avoid any artificial flavour, colour, or sweeteners.

3. Make sure to add in good fat which will balance out any carbs (fruits or veg) you add in.

    Examples of some good fats would be:

    -   Liquid Omega 3 or 369 combo

    -   Flax oil

    -   Hemp oil

    -   Avocado

    -   Coconut oil/chunks, or unsweetened milk

    -   MCT oil

    -   Nut butters

    -   Yogurt

4. Be mindful about the amount of fruit ratio you are using.

5. Be in tune to the portion size of your shake. Liquid nutrients make it harder to gauge satisfaction.

Keep in mind you do NOT need to add in protein shakes. You can get everything you need to be successful with this week's tweak without adding them in.

Please take the time to head over to the Facebook Group or the Livy Method App and watch the quick video that accompanies this post.

LET'S REVISIT BOWEL MOVEMENTS

We have talked a lot about bowel movements over the past few weeks.

At this point, we know when following the Program, it is still normal to have your bowel movements be all over the place. You may experience bouts of constipation which are normal before detox or when making changes in your diet.

It is also normal to have episodes of diarrhea or loose bowel movements, which can occur when the body is in detox and responding to the changes you are making along the way. Once you are done helping the body focus on weight loss and are in maintenance, you will find your bowel movements will normalize again.

LET'S TALK CONSTIPATION:

Constipation is usually the body responding to the changes you are making (change in routine of foods and change in type of foods).

Things to keep in mind if you are experiencing constipation:

- Drink enough water to be properly hydrated.
- Follow the Food Plan consistently and focus on making your meals and snacks as nutrient rich as possible to ensure you are getting enough fiber in your diet.
- Be sure to add leafy greens to meals for added roughage and to support detox.
- Taking a daily fiber supplement such as psyllium and inulin, can help prevent constipation.
- Consider adding in the suggested supplements that can aid in digestion (Vitamin D, Omega 3, Calm Magnesium, digestive bitters, probiotic and/or prebiotic).

LET'S TALK LOOSE BOWEL MOVEMENTS:

Loose bowel movements are a normal and expected part of the process. All of the water you are drinking, the fiber rich foods like fruit, vegetables, and leafy greens you are eating, all contribute to your body's natural way of detoxing.

Things to keep in mind if you are experiencing loose bowel movements:

- Bowel movements are the number one way your body detoxes and releases fat, which can lead to loose bowel movements for some people, especially when the scale is moving.
- Keeping a journal and recording how you are feeling after eating meals and snacks can give you insight into food sensitivities that can cause loose bowel movements and discomfort. Dairy and gluten are the most common sensitivities. This can also include other types of foods and even spices used to prepare foods.

- If you are taking Calm Magnesium, try adjusting the dose. Although it is rarely the sole issue for loose BMs, decreasing it slightly may help.

The body has been working hard to address digestive and BM issues and will continue to make improvements. Although usually nothing to be concerned about, when it comes to bowel movement issues, it is always recommended to check in with your healthcare provider if you have any concerns.

LET'S REVISIT LEAFY GREENS

Leafy greens continue to be an ideal addition to meals because they are not only packed with tons of nutrients that are great for your health and cellular function, but they are also an excellent source of fiber and help the body process food through your digestive system.

Leafy greens can help to increase the glucagon-like peptide-1 hormone that keeps blood sugar more stable and can keep you more satisfied.

Darker leafy greens are also rich in sulfur-containing compounds that support your body's detoxification process.

Plus, all of the changes you have been making in your diet can affect your bowel movements. Leafy greens provide the roughage your body needs to keep you regular throughout this process.

Leafy greens can be added to meals raw, like in a salad, or you might find them more appealing cooked or sautéed and/or added to soups, stews & stir-frys.

The general rule is…if it's green and leafy it works!

Please Note: Leafy greens are not considered a veg on plan. An exception would be Brussel sprouts, cabbage and bok choy, among others which are listed in the Let's Talk Groceries post, that are also classified as a veg and can be used as one or the other or both in your meals.

If you are not a fan of eating your leafy greens, it is still key to get them in. Although they are suggested at lunch and dinner, they can also be added to breakfast and even your snacks.

FOOD FACTS - BEANS & LENTILS

Are you familiar with this rhyme?

"Beans, beans the musical fruit, the more you eat, the more you toot?"

Or is it,

"Beans, beans the musical fruit, the more you eat, the less you toot!"

You may have heard it both ways! But did you notice how the 2 variations say opposite things about gassiness?

SO, WHICH ONE IS IT?

Well...sort of both. Beans and lentils *can* cause an increase in gassiness after eating. This is because of a complex sugar called raffinose, which the body can have trouble digesting. Raffinose passes through the small intestine, undigested, and into the large intestines where your gut bacteria breaks it down. This produces gas that eventually you pass.

However, slowly incorporating more beans and lentils into your diet allows your system to get used to them, making them more easily digested, and decreasing gassiness. Beans and lentils may also help enhance overall gut health by improving intestinal barrier function and increasing beneficial digestive bacteria. If you are new to adding beans and lentils to your diet, start slowly to allow your digestive system to get used to them.

WHAT ARE BEANS AND LENTILS?

Examples of beans and lentils include chickpeas, beans (kidney, pinto, navy, black, etc.), dried peas (split peas) and lentils. These are all the edible seeds of the plants in the legume family and are called "pulses".

Technically, a "legume" is the name of the whole plant including the leaves, stems, and pods. For example, a pea pod (think snap peas) is a legume but the pea inside the pod is a pulse.

Legumes and pulses are a nutritious staple of many diets around the world and have been cultivated by humans for approximately 6000 years!

Check out all the nutrients these pulses are jam-packed with:

- Protein
- Fiber
- Folate
- Calcium

- Iron
- B vitamins
- Vitamin C
- Complex carbohydrates
- Potassium
- Antioxidants

Beans and lentils are digested slowly which gives a feeling of satiety. They also promote a slow burning, steady energy while the iron content helps transport oxygen through the body. This can help to increase your energy and support your metabolism. The high amount of fiber can be beneficial in managing cholesterol, digestive health, regulating energy levels, as well as helping to stabilize blood glucose levels.

CANNED OR DRIED?

CANNED beans and lentils are definitely more convenient but also have a higher price tag. They are already soaked and cooked so are ready to be used in fresh or cooked dishes. Just rinse and go! Canned beans can be high in sodium so something to watch out for when purchasing. Be sure to rinse them well to remove as much sodium as possible but keep in mind they will have absorbed a lot of it. Look for low or no-sodium canned beans and lentils as a better alternative.

DRIED beans are much less expensive but involve some labour. They also take up less space in your pantry. Preparing them can be a bit time consuming as they require soaking and then simmering for up to a few hours, depending on the bean. It can be helpful to prepare a whole bag at once and freezing whatever you aren't using. They freeze perfectly and are ready to use for whatever you are making. Lentils, on the other hand, don't require soaking therefore take less time to prepare.

EASY WAYS TO ADD THEM IN

Beans and lentils are versatile. Because they have a benign flavour, they go along well with virtually any ingredients, herbs, and spices. You can add them to almost anything.

- **Enjoy them as a quick salad topper** - Try roasting them with a bit of olive oil and your favourite spices to enhance their flavour.
- **Add them to soups** - Use them whole or pureed. Pureeing acts as a thickener.
- **Add to chili, curry, stew, and stir-fries** - You can use all beans for a meatless meal, or a combination of meat and pulses to cut down on your meat consumption and make it more nutrient rich.
- **Mash up** chickpeas and mix with your favourite tuna salad ingredients for a vegetarian version.

- **Use them to make tasty and nutritious dips and spreads** - Hummus is the classic,, but you can puree any cooked beans or lentils, add some seasonings to make a dip or spread for a leafy green wrap.
- **Have them for breakfast with or without eggs** - Fry up some black beans with a bit of chili powder and top with cheese, salsa and avocado.

ENVIRONMENTAL HEROS

Not only are they powerhouses in the nutritional department but did you know they are also good for the environment? Legume crops have a lower carbon footprint than almost any other food group. They are considered one of the most sustainable proteins in the world as they have the ability to enrich the soil, reducing the need for chemical fertilizers, and compared to other proteins, they need only one tenth the amount of water to grow. They are also frost and drought resistant which makes them almost indestructible!

LET'S REVISIT SUPPLEMENTS

It is a great idea to revisit the supplement conversation since it is never too late to add them in and it is always a good idea to review them relative to where you are now in the Program.

For more detailed information on each supplement, be sure to visit the original Let's Talk Supplements post in Week 2 and the Let's Talk Secondary Supplements post in Week 6.

Always remember that if you have any concerns adding in any supplements in regards to health issues you have or medications you take, be sure to check in with your healthcare provider.

LET'S REVIEW THE BASIC SUPPLEMENTS:

The following are basic supplements that can be helpful to aid in deficiencies in the body that may affect your ability to focus on fat loss. They can also help support your efforts with this process by addressing the body's needs and have it function at more optimal levels.

VITAMIN D, D3:

Vitamin D is essential in supporting the body's metabolism. Low levels of vitamin D are often found in people who have weight to lose. When someone is lacking vitamin D, the hypothalamus (the very small part of your brain that regulates hormonal functions, amongst other things) senses the lower levels and responds by increasing body weight.

OMEGA 3:

One way you can support the fat loss process is to add in more good fat. Without enough good fat in your diet, your body can be reluctant to let go of your stored fat.

30% of your diet should come from fat and ideally 10% of that should come from omega 3. The primary source of omega 3 is fish and unless you are eating a lot of it, it can be difficult for the body to get enough.

PLEASE NOTE: If you are on prescribed blood thinners or have any other health issues, consult with your healthcare provider before adding in.

CALM MAGNESIUM (MAGNESIUM CITRATE):

There are many forms of magnesium. Calm Magnesium is specifically suggested because it is easily absorbed by the body and supports the detox process. Although magnesium is responsible for 300 actions in the body, it is specifically important while losing weight because it not only helps to convert your foods into usable energy, it also helps calm the nerves and address cortisol levels (caused by stress). This helps your body to relax, which can help with getting deep & REM sleep. Deep sleep is important because that is the kind of sleep you need for the body to best repair, rebuild, and detoxify.

PROBIOTICS:

A probiotic is good bacteria added to your digestive system that helps promote a healthy immune system and can help with weight loss by improving digestion.

PLEASE NOTE: If you're following SIBO or the FODMAP diet while also following the plan, you might be advised NOT to add in a probiotic. If unsure, always check in with your healthcare provider.

PREBIOTIC WITH ADDED CLEAR FIBER:

Prebiotic helps to feed the good bacteria in your gut which can be beneficial in addressing inflammation, digestive issues and helps to promote healthy bowel movements.

DIGESTIVE BITTERS:

If you have known digestive issues, are missing your gallbladder, or simply feel bloated after eating raw vegetables or nuts and seeds, you may want to add in some digestive bitters.

Look for Canadian bitters which is specifically a digestive aid, as opposed to Swedish bitters which contain an added laxative (senna).

COLLAGEN:

Collagen can help with tissue repair, improving the quality of hair and nails, but more importantly skin, which is important when it comes to weight loss.

LET'S REVIEW THE SECONDARY SUPPLEMENTS:

This list is for those of you who may be interested in taking things to the next level when it comes to your health and wellness.

MCT OIL:

MCT oil is a medium-chain triglyceride. Unlike other fat sources that need to be broken down, digested, and stored before it is used by the body, MCT oil is sent directly to your liver where it has a thermogenic effect and the ability to support your metabolism (the rate at which your body functions and burns calories).

Because MCT oil is instantly utilized for fuel instead of being stored as fat, it can help to calm the mind (since your brain is floating in cholesterol, it needs good fat for energy to function) and keep the body revved up and working extra hard.

ADAPTOGENS:

Adaptogens are supplements derived from plants that can help our bodies cope with stress by decreasing sensitivity to stressors, and can help it return to a balanced state when experiencing stressful situations. This can help to decrease your body's cortisol levels.

Cortisol is known as the stress hormone because of the body's stress response. When you are stressed, your adrenals can produce too much or not enough which can signal the need to store fat in the body. Most of the cells in your body have cortisol receptors that use it for a variety of functions including: regulating blood sugar, reducing inflammation, regulating metabolism, and memory function.

Take as directed and be sure to check with your healthcare provider, especially if you are taking medications as there can be interactions.

B COMPLEX:

Vitamin B complex is a group of water-soluble vitamins, which play a very important role in maintaining the growth and the metabolism of cells in the body.

When it comes to weight loss, B12 is especially important because it helps the body convert fats and proteins into energy. B12 is mainly found in red meat, chicken, fish, dairy and eggs.

A B Complex can help the body maintain sufficient levels of a variety of B vitamins so that it can efficiently utilize carbohydrates, fats, and proteins and help the body maintain energy, stamina, and control appetite.

Typically, it is B1, B6 and B12 deficiencies that are an issue. Your healthcare provider can order a blood or a urine test to assess and provide recommendations.

COQ10:

CoQ10 is an antioxidant that also plays a fundamental role in the production of energy by the cells. A deficiency can contribute to lower energy levels and a slower metabolism. It is believed that CoQ10 production decreases with age, which may help explain one of the reasons why it can be harder to lose weight as you get older.

CoQ10 can enhance healthy weight loss because it helps to support increased metabolic function. In addition, it can work to decrease body fat while boosting energy levels by maximizing your body's ability to convert food to fuel.

It's also great for skin. Lack of CoQ10 results in decreased production of collagen and elastin. The loss of collagen and elastin can cause your skin to wrinkle and sag.

NOTE: Check with your healthcare provider before taking CoQ10 if you are on blood thinning or blood pressure medications.

L-THEANINE:

L-theanine is an amino acid found in both green and black tea leaves and also mushrooms. It is thought to be effective in decreasing brain chemicals that contribute to stress and anxiety while increasing brain chemicals that encourage a sense of calm.

Some research also suggests that L-theanine may improve the function of the body's immune system and help to improve inflammation in the intestinal system.

Due to its calming effects, L-theanine may also help lower blood pressure so you may want to keep that in mind and consult with your healthcare provider if you have low blood pressure.

Women who are pregnant or breastfeeding should consult their healthcare practitioner before adding L-theanine or supplementing with green or black tea.

TURMERIC:

The primary antioxidant in Turmeric the spice is curcumin, which is an anti-inflammatory. While increasing your intake of turmeric isn't a lone strategy for weight loss, it may help you address the inflammation and help with metabolism.

The best curcumin supplements contain piperine, which substantially increases the absorption and therefore effectiveness.

Check with your healthcare provider before adding this in, especially if you are taking medications as there can be interactions.

TRACE MINERALS:

Minerals are needed for important metabolic functions in the body. Even though trace minerals are only required in small amounts, they are indeed essential. Not only for good health, but also weight loss.

There are two classes of minerals:

1.   Major
2.   Trace

Major minerals include: calcium, potassium, chloride, phosphorus, magnesium, sodium, and selenium.

Trace minerals include: chromium, germanium, manganese, rubidium, vanadium, cobalt, iron, molybdenum, zinc, copper, lithium, nickel, and silica.

Adding in trace minerals that include sodium are beneficial in preventing low sodium levels caused from changes in your diet, taking medications, excessive sweating, and electrolyte loss.

For More information on these supplements please visit the Let's Talk Supplements post in the Week 2 Guide and the Let's Talk Secondary Supplements post in the Week 6 Guide. As with all the suggestions, be sure to check with your healthcare provider if you have any concerns.

LET'S REVISIT CRAVINGS

At this point, if you are following The Program, you should find any cravings you had or have are minimal. And if you do have them, they are nothing to be feared and can actually be your body giving you a heads up on its needs.

If you are consistently following the Food Plan and drinking the water, any cravings should be few and far between. And if they do pop up, it's usually just a matter of making a few tweaks.

LET'S TALK SUGAR:

The key to addressing sugar cravings is to understand that it's not actually sugar your body wants. It's the increase in insulin as a result of having it that has your body asking for more.

When you reach for sweets or foods with high sugar content, your body increases insulin production, which can cause your blood glucose levels to drop. This can create a dip in energy and a desire for even more sugar. So, when you have sugar your body will immediately want more sugar.

REASONS WHY WE CRAVE SUGAR:

More is more.

When you have sugar, your body tends to want more sugar. These cravings can be so intense that if you create a habit of having sugar at the same time every day, your body will begin to crave and expect it at that same time each day. This is also the reason you end up eating that whole box of cookies in one sitting!

THE FIX:

- Making sure to add in healthy fats to your meals along with protein, which will help feed into your satiety hormones, have you feeling more satisfied, and prevent any cravings along the way.
- If you do find yourself indulging, you can decrease sugar cravings by having some protein and fat with your sweet treat. For example, if you indulge in a cookie, you can minimize the desire to eat another cookie by having a slice of cheese, a handful of nuts, or a glass of milk.

Dehydration is a factor.

When you are dehydrated and not picking up on the cues from your body to drink enough water, your body's next best bet is to crave foods with a high water content, like fruit. Fruits are also sweet, so you may mistake your body's cue to consume more water and instead find yourself reaching for processed carbs and sugar.

This is why you may hear the advice to drink a glass of water before you eat to satisfy your appetite. Drinking water doesn't actually satisfy your appetite. So if you drink it and feel satisfied, chances are you were never hungry and didn't need that sweet treat in the first place.

THE FIX:

- Drink more water.
- Sip water throughout the day, aiming for a minimum of 2.7 - 3.5 L a day and even more on days you exercise, are more active, sweating a lot or when the climate is hot and/or dry.

You are tired.

When you are tired, your body goes looking for a pick-me-up so you may find yourself reaching for something sweet.

The same thing happens around 3 or 4 p.m. each afternoon when the body is wired to take a dip in energy and slows your circadian rhythm. What your body is really looking for is a nap. (There are places in the world that do just that: think of the siesta.) In our fast-paced, high-stress world, it's not always possible to have an afternoon nap, so the body goes looking for easy energy by way of higher sugar to pick it up and keep it going.

THE FIX:

- Make sure to eat all your meals and especially your snacks. This will help to avoid energy levels that dip when you go for long periods of time without eating.
- Your mid-morning snack of fresh fruit will top up your energy reserves in the morning and your vegetables, nuts and seeds in the afternoon will keep your body working hard throughout the afternoon.
- These foods have a high nutrient value and are harder to digest, which will keep your digestion stimulated and your body awake and functioning when it's craving a nap.

With a few adjustments, you can easily beat the need for sweets and stay on track to reach your goals and not be held captive by sugar cravings anymore.

REASONS WHY WE CRAVE SALT:

You need more salt.

Salt is one of the electrolytes quickest to deplete through sweating. When exercising, living in a hot climate or taking some medications that can cause dehydration, sometimes in extreme cases, when you crave salt, it means you need salt.

THE FIX:

- Add salt to your diet
- Add trace minerals to your water
- Check out the Let's Talk Low Sodium post for more information

You need more good fat.

When you crave salt, it generally means that the body is asking for more good fat. When you are stressed, your body is revving high, you burn lots of calories, your brain works really hard and your body quickly gets depleted of its nutrients. Periods of high stress can rapidly deplete your vitamin and mineral reserves. So, when you are stressed, your body is looking for more sustaining energy by way of good fat. You don't have to be stressed for the body to need more good fat. Fat is essential for cellular function as well as brain and heart health.

THE FIX:

- Your body would rather get that fat from the foods you eat than to utilize its emergency reserve. Without enough good fat coming in, your body will be reluctant to release fat. So, one way you can speed up that fat loss process is to make sure you are adding healthy fats to your meals. It's also beneficial to add in an omega 3 or 3-6-9 supplement.

LET'S TALK TUMMY RUMBLINGS & HUNGER PAINS:

We are taught to believe if your tummy rumbles you must be hungry, when in fact that's not what the noise and rumblings are about. It's actually your body's natural MMC or Migrating Motor Complex, a self-cleaning mechanism where in between meals and snacks, it works to clear bacteria and food particles out of the stomach and small intestine.

Because we are eating so often during the day, the body is doing most of this work at night. As we move through the Program, we will be phasing you into more natural patterns of eating which will be more in tune to your body's needs, which include the downtime it needs in between meals to self-regulate.

TO RECAP:

Cravings continue to be nothing to stress about. As you progress through the Program, and find your hunger levels fluctuating, and your body's needs changing, cravings can give you insight into any adjustments you need to make.

As you continue this process, you will become even more in tune and able to differentiate between the body's needs and your wants.

LET'S REVISIT TRAVEL

If you haven't traveled up until this point, or you are thinking about traveling soon, let's revisit travel so you can make the most of it so you can hit the road.

LET'S START WITH VACATIONS:

Vacations can do wonders for weight loss. Change in environment, less stress, abundance of fresh food, and some decent sleep can be exactly what the body needs to get the scale moving. So, don't stress if you can't follow the Food Plan perfectly while away. It's ok to have your food choices be off routine if your schedule is off from your normal weekly routine.

No one is expecting you to deprive yourself of any of the joys that come with being on vacation to be successful. Feel free to indulge, just be mindful to balance it out. Focus on your water and try to get in fresh fruits, vegetables and leafy greens when you can.

One of the biggest challenges while vacationing is flying. Here are some tips:

- Resist the urge to indulge in treats before you fly. Flying is super dehydrating and combined with high sugar is a recipe for craving carbs, serious bloating, and constipation once you land.
- Spend the money on healthy snacks so you are not inclined to eat the crackers and cookies or heavily salted meal they serve during the flight.
- HYDRATE! The altitude when flying is very dehydrating. So, before, during and after you land, focus on getting your water in.

While it's not unusual to lose weight while away on holiday, most people will find their weight will go up. This can be due for a variety of reasons. Have faith that after a few days of getting back at it and following the Program, your weight will drop right back down again. Have fun and focus on making choices that make you feel good and you can't go wrong.

LET'S TALK TRAVELING FOR WORK:

Traveling for work can have you here, there and everywhere while making a lot of stops along the way. This can make it challenging when it comes to following the Food Plan. Whether you are hitting the road for long hours, or just driving to and from work, having a plan and being prepared can make all the difference.

One of the biggest challenges while traveling for work is the inconsistencies of being on the road. Here are some tips:

- Assess your day before it starts and make a plan.

- Be prepared with extra snacks and keep water on hand.

- Look for quick and easy snacks that work on the go.

- Try to keep the routine of the Food Plan the best you can.

- Set timers and alarms to help keep you on track.

- Don't worry about a few off meals or snacks.

- Stop at grocery stores instead of fast food restaurants.

- Make the best choices you can, when you can if the choices are limited.

- Focus on the water.

- Bathroom visits can be inconvenient, get the water in when you can and hold off when you need to.

Traveling for work is not as fun but can be just as effective, as travel in general is very stimulating for the body. Try to stay on plan the best you can and don't stress. It's all about being mindful, planning ahead, and making choices that fall in line with your goals to set yourself up for success.

LET'S REVISIT CELEBRATORY WEEKENDS

You can be hard core about your journey and still enjoy those special moments in life on the way to reaching your goal.

Let's revisit some top tips for navigating and staying on track:

1. **Take some time to set your intentions before the weekend. Are you going to focus on following the Food Plan, choose to indulge, or take each day as it comes?**

    There is no right or wrong answer to this, it's all about how you want to feel when it's time to get back at it. Regardless, make a plan so you are prepared.

2. **Make a point of eating normally the day of any big event, or in anticipation of a big/ festive meal.**

    Follow the Food Plan leading up to your event as consistently as possible. This will help keep your digestive system stimulated so you are able to digest your meal better and feel less bloated after eating a bigger meal and prevent you from overindulging.

3. **Start your day higher in protein and fat and minimize carbs. For example, choose eggs over oatmeal. This will get your body working harder from the get-go and give you more sustaining energy.**

    Also, if you start your day higher in carbs like cereal, oatmeal or bread, you run the risk of setting yourself up to crave more carbs and sugar the rest of the day. If there is a lot of food around, you may be more tempted by it.

4. **Stay on top of your water and start drinking earlier in the day.**

    Staying hydrated helps keep your energy up and your cravings down which will help you continue to make choices that make you feel good, even when off routine. If you are on the road or out and about, make a plan and get it in when you can.

5. **Get right back at it the day after indulging.**

    Trying not to eat or punishing yourself for overeating only makes the situation worse. The more consistent you are with getting back to following the Food Plan, the better you will feel and the quicker you will be back to working towards your weight loss goals.

And finally, keep in mind:

There is nothing you can do that can't be undone by getting right back at it. The Program is designed to keep you moving forward, so all you need to do is pick up exactly where you left off. Keep in mind, what you learn by not following the plan can be just as insightful and as much of a value as following it perfectly. It's all part of the process.

That being said, the more consistent you are in following the Program, and the more you can minimize any indulgences along the way, will help to maximize your efforts and get you closer to reaching your goals.

WEEK 10 GUIDELINES: LEVELLING UP YOUR MIND BODY CONNECTION

The tweak this week is to continue with the Food Plan Revamp while following the guidelines, maximizing your efforts and strengthening your mind body connection. This is also where we introduce the concept of Back on Track.

This week you will want to pay particulate attention to how your body is responding from the changes you made last week. Noticing how the slightest change can affect your hunger and satisfaction levels.

Let's review the basics for the Food Plan Revamp tweak. Refer to the Week 9 Guidelines for a more in depth review of the information.

RECAP OF THIS WEEK'S TWEAK

- **Breakfast** - Protein is still the focus, however, you want to maximize your choices, ideally taking out any carbs like bread, crackers, oatmeals (if you have been having), along with minimizing any fruits, using vegetables instead. This is also where you can start adding in protein shakes.

- **Morning Snack** - This can still be fruit but you will want to add protein and fat to it. You also have the option of switching it up altogether and have just protein and fat.

- **Lunch** - Protein is now the star of the meal with vegetables, leafy greens, and healthy fats.

Although the goal is to minimize any starchy carbs. If you feel you still need them, just be sure to keep the portion on the smaller side.

- **Afternoon Snack (only one)** - There will only be one afternoon snack. You can combine the vegetables and nuts/seeds snack or see Week 9 Guidelines for other ideas/options.

- **Dinner** - Vegetables are now the star of the meal with added protein, leafy greens and healthy fats. Please note, the added carbs by way of the vegetables at dinner will help balance out the day of eating higher protein.

Portion wise you are continuing to eat to just enough so when you walk away you are feeling satisfied not stuffed. You want to continue to be mindful by asking the 4 questions, along with maximizing your efforts while turning up the volume on your internal dialog. This will help to strengthen your mind body connection even more.

INTRODUCING BACK ON TRACK

Weekends, holidays and vacays can be tricky when it comes to staying on plan because we tend to be more off routine, making it a bit more difficult to follow the routine. Add in a long/holiday or celebratory day and it can make it even harder.

Back on Track is the technique you will use after indulging in or having an "off day", "off weekend", or even an "off week" of eating as you continue to work through the rest of the Program to reach your goal, and once you are in maintenance you will use it to help maintain your weight.

Back on Track refers to the original Food Plan formula, the same one you followed during the first few weeks of the Program. The original Food Plan has now become a familiar routine for the body that will help it reset and catch up after indulging.

THE METHOD OF GETTING "BACK ON TRACK":

- Protein for breakfast
- Fruit for snack
- Vegetables with added protein, leafy greens, and healthy fats for lunch
- Vegetable snack
- Nuts and seeds snack
- Protein with added vegetables, leafy greens, and healthy fats for dinner

When eating "Back on Track," you want to be consistent, eating all meals and snacks and be extra mindful of portions. You want to keep lunch and dinner as light as possible with more leafy greens and avoid any starchy carbs.

You will also want to maximize your efforts by:

- Getting in extra water

- Eating as early in the evening as possible

- Getting quality sleep

- Moving your body

- Managing your stress

- Being consistent with any supplements you are taking

If you get on the scale after indulging and your weight is up, it's important to understand that it is not real weight gain. Weight up is just from a backlog of hard to digest foods, salty food, and your body retaining water along with various other reasons.

For that reason, you will want to implement Back on Track for as many days as you need to feel back on track as opposed to waiting for the scale to drop back down. How long you implement Back on Track depends on how off the rails you went. Normally 1 to 3 days is enough.

You may feel inclined to eat less or to skip meals and snacks after indulging thinking this will help you get ahead and Back on Track faster, but it will not. Under-eating after over-indulging will only reinforce the need for the body to hold onto and store fat. It will also under-stimulate your digestive system making it longer to get back on track.

- Back on Track is best reserved for when you really go off the rails for a couple or more days. Not just one off meal, snack, or indulgence.

- It is NOT meant to be used to manage day to day fluctuations on the scale.

It is best to keep any indulgences to a minimum while looking to lose weight. Reserve Back on Track for the times you really need it.

FREQUENTLY ASKED QUESTIONS

1. **For this tweak are we switching our lunch with our dinner?**

   This week, protein is the focus at lunch, and vegetables are the focus at dinner.

2. **When I add protein to my fruit snack, can I add meat protein?**

   Yes, you can add any type of healthy protein and fat to your fruit snack.

3. **Would nuts or cheese be considered both protein and fat? Is having either of them with fruit or vegetables enough to bump up the protein and fat?**

   Yes.

4. **What is the best snack option during this tweak?**

   There are a lot of great options. It is best to focus on protein and healthy fat for this week's tweak. For example, if having fruit or vegetables, be sure to add protein and healthy fat to your snack or you can have protein and fat on its own. Be sure to check what is listed in the Week 9 Guidelines.

5. **Can we begin using Back on Track (BOT) now, or is it meant for the end of the Program?**

    Back on Track is a great technique to use moving forward after over-indulging in or having an off day, weekend or even an off week. This is a technique you will continue to use as needed, keeping in mind, you want to keep any indulgences to a minimum. It is important to note, BOT is not meant to be used to manage day to day fluctuations on the scale or for one "off" meal or snack.

6. **In the case that I do need to use Back on Track, where would I pick up in the Program once I feel back on track?**

    Whether you need to use Back on Track, sickness protocol, or if you have to stop following for any reason, you will pick up where you left off in the Program. For example, if you indulged on Day 71 and 72, and then do BOT for a couple of days, you would then go back and start on Day 71.

7. **Should I track Back on Track days in my Livy Method App or should I keep moving forward with entering my meals and have it run over the 91 days?**

    The Livy Method App is specifically designed to guide you through the 91 days of the Program. Back on Track days, similar to sick days, are counted as extra days and there is no need to track them.

Please take the time to head over to the Facebook Group or the Livy Method App and watch the quick video that accompanies this post.

LET'S TALK BACK ON TRACK

Weekends, holidays and vacays can be tricky when it comes to staying on plan because we tend to be more off routine, making it a bit more difficult to follow the routine. Add in a longer holiday or celebratory days and it can make it even harder.

You may have heard me reference getting "Back on Track." BOT refers to getting back to the basics.

Back on Track is the technique you will use after indulging in or having an "off day," "off weekend," or even an "off week" of eating as you continue to work through the rest of the Program to lose, and once you are in maintenance, to help maintain your weight.

Back on Track refers to the original Food Plan, the same one you had been following the first few months of the Program.

The original Food Plan has now become a familiar routine for the body that will help it reset and catch up after any "off days".

THE METHOD OF GETTING "BACK ON TRACK":

- Protein for breakfast
- Fruit for snack
- Veg, protein, leafy greens, and healthy fats for lunch
- Veg snack
- Nuts and seeds snack
- Protein, veg, leafy greens, and healthy fats for dinner

When eating "Back on Track," you want to eat all meals and snacks, but keep the portions on the smaller side.

This is NOT for the sake of eating less calories, but to help the body stay focused on getting rid of any backlog of food which is attributing to your weight being up.

- You want to keep lunch and dinner light with more leafy greens and avoid any heavier carbs. You want to get in extra water.
- You want to eat as early in the evening as possible. You want to help the body get a nice, deep sleep.
- You want to move your body, go for a walk after dinner, have an Epsom salt bath, and head to bed earlier. You also want to be as consistent as possible with the supplements.

If you get on the scale after indulging and your weight is up, it's important to understand that it is not real weight gain. Weight up is just from a backlog from hard to digest foods, salty food, and your body retaining water.

You will find after being "Back on Track" for a few days, your weight will drop right back down to where it was before you had your off day/s. And then you can carry on and pick up where you left off in the Program.

With that said, Back on Track is not always about the scale coming back down because sometimes your weight can be up for other reasons. In that case, you implement BOT until you "feel" BOT, which usually takes 1-3 days.

You may feel inclined to eat less or to skip meals and snacks after indulging, thinking this will help you get ahead and Back on Track faster, but it will not. Under-eating after over-indulging will only reinforce the need for the body to hold onto and store fat. It will also under-stimulate your digestive system making it take longer to get back on track.

- Keep in mind, Back on Track is NOT to be used unless you overindulged for a day or more.
- It is NOT meant to be used to manage day-to-day fluctuations on the scale or one "off" meal.
- It is best reserved for when you really go off the rails for a couple or more days. Not just one off meal or indulgence.

How long you implement Back on Track depends on how off the rails you went. Normally a day or two is plenty to help the body get back on track. Also, best to keep any indulgences to a minimum while looking to lose weight. Avoid the mentality of making this a lifestyle thing, where you try to have your indulgences and lose weight too. Reserve Back on Track for the times you really need it.

Please take the time to head over to the Facebook Group or the Livy Method App and watch the quick video that accompanies this post.

LET'S TALK PEOPLE'S REACTIONS TO YOUR WEIGHT LOSS

This post is to provide insight into how to manage comments and reactions to your ever-changing body.

First thing is first. You are doing this Program for you. Make sure you remember that each and every day. Let that be the driving force to get you to your "Finally & Forever". Whatever your end game is, it's yours. All of the work that you've put into yourself by doing this so far is amazing, and you deserve to be your best self! Nothing and nobody should get in the way of you achieving your goals.

Always remember that no opinion but yours matters when it comes to your body and your choices. Whether you're bigger, smaller or anything in between, some people will always have something to say.

Positive or negative, you will feel like you are being treated in a different way than you ever have been in the past. These reactions can make you feel so many ways. There are times that people will be celebrating your successes, times where people can be uncomfortably negative or awkward, and even some times where others may try to sabotage your achievements (we all know one or two cookie-pushers!!).

Cheerleaders are the best! Those are the friends and family you need to keep close. People say that it's not during the hard times when you know who your friends are, it's during the great times. The positivity and light that comes from these people is gold – hang on to it for more motivation for you to keep pushing towards your goals!

There has been a lot of discussion recently with members having negative reactions about their weight loss from their loved ones. That negativity can be tough to handle. Even if you are a generally confident person, it can feel hurtful and unnerving.

There are many reasons why friends and family can have negative reactions to your weight loss.

- Jealousy
- Fear, shame
- Genuine concern
- People don't realize how impactful their words and opinions can be
- Social awkwardness, especially post pandemic
- Changing dynamic in a relationship (i.e. you're not the fat friend/sister/brother anymore)

The negative things people do may be different for everyone. Some examples of negative reactions include:

- Not saying anything or pretending not to notice your weight loss
- Asking if you're sick
- Questioning your portions, food choices, supplements, exercise routine…
- Saying things like, "enough already" and "You've lost too much weight – stop now!"

- Pushing unwanted food your way

- Judging you when you don't want dessert, a second portion, finishing your entire meal, etc.

- Offering other weight loss programs/tips/advice

- Telling you that you were more fun (or cuter, or funnier…) when you were bigger

Sometimes, the negativity can even come from the people you trust the most in the world - like your spouse or immediate family. Comments can be direct or indirect, like questioning portions or making small body-shaming jokes or remarks. This can be hurtful from anyone, but can be even more so for someone you are meant to trust or be vulnerable with. It can make you question what you're doing and everything you have done so far.

Here are some ideas to help you navigate these conversations:

1. **Be yourself!!** Such a cliché, but it is the best advice anyone can hear! You are on the road to your Finally & Forever – your life, thoughts, feelings and day to day will change. This is wonderful! No better time than now to practice being yourself and becoming your most confident you!

2. **Don't take it personally.** There are many people right now who have gone through their own dark times, including gaining a lot of weight, especially while trying to navigate through this global pandemic. They can be socially awkward because of the lack of social situations, and their own insecurities. It can be hard for them to handle your new positive outlook and healthy new look. This is them. Not you. Enjoy your new self and move on.

3. **React with kindness and stay calm.** Take a moment to carefully think about what you want to say, and breathe. Be polite, make sure you are expressing yourself in a respectful voice, and smile. Sometimes it's not worth it to stoop down to their level; it's nice to leave a negative situation feeling like the bigger person.

4. **Remember that no two situations are the same.** Think for a moment about how you want to handle this particular situation, because it may be different from others that you've encountered in the past.

5. **Diffuse the situation with humor.** It can sometimes release the tension of an awkward conversation.

6. **Talk to the person to tell them how you are feeling.** If you are not able to have a discussion in the moment, you can always take a step back, think about what happened, and pull the person aside to tell them how you feel. Be direct. Sometimes the conversation can be difficult, but it can be just as difficult for you if you are constantly hearing negative comments from those you love.

7. **Don't overthink it.** If you've confronted someone about their behaviour and they do not respond well, remember that it is not your responsibility to change people. You've done the

best you can to resolve the situation. Sometimes you have to accept that they have their own issues, realize that it is no fault of your own, and let them find their own solutions.

8.   **If you need a cheerleader – reach out!** If you are a member of our Facebook Support Group, our team and many of our past and current members are happy to help to give you the boost you may need!

Experiencing negative reactions is never fun, but remember that positive reactions are far more common. Be sure to make time for those positive people in your life. However, you want to navigate the negative situations is up to you, just be strong and remember that you are working towards becoming your best you!

FOOD FACTS - FOOD FOR A HEALTHY GUT

As soon as you began The Livy Method, you started improving your gut health. You did this just by implementing the Food Plan.

- Eating lots of fresh fruits and veggies
- Regularly eating leafy greens
- Increasing healthy fats
- Eating raw nuts and seeds
- Taking apple cider vinegar
- Adding in pre & probiotic supplements
- Eliminating, or significantly decreasing, the amount of processed foods and sugar you are consuming

LET'S TALK MICROBIOME

Microbiome is a word you may be hearing more and more these days.

The gut microbiome refers to the microbes found in your digestive system and can affect many aspects of your health. Microorganisms or microbes are microscopic living things like bacteria, viruses, and fungi. There are about 100 trillion bacteria, good and bad, that live in your digestive system.

We all have healthy and unhealthy microbes in our gut but when things get out of whack and the unhealthy ones start to take over, it can have a negative impact on your health. An unhealthy balance can contribute to weight gain, increased blood sugar levels, chronic inflammation, decreased cognitive function, heart disease, as well as many other areas that are currently being studied. Many things, including the foods we eat, can impact the balance of bacteria found in the digestive tract.

HOW CAN I CONTINUE TO IMPROVE OR SUPPORT MY GUT HEALTH?

If you want to go further in improving your gut health, or supporting what you've already done, there are some specific foods that can help you level up your gut microbiome. These foods help to increase healthy bacteria and decrease the ones we want less of.

EAT A VARIETY OF FOODS, ESPECIALLY PLANT FOODS - Different foods lead to a more diverse microbiome. Maybe it's time to start experimenting with different foods you have never tried before. Also decreasing meat consumption and replacing it with plant-based proteins can help increase healthy bacteria in the gut.

EAT CRUCIFEROUS VEGGIES - So many benefits to these super veggies including healing your gut. High levels of prebiotic fibers and the powerful antioxidant, sulforaphane help to increase the healthy bacteria in your gut. Eating a variety of these veggies raw, or cooked, contributes to a diverse microbiome.

EAT FERMENTED VEGETABLES - sauerkraut, kimchi, miso, tempeh and naturally fermented pickles (found in the refrigerated section and should say "fermented". Not the same as pickled pickles found in the aisles). Fermented foods contain more lactobacilli which is a type of bacteria that can benefit the health of your gut.

EAT OTHER FERMENTED FOODS - Yogurt, kefir & kombucha. When it comes to yogurt, look for "contains live active cultures" and avoid products with high amounts of sugar.

EAT FOODS THAT ARE HIGH IN PREBIOTIC FIBERS - Apples, asparagus, bananas, barley, dandelion greens, garlic, leeks, oats, onions & seaweed to name a few.

INCORPORATE WHOLE GRAINS - Whole grains contain lots of fiber and nondigestible carbs that make their way to the large intestine promoting the growth of beneficial bacteria.

EAT PULSES - Beans and lentils are high in prebiotic fiber and help promote a healthy digestive system.

You are already doing wonders for your gut microbiome just by following the plan. These are just some tips for those of you looking to level up or maybe just make some improvements. Every little bit adds up.

To read more about gut health, refer to the Science Guide and check out the Issues with Digestion and the Maintenance and the Microbiome posts.

WEEK 11 GUIDELINES: PERSONALIZING THE FOOD PLAN

This week is where you are doing all the things you can do to help get and keep the scale moving while levelling up your efforts to be even more in tune to your body's needs.

This is an exciting place to be in your Weight Loss journey! This stage of the Program is about having faith in all the hard work you have done and trusting the foundation you have built.

It's also about continuing to MAXIMIZE your efforts to keep the body focused on fat loss until you reach your goal.

WHAT DOES PERSONALIZING THE FOOD PLAN LOOK LIKE?

You are still following all of the basic guidelines:

- Continue to check in at the original meal and snack times
  - Breakfast
  - Morning snack
  - Lunch
  - Snack
  - Snack
  - Dinner
- Ask yourself the 4 Mindfulness Questions
- Be mindful and in tune to portions, continuing to eat just enough
- Avoid going longer than 3.5 to 4 hours without eating

- Continue to focus on higher protein at breakfast

- Continue to make your food choices nutrient rich

- Stay on top of your water intake

- Take your supplements

- Avoid eating too late in the evening

- Maximize your efforts by reviewing the 20 Questions in the Let's Talk Maximizing Your Efforts Checklist post

- Manage stress levels

- Focus on sleep

- Move your body

When it comes to what to eat and when, you will still be checking in at each meal and snack time. **Breakfast, snack, lunch, snack, snack, dinner.** The difference is you will be making your food choices based on the following:

1. **WHEN TO EAT:**

    - Before each meal and snack time, check in and ask yourself if you are hungry and need to eat. If so eat.

    - If you feel you are not really hungry but could eat, be sure to have a token amount.

    - If you are not hungry, you no longer need to force yourself to eat token amounts, so you can skip that meal or snack. However, if you run the risk of going longer than 3.5 - 4 hours, you should still have a token amount.

    - Keep in mind that hunger levels can change day to day. Some days you may need to eat all of the meals and snacks, while other days you may feel the need to eat less often.

2. **WHAT TO EAT:**

    - Although there is no longer a star of the meal at lunch and dinner, you still want to make sure you have the necessary components for your meals. Protein, vegetables, leafy greens and healthy fats.

    - Lunch is still the best time to add in any heavier or starchy carbs as needed.

    - The focus at breakfast is still higher protein.

    - You want to choose options from the same kinds of foods included in the grocery list that you have been eating all along.

    - Rather than eating specific foods at specific times, you now have a bit more flexibility when it comes to what you are eating and when.

- Make your choices based on what is most appealing in the moment, for example, you may choose to have nuts in the morning and fruit in the afternoon.

- When you are hungry ask yourself, what exactly am I hungry for and what's the best choice for me to maximize my efforts.

3. **HOW MUCH TO EAT:**

- Continue to ask the 4 Mindfulness Questions and be super in tune when it comes to portions.

- You want to continue to eat just enough, where 15 minutes later you are feeling satisfied, and not stuffed.

- Keep in mind that portions are what they feel like and not what they look like. Some days you may need more or less to eat than others.

NOTES:

- Breakfast is still optional, however, it is beneficial to have when it comes to maximizing your efforts. Stick with high protein to start your day.

- Morning snack can be optional, depending on if and when you had breakfast and you now have more options to choose from when it comes to your morning snack.

- There is no longer a "star of the show" for lunch or dinner. Choose foods that are appealing to you in the moment. Be sure to include vegetables, protein, leafy greens, and healthy fats.

- At lunch, you can add starchy veg and heavier carbs back in as needed.

- Leafy greens are still a benefit to add to your meals.

- You can have one or both of your afternoon snacks, or you can skip them altogether depending on when you had lunch, and what time you are eating dinner.

- Ideally, dinner should be the smallest meal of the day. At this point, you can skip it if you are not hungry, depending on the time of your last meal or snack.

- It is still best to minimize heavier carbs at dinner when looking to lose weight.

The biggest change this week is you no longer have to force yourself to eat token amounts when you are not hungry. And you have more flexibility with your snacks and snack times, allowing you to be even more in-tune to your body's changing needs.

The purpose of this week is to transition your body into a style of eating more conducive to helping it focus on fat loss, while feeding into its need to function more efficiently and at optimal levels. At this point, the body wants the fat gone as much as you do. So, continue to maximize your efforts, while you lean in and trust in the mind-body connection that you have been working so hard to build.

FREQUENTLY ASKED QUESTIONS

1. **Can we add bread and pasta back in?**

    If you still have weight to lose, it is still best to keep bread and pasta to a minimum.

2. **Is it better to skip lunch or dinner?**

    You do not want to be skipping any meals "just because". If you are not eating a meal, it would be because you are not hungry for it. If you do skip a meal, be sure to follow the guidelines of when to eat, not going longer than 3.5 - 4 hours between meals and snacks.

3. **If I skip meals and snacks will my body go into starvation mode?**

    Not if you are following the 30 minutes to 3.5 hours between meals and snacks rule. If you go past 3.5 hours and you are not hungry, then this is a case of where you should eat at least a token amount of the next meal or snack.

4. **Can I have a protein shake for my lunch or dinner?**

    Protein shakes are best to have at breakfast or at snack time. If you do choose to have one at lunch or dinner, be sure to still include all of the necessary components of your meal, like protein, vegetables, leafy greens and healthy fats.

5. **Are we still making meals nutrient rich?**

    Absolutely, nothing changes there! Be sure to add good fats to your meals and make them as nutrient rich as possible.

6. **Is there a 'star of the show' for lunch and dinner?**

    A high protein breakfast is still encouraged as a benefit, but there is no longer a star of the show for lunch or dinner. You want to choose what is appealing to you in the moment. Ideally, you still want to include protein, vegetables, healthy fats, and leafy greens and make your meals as nutrient rich as possible. It is still best to have heavier carbs at lunch over dinner.

7. **What snack combinations can I have?**

    You still want to choose your snack options from the same kinds of foods you have been eating all along. But rather than eating specific foods at specific times, you can now make your choices based on what's most appealing in the moment when you are hungry.

    For example, you may choose to have nuts in the morning and fruit in the afternoon. It is still a great idea to add protein and fat to any carbs like fruits or vegetables.

Please take the time to head over to the Facebook Group or the Livy Method App and watch the quick video that accompanies this post.

LET'S TALK MAXIMIZING YOUR PERSONAL FOOD PLAN

Now that you have had some time to work on Personalizing the Food Plan with Week 11, let's talk things you can do to Maximize your efforts more and take things to the next level.

LET'S TALK: FOOD CHOICES

When it comes to digestion, some foods are easier to digest than others. This is something to keep in mind when you are looking to lose weight and be in tune to your body's needs. In understanding how your body processes and digests certain foods, you can take things to the next level with your food choices.

For example:

Water (immediately digested)

Juice and other liquid nutrients (10 - 15 min to digest):

- Juice can be an issue because it lacks fiber and increases your blood sugar.

- When it comes to liquid nutrients, it can be hard to gauge portions as they skip the digestive breakdown process.

- Natural juices can be an ideal addition in the summer when it is super hot or when you overexert yourself so much you need to replenish your glycogen (energy) stores fast. (Note: these occasions are rare.)

Fruits (20 - 40 min to digest):

- Fruits are easy to digest so they are perfect when you need quick and easy energy.

- Fruits are also nutrient rich and high in fiber.

- If you are looking for more sustaining energy, it is a great idea to combine your fruit with protein and fat.

- If you are not looking for quick energy or are mindful of insulin levels, it is a good idea to pair your fruit with protein & fat to neutralize.

Vegetables (40 - 90 min to digest):

- Vegetables are harder to digest than fruits, especially if eaten raw. Therefore, they are good for stimulating the digestive system and have a high nutrient value.

- Vegetables are a good source of fiber and serve as an energy food, giving the body the carbohydrates it needs without the added sugar.

Nuts and Seeds (2 - 3 hours to digest):

- Harder to digest but contain protein and fat which can give you more sustaining (lasting) energy.

Eggs (45 min to digest)

Fish and seafood (40 - 90 min to digest)

Beans and legumes (1.5 - 2 hours to digest)

Starchy Vegetables (1.5 - 2 hours to digest)

Grains (approximately 2 hours to digest)

Chicken/poultry (approximately 2 hours to digest)

Red meat and pork (can take 5+ hours to digest)

Dairy (can take 2 - 5+ hours to digest)

HOW YOU CAN USE THIS INFORMATION TO YOUR ADVANTAGE

1. **"I'm feeling low on energy and need a quick snack, so I'll grab some nuts."**

    Nuts take 2 - 3 hours to break down, whereas fruit takes 20 - 40 minutes. So, if you are looking for quick and fast energy, fruit is a better choice than nuts.

    Nuts are hard to digest, which is why in the beginning of the Program, we added them as a second snack in the late afternoon, to purposely make the body work hard and keep you more satisfied longer. So, when grabbing something easy but looking for more sustained and longer lasting energy, you may want to have some nuts.

2. **You are going out for a night on the town or a late event.**

    Instead of having something like steak, which is harder to digest, have fish or seafood, which is much faster and easier to digest. That will give you the energy you need to enjoy your night out without feeling bloated and heavy, as well as interrupting your sleep later.

LET'S TALK: TOP TIPS FOR GOOD DIGESTION

1. **Check in at scheduled meal and snack times.**

    Life can get busy and it's easy to get sidetracked and forget to eat. While looking to lose weight, it is a great idea to check in on yourself until it becomes second nature and you are more in tune with when, what, and how much to eat.

2. **Be conscious of what you eat and your portion sizes.**

   If you are still looking to lose, it is key to be mindful of portions and continue to ask the 4 Mindfulness Questions.

   Although you can use Back on Track if and when needed, overindulging stresses the body out, signals weight gain, and can cause indigestion, so it is best to keep to a minimum.

3. **Chew your food completely and try to minimize talking while eating.**

   Incomplete chewing and talking while eating can cause premature swallowing. Our digestive systems are not designed to digest large pieces of food. When we put large pieces in our stomach, it can lead to incomplete digestion and digestive discomfort.

4. **Relax while eating your meal.**

   This may seem super simple, but many of us are always on the go and always on the clock rushing through everything we do.

   Eating when you are rushed increases your stress and slows down the digestive process. Try to create a calm atmosphere when eating.

5. **Practice good posture.**

   This is key especially with your ever-changing body, just from a structural point of view and making sure muscles are supporting proper alignment.

   When you slouch or hunch over, extra pressure is put on the digestive organs in your abdomen. This extra pressure can cause poor digestion. You should practice sitting with your shoulders back and your chin tucked in. This will allow more room for the digestive organs and will help improve digestion.

6. **Avoid eating after dinner and late at night.**

   Worth repeating, our bodies, including our digestive system, slow down in the evening hours as it gets ready to rest and rejuvenate. When we put food into our stomach at these late hours, it disrupts your wind down process, can interrupt your sleep, and can prevent the body from focusing on detox.

7. **Take a brisk walk after eating.**

   Increased physical activity after a meal actually helps with digestion, improves gut health, and increases the production of digestive enzymes. This will lead to more complete digestion of your food.

8. **Try a spinal twist.**

   Spinal twists allow excess toxins in the digestive system to be released, which has a calming effect. While in a cross-legged sitting position, slowly turn to the right and hold while taking 5 deep breaths, then repeat this process on the left side.

9.   **Avoid ice cold drinks while eating.**

Although a nice cold glass of water can be refreshing in the warmer months, ice cold drinks can slow down the digestive process.

Think of it as putting ice on a muscle. The muscle stiffens and does not function as well. Warm or room temperature water or teas will encourage proper digestion even in the warmer months.

Now, this isn't to say you can't drink cold water while eating, just be in tune to how it may be affecting your digestive system in the moment.

REMEMBER:

These tips are not meant to stress you out or to complicate the process, but give you more options when it comes to Maximizing your efforts and taking things to the next level.

Rest assured, you are doing enough by being mindful and following the Program as designed.

We hope you are enjoying this week of Personalizing the Food Plan. Try to have fun with it as you work to take things to the next level.

HOW NOT TO GAIN WEIGHT

Let's talk about how not to gain weight back after putting all of your time and energy into losing it.

It is key to understand that the way you have gone about losing weight with this process is different from any past attempts at fat burning.

When you force your body to utilize its fat reserves by restricting energy foods or starving and depriving it of nutrients, you leave the body with no choice but to burn its stored fat for fuel. Although it's effective for weight loss, it also immediately reinforces the need for your body to hold onto and store fat.

Simply put, if you use your body's stored fat for energy as a method for weight loss (fat burning), your body will store it all back plus more the first chance it gets, and it will do so thinking it's doing you a favour! Which is why you can lose weight with a fat burning diet, but you can't maintain the loss after you go back to normal eating.

With The Livy Method, because you have lost weight in a way that's not only healthy for your body but also for your mind, if you follow the 4 Stages of Finally & Forever, gaining weight back is not as much of a concern.

However, there are a few reasons why someone might gain weight back after this process that you need to be mindful of:

1. **NOT PUTTING TIME INTO MAINTENANCE**

    *   Maintenance is key. You have got to give your body time to get used to functioning at your new weight. You want your new weight to become your new norm/set point.

    *   Even though you may have hit your goal and are done losing, your body is not done solidifying the weight you have lost.

    *   Things like metabolism, blood flow, body temp and hormones are just a few of the things the body will need to address & adjust to be able to stabilize at your new weight.

2. **NOT CONTINUING TO BE MINDFUL**

    *   This is also where the concept of "Check Yourself Before You Wreck Yourself" comes in. You don't gain 10 or 20 lbs without noticing. Continue to be mindful and when you notice, simply check yourself and implement Back on Track.

    *   Be mindful of falling back into old habits like thinking less is more and trying to control your body instead of being in tune to it.

3.   **NOT ADJUSTING TO SITUATIONAL CHANGE**

- For example, losing your weight at home where your routine, environment and stress levels are different than if you went back to work. The situation being you were at home all day and now you are at your place of work.

- Another example of this would be to have a change in job, where your stress levels are different. Helping the body manage new stress by bumping up omega 3, adding in more movement, or being mindful to get to bed earlier to adjust to your new schedule, are a few examples of what you can do to help minimize the impact of situational change.

- It's key to help the body adjust and adapt to change. Change in environment for example; needing more water in a dryer environment than you are used to. Adjusting to stress as noted above, or even a change in the times you are able to eat. For example, having more business meetings or a job that restricts when you can eat.

- The goal is to minimize the impact on the body by helping it adjust to physical or emotional stress/change.

4.   **SEASONAL CHANGE**

- This one is all about not forcing yourself to eat salads when you are craving something heartier. In the cooler months, for example, be sure to be in tune to your body's needs. Grains and starchy vegetables, fatty meats, along with hot and spicy foods are more appealing for a reason. They help to create heat in the body which helps to eliminate the need for the body to store extra fat to keep you warm.

- Alternatively, be sure to decrease the starchy carbs and bump up cooling and easier to digest foods such as salads, fruits and vegetables in the warmer months.

- Try to eat a seasonally sourced diet or incorporate seasonal foods when possible.

ADDITIONAL THINGS TO AVOID TO PREVENT WEIGHT GAIN:

- Making a habit of going all day without eating. If this happens every now and then, it is not a big deal. But if you make it a habit (like for weeks and months) the body will pick up on this and feel the need to start storing fat.

- Not eating all day in anticipation of having a bigger meal later in the day. Starving the body followed by overeating reinforces the need for it to store fat.

- Not eating the next day after indulging. Although you may not feel like eating much after a day of indulging, it's key to help stimulate the digestive system to help get rid of any backlog.

- Over exercising and not giving the body enough rest in between workouts can lead to overtraining and the body feeling a need to store fat to compensate.

- Not prioritizing your body's needs like managing stress and getting enough sleep.

- Not replenishing the body or helping it heal after illness. For example, pushing the body to recover too soon.

- Not drinking enough water. Although you don't need to be drinking as much water, you still want to be mindful of being hydrated so your body can function properly.

- Not being mindful of your body's ongoing and ever-changing needs.

As you can see, easily maintaining your weight truly is about being mindful and continuing to be in tune to your body's needs while you navigate and enjoy life.

It's not as hard as you think and a little effort goes a long way in terms of living a worry-free life when it comes to your weight.

Please take the time to head over to the Facebook Group or the Livy Method App and watch the quick video that accompanies this post.

WEEK 12 GUIDELINES: MAINTENANCE AND MINDFULNESS

This week we will be having discussions on moving forward after you are done losing and how to proceed if you have more weight to lose after the group is done. But for now, let's focus on this week and finishing strong.

As we enter the final week of the Program, it is time to talk about maintenance for those of you who have reached your goal, or are getting close. To be clear, maintenance is for those of you who are done losing and have reached your goal weight.

There are four stages when it comes to losing your weight Finally & Forever:

STAGE 1 - LOSING WEIGHT AND REACHING YOUR GOAL

Timeframe: As long as you need

This is where you are working towards your weight loss goals using The Livy Method.

STAGE 2 - SOLIDIFYING THE WEIGHT YOU HAVE LOST

Timeframe: 2 - 3 months

This is when you have reached your goal and are now looking to solidify the weight you have lost so you can easily maintain it moving forward.

You have two choices when it comes to solidifying your weight:

1.   Continuing with Personalizing the Food Plan
2.   Repeating the Program

During this stage you will continue with Personalizing the Food Plan or repeating the process, but in a more relaxed manner because you are not looking to lose weight.

With your body now minimizing its focus on fat loss, it can allocate resources to other areas of the body when it comes to repairing, rebuilding, regenerating, and rejuvenating.

STAGE 3: TESTING THE WATERS

Timeframe: As long as you need

This is where you are learning what maintenance looks and feels like to you, and learning to trust the changes you made.

- Here is where you may start to mindfully indulge here and there using Back on Track as needed.
- Continuing to support the new habits you have created and be aware of how your body is responding to the choices that you are making.
- Just because the body is done dropping fat, doesn't mean it is done doing the work to support it.

STAGE 4: FINALLY AND FOREVER

Timeframe: Lifetime

This is where you wake up, look good, feel good and go about your day without worrying about what to eat and when, mindfully making choices in tune to your body's needs.

- You should now have faith in all your hard work and trust the mind-body connection that you have established.
- You should be in a place where your internal dialogue, and that space in your brain reserved for obsessing about what you eat and don't eat, is non-existent or getting close to it.
- You will continue to use Back on Track as needed and support the habits you have created as part of your new healthy lifestyle.

But, with that said, this is also where you implement the concept of "Check Yourself Before You Wreck Yourself."

CHECK YOURSELF BEFORE YOU WRECK YOURSELF

Although you have lost weight in a healthy way that has you in tune to your body's needs, moving forward, you will always need to be mindful of the choices you make, understanding how your choices will affect your body, and then self-correcting, balancing out, and getting Back on Track to minimize the effect.

I have been able to easily maintain my weight for over 30 years. My weight has fluctuated up and down naturally and sometimes more than others, but for the most part, it's just a matter of going by how I feel.

If I make crappy food choices, I feel crappy, then I just get Back on Track. I never indulge without understanding how I will feel after. This may seem like work, but after a while it just becomes second nature.

Continue to be in tune to your body's needs and be mindful of the messages you are sending and receiving.

LET'S TALK SUPPLEMENTS AND WATER IN MAINTENANCE

Once you reach Maintenance, you can re-evaluate the supplements you are taking. You may choose to leave some in or switch some of them up. Please note, taking out the supplements WILL NOT cause you to gain weight. At this point, you will just be keeping them in for their health and wellness benefits.

With regard to water, you only need to drink enough to keep you hydrated.

STILL LOOKING TO LOSE??

If you are still looking to lose weight, you want to continue with Personalizing the Food Plan and maximizing your efforts this week to complete the 91 Days of the Program.

If you are looking to continue your weight loss journey, be sure to review the post on options for continued weight loss.

For now, focus on completing the Program and finish just as strong, if not stronger than the day you started.

Please take the time to head over to the Facebook Group or the Livy Method App and watch the quick video that accompanies this post.

4 STAGES OF FINALLY & FOREVER

It's time to have a conversation about Maintenance and the 4 Stages of Finally & Forever.

This is one of our favorite things to talk about because it is what sets The Livy Method apart from other weight loss programs. It is not just about losing weight in a healthy way physically and mentally, it's about losing weight in a way that's going to be Finally & Forever.

Let's talk about the 4 Stages of Finally & Forever:

1. **The first stage is losing your weight and reaching your goals.**

2. **The second stage is Solidifying Your Weight.**

   - This is where you are helping your body to solidify the weight you have lost. Meaning, giving your body time to make your new weight your new norm.

   - You can solidify your weight by using Option 1 – Repeating the Program because there are so many benefits to leveling up your health and wellness, even though you don't have any more weight to lose. Or you can use Option 2 – Personalizing the Food Plan.

   - This stage takes about 2-3 months, depending, everyone's a little different. Some people can lose their weight and just move on. However, sometimes even though you lost your weight physically, you might still have work to do mentally. For example, working through issues and associations and reinforcing the new habits that you have created for yourself.

3. **The third stage, Testing the Waters.**

   - This is where you are learning to trust yourself and the changes you have made. It is also trusting your body, and having a more clear understanding of what maintenance looks like and feels like to you.

   - This is where you might start indulging more like eating the pizza on pizza night, or having a few chippies here and there, and using Back on Track as needed.

   - This is where you move forward understanding your weight is going to continue to fluctuate but it's not real weight gain. It's learning to trust that you've got this and this really is going to be forever.

   - It's about continuing to be mindful and in tune with your body and being aware of how it reacts to certain or new foods and listening to the messages it is sending you.

   - This stage can take weeks for some and months for others. Only you will know when you are ready to move on to the fourth and final stage.

4. **The fourth stage is Finally & Forever.**

- This is where you wake up, you look good, and you feel good. You just go about living your life.

- This is where you truly get to move on from your weight loss journey.

Even after completing the stages you will have to continue to be mindful. But this is where all of your hard work will pay off so you can move on from your weight loss journey and truly live your best life.

Please take the time to head over to the Facebook Group or the Livy Method App and watch the quick video that accompanies this post.

CONTINUING TO LOSE - OPTION 1 - REPEATING THE PROGRAM

LET'S TALK OPTION ONE - REPEATING THE PROGRAM!

Repeating the Program means doing a complete reset of the Program and re-doing the process over again week to week from the beginning, which is an effective option. The idea being that you are restarting the process with your body now functioning at a more optimal level.

Some of you who have more weight to lose, may have to complete another few rounds to reach your goal. Have faith that each time your body will be working just as hard to help you reach your Finally & Forever weight loss goals.

The first time around, you will find yourself more focused on the physical elements of the Program, like what you are eating and how your body is responding.

You will find when you repeat the process, it becomes more of a mental game. So, it is key to approach each new group with Fresh Eyes. If this was your first time through the Program and you are considering doing a reset, I would suggest reviewing the Let's Talk Fresh Eyes post.

Keeping in mind each time you repeat the process, it's key not to assume your body will respond in the same way because your body next time around will be functioning on a whole other level.

You will want to continue repeating the process until you have reached your goal. Once you reach your goal, you can continue to follow through on the steps to help solidify your weight and finish the Program, or start the maintenance phase.

You can redo the Program by signing up for the next group session or follow along on your own.

For those of you who may be behind in the group and following on your own timeline:

- Do your best to complete as many weeks as possible before Repeating the Program.
- If you are doing the Program on your own, then be sure to complete the full 12 weeks before you start again.
- If your plan is to do the next group, then keep following along as far as you can and then reset with the new group.

Repeating the Program is an effective method to continue to lose for many reasons. It gives the option for the body to level up your health and wellness as it challenges the body to address issues and continue to make change. There is an advantage in knowing what's to come and how to set yourself up for success to capitalize on the process.

CONTINUING TO LOSE - OPTION 2 - PERSONALIZING THE FOOD PLAN

LET'S TALK OPTION 2 - PERSONALIZING THE FOOD PLAN!

Personalizing the Food Plan is the tweak you have been following for the last two weeks.

When Personalizing the Food Plan, you need to be as diligent and as consistent as possible and use all of the tools you have learned along the way to keep the scale moving.

Remember that Personalizing the Food Plan is checking in at every single meal and snack and making the best food choices based on the guidelines. It's being super in tune to portions, and it's making sure to consistently Maximize.

When Personalizing the Food Plan, you can still implement Back on Track when you find yourself indulging, although it is best to keep it to a minimum while looking to lose.

Personalizing The Food Plan is an effective method for reaching your goal, so continue to stay focused and visualize the end game. Think of Personalizing the Food Plan as following a diet specifically designed for you.

The benefits of following your Personalized Food Plan to continue to lose weight over Repeating the Program, is that it gives you more flexibility in your day-to-day food choices.

BRIDGING THE GAP BETWEEN GROUPS

Let's talk bridging the gap between the end of this group & repeating the process again in the next Program.

If you are planning on doing the next group, it is ideal to continue to follow Personalizing the Food Plan until the start date.

If you do find yourself indulging/enjoying/partaking in the weeks in between groups, be sure to use Back on Track as often as you need and then continue on with Personalizing the Food Plan.

If you find you are at capacity and still want to lose, but know you won't have the same kind of time and energy to give to the process on your own, you might want to consider using the Back on Track Method to bridge the gap.

Back on Track is ideally reserved for when you find yourself indulging and needing help to get back on track. However, if you feel at capacity or are dealing with added stress in your life, it could be exactly what you need to help keep the body calm and maintain status quo until you start the next group.

ON A FINAL NOTE:

If you are behind in the group and working through any of the previous weeks, continue to work at your own pace and be sure to use the search feature in the Livy Method App to help answer your questions. Keep in mind, you will still have access to all the information in the support group as well if you need.

If you have signed up for the next group, you can continue with moving forward from where you are at and then reset when the new group starts.

At the end of the day, it is all about what feels best for you.

MAINTENANCE - OPTION 1 - REPEATING THE PROGRAM

LET'S TALK OPTION ONE - REPEATING THE PROGRAM!

Repeating the Program means doing the Program again by following the Guidelines as designed week to week from the beginning to the end.

This is an effective way to solidify the weight you have lost, along with continuing to work on addressing any health issues and strengthening your mind-body connection. It is also a benefit as it allows more time to specifically focus on working through your old issues, associations and habits to further solidify the new ones that support your new lifestyle.

You can Repeat the Program by signing up for the next Weight Loss by Gina Program which is a benefit as you will have access to all of the most current information, seasonal tweaks, guest segments along with day to day guidance and support.

The other option is by Repeating the Program by following along on your own using the information from your current group. Although we stop posting and answering questions, you will still have access to all of the information, including all of the posts, videos, live segments, and the Livy Method App.

It is advised when Repeating the Program to help solidify your weight, that you be sure to complete the full 91 days before you move on to the Third Stage of Finally & Forever, Testing the Waters.

When Testing The Waters, you will use Personalizing The Food Plan until you feel confident moving on to the fourth and final stage of Finally & Forever.

Regardless, if your plan is to redo the Program on your own or by signing up for the next group, you can ask all the questions you have along the way in the Maintenance and Mindfulness group.

If you choose this option, this is how the 4 Stages of Finally & Forever will look:

- **Stage 1** – Losing your weight and reaching your goal
- **Stage 2** – Solidifying your weight by Repeating the Program
- **Stage 3** – Testing the Waters using Personalizing the Food Plan (using Back on Track as needed)
- **Stage 4** – Finally & Forever, eating in tune to your body's needs. (continuing to use Back on Track as needed.)

MAINTENANCE - OPTION 2 — PERSONALIZING THE FOOD PLAN

LET'S TALK OPTION TWO — PERSONALIZING THE FOOD PLAN

Repeating The Food Plan (PTP) is doing all of the things that were posted in the Week 11 Guidelines of the Weight Loss Program.

The benefit of following your Personalized Food Plan over Repeating the Program to solidify your weight, is it gives you more flexibility in your day-to-day food choices.

PTP to maintain your weight is a bit different from PTP to lose weight. When looking to maintain, you don't necessarily have to be as diligent or as consistent when following, but it is still a good idea to use all of the tools you have learned along the way when you were trying to lose.

Continuing to be mindful is truly the key to maintenance and a life beyond weight loss. So it's good practice to keep up with being in tune to your body's needs to help it focus on solidifying and adjusting to your new weight, so your new weight becomes the new normal for you.

When PTP, you should still use Back on Track when you find yourself indulging and not feeling your best.

Remember that PTP is checking in at every single meal and snack and making the best food choices based on the Guidelines of the Weight Loss Program even though you are no longer looking to lose. It's about continuing to be super in tune to portions, and asking the four questions until it becomes second nature and you no longer need to ask.

If choosing PTP, you will continue to use it in the final 3 stages of maintenance, Solidifying Your Weight, Testing the Waters and Finally & Forever.

Being clear about next steps is key, as you don't want to find yourself flip flopping from one Option to another. So be clear about your intention if Personalizing The Food Plan is the method you plan to use to solidify your Finally & Forever weight.

If you choose this option, this is how the 4 Stages of Finally & Forever will look:

- **Stage 1** – Losing your weight and reaching your goal
- **Stage 2** – Solidifying your weight by Personalizing The Food Plan
- **Stage 3** – Testing the Waters continuing to use Personalizing the Food Plan (using Back on Track as needed.)
- **Stage 4** – Finally & Forever, eating in tune to your body's needs. (continuing to use Back on Track as needed.)

MAINTENANCE FAQS

Here are some of the frequently asked questions about maintenance:

1. **I'm enrolled in the next Weight Loss Group. Not quite at my goal weight. Can I belong to both?**

   You can totally be a member of both, however, if you still have weight to lose, best to continue with the weight loss group until you have lost your weight. The maintenance group is continuous so it will always be there for you to check out when you're ready.

2. **If Repeating the Program, can I be a member of both groups?**

   Yes, this can be an advantage for you. You can follow along in the current weight loss group for each week's tweak and also participate in the conversations that take place in the Maintenance & Mindfulness group.

3. **If I am Repeating the Program for maintenance should I still be eating all of the meals and snacks and follow all the tweaks such as downsizing?**

   If you are going to re-do the Program to solidify your weight, you still want to follow the Food Plan and each week's tweaks as designed. You do not have to be as strict, but it is still best to follow along with the Program as it's laid out.

4. **If I am Personalizing the Food Plan for maintenance, do I continue to eat multiple snacks per day?**

   You want to follow the same guidelines for Personalizing the Food Plan that you did while losing weight. Be sure to check in at all meal and snack times, assess your hunger levels and continue to choose from the same kinds of foods you have been eating. Also, be mindful of not going longer than 3.5 - 4 hours without eating.

   While in maintenance you want to continue to be in tune with how you are feeling when it comes to your meals and snacks. Remember that your hunger levels can change day to day. You may find that some days you are hungrier and may need multiple snacks and some days not as many.

5. **Will we be able to use the Livy Method App when we are in the Maintenance & Mindfulness Group?**

   Yes, after completing the 91 days of the weight loss program, the Livy Method App turns into a general tracking mode that you can use in maintenance.

6. **Do I need to continue taking the ACV/lemon water in the morning?**

   There are benefits to starting the day with ACV or lemon water, however, it is your choice whether you want to continue. You don't have to continue using it in maintenance.

7. **How much water should I drink now that I'm in maintenance?**

While in maintenance you just want to drink enough water for basic body function. Be sure to continue to assess your body's hydration needs by paying attention to its cues, such as if you are feeling thirsty.

8. **What supplements should I continue to take now that I've reached my goal?**

That is a personal choice. Although they are still a benefit for basic health and wellness, this is a good time to reassess the supplements you are taking and why. It is a great idea to discuss this with your healthcare provider or pharmacist to ensure your body's needs are being met.

9. **Should I still weigh myself every day while I'm in maintenance?**

It is your choice. It is a good idea to continue to use the scale as a tool to better understand your body's natural fluctuations and what maintenance looks like and feel like to you. The goal is to eventually stop using the scale and go by how you look and feel.

10. **What is the difference between real weight gain and the scale being up?**

The scale can be up for so many reasons, and will continue to fluctuate even in maintenance. It is much harder to gain weight than you think. If you continue to make the choices that align with your goals, you can be confident you are not gaining weight. Real weight can also be felt more than it can be seen on the scale. You may feel it in your digestion, energy levels and how your clothes fit coinciding with the choices you are making.

11. **How much time should I put into maintenance? Do you add more time if you had more weight to lose?**

After reaching your goal weight, you want to put approximately 2-3 months into the second stage of Finally & Forever which is solidifying your weight. You don't necessarily need more time if you have lost a lot of weight or it took you longer to lose as you have been solidifying your weight along the way. When you begin the third stage, Testing the Waters, you may need more time to solidify your new habits and routines, so this could keep you in maintenance longer. It is more about frequency, consistency and how you feel rather than the amount of time you might need.

END OF PROGRAM FAQS

With the Program coming to an end, we have compiled a list of some of the most frequently asked questions.

1. **Will we have access to this group when it's done?**

   Yes! Although we stop posting and answering questions on Sunday July 23rd, you will still be able to access the group to review the information after we are done.

2. **What if I have feedback about the Program I would like to share?**

   We want to hear from you, so please fill out the survey posted in the group and share your thoughts.

3. **Will I still be able to listen to the podcasts between groups?**

   Yes, the Weigh In with Gina Podcast is available at any time on all podcast platforms.

4. **Do I need to keep taking the supplements?**

   If you have reached your goal and you are ready for maintenance you can decide what you want to continue to take for health benefits. Otherwise, you don't need to keep taking them to maintain your weight.

   If you are still looking to lose weight you have options. You can take a break from the supplements between groups or keep taking them. There are benefits to both options so it's really a personal preference.

   Same rules apply for the ACV or Lemon water

5. **I'm concerned about gaining weight in between groups. How do I avoid that?**

   Be sure to review the post on "How Not To Gain Weight"

   Be sure to have a plan and be clear on next steps by reviewing the next steps options Posts.

   Be sure to use Back on Track when you indulge for as many days as you need until you feel back on track.

6. **How do I find you in between groups?**

   • You can follow Gina over on her social media pages.

   • Facebook: https://www.facebook.com/ginalivy

   • Instagram: https://instagram.com/ginalivy

   • If you have reached your weight loss goals, register for our WLBG: Maintenance and Mindfulness Group on Facebook. Register on www.ginalivy.com

7. **Will the Fall 2023 Group have its own Support Group?**

Yes, each new group has its own separate support group. At time of purchase, you will be sent a link to the new group.

8. **How do I register for the next Group?**

Visit the sign up page on the website: www.ginalivy.com

9. **What if I didn't get a code for the new Facebook Group or Livy Method App?**

Any administrative questions should be sent through the website www.ginalivy.com or email weightloss@ginalivy.com as they have the resources to help.

Any App specific questions can be directed to techsupport@ginalivy.com

10. **Do I need Facebook to sign up for the new Group or can I just use the Livy Method App?**

-   All of the same posts and instructional videos that are posted in the Facebook Support Group can be found in the App, including the Daily Check In Video. You can access and to listen to the LIVE segments by way of our podcast.

-   There is a database in the App where you can search information. However, the Facebook group is where the team is available to answer any questions you may have.

-   Essentially you would only need to join the Facebook Support Group to participate in our live segments or have your questions personally answered by our team of Program Specialists.

11. **Where do I download the Livy Method App?**

You can follow the directions sent by email at the time of purchase or download from the Apple App Store or Google Play Store.

If you have already downloaded the App, there is no need to download it again. Simply select the program that you wish to unlock with your new code.

For more information about the Livy Method App, head over to our App Help Guide on our website: https://www.ginalivy.com/appguide

12. **Is there a new book for the Fall 2023 Group?**

Yes! There will be a new updated version of the book available specifically for the Fall Group.

WLBG RECIPE GUIDE

This section includes just some of the easy and delicious recipe ideas you can make while doing the Program. There will be more recipes and meal ideas posted within the Group.

BREAKFAST RECIPES

WLBG SPECIAL BLEND CEREAL

Looking for a high protein breakfast to start your day off right that doesn't involve eggs, dairy or gluten? Here's the recipe you've been waiting for!

Servings: 32

Prep & Cook Time: 20 minutes

INGREDIENTS

TOASTED QUINOA

- 1 cup quinoa, rinsed well and drained
- 4 cups water
- 1 tbsp olive, avocado, coconut, or grapeseed oil
- 1/2 tsp salt

WLBG SPECIAL BLEND CEREAL

- 1 cup toasted quinoa
- 1 cup chia seeds
- 1 cup raw buckwheat, whole kernels, or groats
- 1 cup hemp hearts/seeds

SUGGESTED TOPPINGS

- Nuts, seeds, and extra hemp hearts
- Coconut, almond, soy milk, or any milk or cream you like
- Unsweetened toasted coconut
- Yogurt
- Nut butter
- Any type of fruit

DIRECTIONS

FOR THE TOASTED QUINOA

1. Rinse quinoa in a mesh sieve over cold running water for about 2 minutes. Let drain.
2. Bring 4 cups of water to a boil and add quinoa. Turn down to a simmer and cook for 10 minutes. Drain well.
3. Turn the oven broiler to high and position a rack in the top third of the oven.

4.   Put well drained quinoa back in the pot and mix in olive oil and salt. Spread thinly and evenly on a baking sheet.

5.   Broil for 8-10 minutes (times may vary depending on your oven). Watch it carefully and stir halfway through. You will hear it pop and it will start to toast. Keep a very close eye in the last half of broiling. There should be no moisture left so if necessary lower the oven rack and toast a little longer until it is dry and crispy. For extra insurance, turn off the oven and let the quinoa cool down in the oven.

6.   When done, let cool completely on the tray. It must be cooled completely before mixing with the other ingredients.

7.   Store any extra toasted quinoa in an airtight container in the fridge and use it to top breakfast cereals, yogurt, salads, grilled vegetables etc.

WLBG SPECIAL BLEND CEREAL

1.   Mix together all 4 ingredients and keep in an airtight container in the fridge.

2.   To make cereal, add 1/4 cup of boiling water to 2 tbsp cereal mix (use more or less water for a thinner or thicker texture). Let stand, covered with a plate, for 3-5 mins or until desired softness is reached. Serve topped with any combination of the suggested toppings above or create your own!

NOTES:

STORAGE: Store in an airtight container in the fridge for up to 1 month.

Extra toasted quinoa is delicious on top of yogurt, other cereals, salads, grilled vegetables, popcorn etc. You will soon be addicted!

EASY HOMEMADE EGG BITES

Homemade egg bites are a perfect make-ahead breakfast and a great way to use up leftover vegetables and other ingredients.

Servings: 12 pieces

Prep & Cook Time: 40 minutes

INGREDIENTS

EGG BASE

- 10 large eggs
- 1/4 cup plain yogurt or sour cream, full fat
- Salt and pepper to taste

SPICY RED PEPPER & PEPPER JACK

- 1 cup red pepper, small dice
- 1 cup pepper jack cheese, grated or cubed
- Your favourite hot sauce, to taste

BROCCOLI & SMOKED CHEDDAR

- 1 cup broccoli, cooked, chopped into small pieces
- 1 cup smoked cheddar, grated
- 1 tbsp grainy Dijon mustard

DIRECTIONS

1. Preheat oven to 325°F. Generously grease a 12-cup muffin tin and place inside a larger baking pan.

2. Divide your chosen ingredients between the cups, they should be about 2/3 full.

3. Whisk together eggs, yogurt, salt, and pepper and pour evenly over each cup.

4. Pour about one to two inches of hot tap water into larger pan. Grease a piece of foil large enough to cover the pan and cover with greased side down. If you don't have a larger pan, you can bake these directly in the oven leaving off the greased foil. Check for doneness after 15 minutes.

5. Bake for 25-30 minutes or until set. Remove from oven and remove muffin tin from pan. Let cool. Use a butter knife to loosen from pan. Serve warm or refrigerate or freeze for later.

NOTES:

STORAGE: Let cool completely and store, covered, in the fridge for 5 days. Or wrap individually and store in the freezer for up to 3 months. Let thaw in fridge overnight.

SUBSTITUTIONS: Use any combination of vegetables or cheese you like.

HAVE IT FOR LUNCH OR DINNER: These make a perfect protein addition to any veggie packed lunch with some leafy greens! Eggs are great for dinner! Serve with a side salad or just some leafy greens.

BAKED AVOCADOS WITH EGGS, CHORIZO AND A SIDE OF GUACAMOLE

Servings: 2

Prep time: 10 min

Cooking time: 20 min

INGREDIENTS:

- 1 large avocado
- 2 eggs
- 1/2 chorizo sausage
- 1/2 medium tomato
- 1 green onion
- 1/4 lime juice
- 2 tbsp chopped cilantro
- Olive oil
- S&P
- Chopped chives for garnish

DIRECTIONS:

1. Preheat oven to 450°F

2. Remove sausage from the casing. Heat a frying pan over medium high. Add sausage and break it up into small bits using a wooden spatula. Cook until browned all around, 3-5 min. Set aside.

3. Halve the avocado lengthwise and remove the pit. Using a spoon, scoop out the flesh leaving about a 1/2 inch border around.* The hollow should be large enough to fit an egg. Set the scooped out avocado flesh aside.

4. Place the avocados into an ovenproof dish, cut side up.** Break the eggs into the hollow and top with cooked chorizo. Bake until the egg whites are set, about 15 min.

5. While the avocado bakes, chop the tomato, green onions, and cilantro. Combine the remaining avocado flesh, tomatoes, green onions, cilantro, lime juice, and olive oil. Salt to taste and mix well. Set aside.

6. Garnish the avocados with some chopped chives and serve with the guac on the side. Enjoy!

NOTES:

*Try to choose large avocados so the eggs easily fit in. Make the hollows shallow – the eggs will cook through more evenly.

**If your avocado halves do not stay upright, before you add the eggs, make small nests using strings of tin foil. Roll and squish the foil into a tube and close the two ends together into a ring. Place the avocados in the middle for more stability. Alternatively, you can use small and shallow ovenproof bowls.

MATCHA OVERNIGHT OATS WITH HEMP HEARTS & CHIA SEEDS

Servings: 3

Prep time: 5 min

Additional time: 3-8 hours

INGREDIENTS:

- 1 cup old fashioned oats
- 1 cup yogurt
- 3 tbsp hemp hearts
- 3 tsp chia seeds
- 1 tbsp matcha powder
- 1/4 cup strawberries
- 1/4 cup raspberries
- honey
- toasted coconut
- macadamia nuts

DIRECTIONS:

1. To portion overnight oats, grab three mason jars or containers of your choice. Alternatively use a bowl to make one batch.

2. In a mason jar, combine 1/3 cup of oats, 1/3 cup of yogurt, 1 tbsp hemp hearts, 1 tsp of chia and 1/3 tbsp of matcha. Add a splash of honey and about 1/4 cup of cold water. Mix well and cover. Repeat for the remaining jars.

3. Refrigerate overnight or at least 3 hours.

4. When ready to eat, remove from the fridge and top with sliced strawberries, raspberries, toasted coconut, and macadamia nuts. Sprinkle with hemp hearts and drizzle with some honey. Enjoy!

NOTES:

Make sure to use old fashioned rolled oats for the best texture. Quick oats will become quite mushy when soaked overnight.

Feel free to swap the topping for nuts of your choice, add bananas and other fruit, or nut butters. Overnight oats are great to make ahead in batches. They keep well in the fridge for up to four days and are fantastic on the go meal!

LUNCH RECIPES

GARLIC SHRIMP ZOODLES WITH GREEN GODDESS DRESSING

Servings: 2

Prep time: 15 min

Cooking time: 10 min

INGREDIENTS:

- 3 zucchinis
- 20 large shrimp, deveined
- 3 garlic cloves
- 1/2 bunch cilantro
- 1/2 bunch parsley
- 1 shallot
- 1/2 avocado
- 2 tbsp Greek Yogurt
- 1 tbsp lemon juice
- 1 tbsp butter
- olive oil
- S&P
- Sesame seeds and chili flakes for garnish

DIRECTIONS

1. Trim and spiralize the zucchini.*
2. In a small bowl, combine deveined shrimp, minced garlic and a splash of olive oil. Salt slightly, mix well and set aside.
3. In a blender or a food processor, combine parsley, cilantro, avocado, shallot, Greek Yogurt and lemon juice.** Salt to taste and process until smooth.
4. In a large frying pan, over medium high, heat the butter until it starts to bubble. Add shrimp, cook stirring often, until it turns pink, 2-3 min.
5. Add the zucchini noodles. Toss the noodles with tongs and cook until "al dente" – they should be wilted, but still have a crunch, 4-5 min.
6. Serve the zoodles with a drizzle of the green sauce. Sprinkle it with sesame seeds and chili flakes. Enjoy!

NOTES:

*Vegetable spiralizer is a fantastic tool to have in a kitchen, however, it is not the only way to make zoodles. You can use a julienne vegetable peeler or a mandolin, as well as a standard vegetable peeler to make wide zoodles or ribbons.

**You can use any fresh herbs for your green goddess sauce! Not a big fan of cilantro? No problem! Swap for chives, dill, tarragon, spinach…If you enjoy some heat, throw in a Jalepeno or a chili pepper. This sauce keeps well in the fridge for a few days and is great for salads or as a dip.

HUMMUS BOWL WITH QUINOA SALAD AND HEMP HEARTS

Servings: 4

Prep time: 15 min

Cooking time: 20 min

INGREDIENTS:

- 1 cup uncooked quinoa
- 2 cups chicken stock
- 2 medium tomatoes
- 1/2 english cucumber
- 1 bunch cilantro
- 1 bunch parsley
- 1/4 red onion
- 1 lemon juiced
- 2 garlic cloves
- hemp hearts
- olive oil
- Salt
- Cumin
- smoked paprika

DIRECTIONS

1. Rinse the quinoa under cold water. Drain well. Combine quinoa and chicken stock in a small pot. Bring to a boil, then turn the heat down to maintain a gentle simmer. Cook until the quinoa has absorbed all of the stock, about 15-20 min, cover, remove from heat and set aside to cool.

2. While quinoa cooks, chop the tomatoes, cucumbers, onions and herbs finely.

3. Drain the chickpeas. In a food processor combine the chickpeas, tahini, 1/4 cup olive oil, garlic and half of lemon juice. Add 1 tsp of cumin and salt to taste. Add 1 cube of ice (this will help to create smoother and silkier texture). Process until smooth.

4. In a large bowl, combine chilled quinoa, tomatoes, cucumbers, red onions and chopped herbs. Salt to taste. Add the rest of the lemon juice and about 1/2 tsp cumin. Mix well.

5. To serve, spread about 2 full tbsp of hummus in a bowl. Drizzle with olive oil and smoked paprika. Add quinoa salad on the side. Sprinkle with hemp hearts. Enjoy!

CURRIED RED LENTIL SOUP

Curried Red Lentil Soup is flavourful, hearty, and nutritious. It's easy to make and has been a family favourite for many years. Even your kids will love it!

Servings: 10-12

Total Cook & Prep Time: 45-30 minutes

INGREDIENTS:

- 1 lg white onion. approx. 2 cups diced small
- 1 lg celery stalk. approx. 1 cup diced small
- 1 jumbo carrot, approx. 1.5 cups diced small
- 1 small sweet potato, 2 cups diced small
- 2-3 cloves garlic, 1 tbsp minced
- 8 cups baby spinach leaves, or greens of your choice
- 1 tbsp curry powder
- 1 1/2 cups red lentils, rinsed
- 3 tbsp olive oil
- 4 cups chicken stock, low sodium
- 1 – 400 ml can coconut milk
- 1/2 cup packed cilantro or parsley leaves, chopped
- 1/2 lemon, juice of
- Salt and pepper to taste

DIRECTIONS

1. Peel, rinse, chop and measure out all of your ingredients first.
2. In a large pot heat olive oil over medium high heat. Add onions and cook, stirring occasionally, for 3-5 minutes or until soft and translucent. Turn down the heat if they are browning before softening.
3. Add the celery, carrot, sweet potato, lentils, and garlic, stir to combine. Add curry powder and continue stirring for one minute.
4. Stir in stock and coconut milk. Increase the heat and bring to a boil. Once boiling, reduce heat and simmer, covered, for 15 minutes.

5. Stir in spinach. It will seem like a lot, but it wilts and reduces as it cooks. Cover and simmer for 5 more minutes.

6. Remove from heat and add lemon juice and cilantro or parsley. Add salt and pepper to taste. You can also add a bit more stock or water if it's too thick for your liking.

NOTES:

STORAGE: This soup will keep in the fridge for 5 days or in the freezer for up to 6 months.

SUBSTITUTIONS: You can use any type of lentils but cooking time may need to increase slightly. Continue cooking until the lentils are soft. Use vegetable stock instead of chicken stock and heavy cream instead of coconut milk.

HAVE IT FOR DINNER: This soup is well balanced with both vegetables and protein, but if you'd like to bump up the protein a bit more, sprinkle with hemp hearts, toasted seeds or nuts. Top it with a dollop of sour cream or plain Greek yogurt or a boiled egg!

MAKE IT VEGETARIAN: Replace the chicken stock with vegetable stock.

THAI STYLE SLAW WITH PEANUT DRESSING

A crunchy and delicious Thai style slaw. It's easy to prepare and keeps for days in the fridge! This salad has everything you need for a perfectly balanced lunch on plan. Or have it for dinner as a side to your favourite protein!

Servings: 6

Prep Time: 30 minutes

INGREDIENTS:

- 1 cup edamame beans, steamed
- 4 cups (1/2 a head) savoy cabbage, thinly sliced
- 1 bell pepper, thinly sliced
- 1 medium-large carrot, shredded
- 2 green onions, thinly sliced
- 1/2 cup cilantro, chopped
- 1/2 cup chopped peanuts, for garnish
- lime wedges, for garnish

PEANUT DRESSING

- 2 cloves garlic, minced
- 4 tbsp fresh squeezed lime juice
- 3 tbsp soy sauce
- 1/2 cup peanut butter, all natural
- 2 tsp avocado or olive oil
- 2 tsp brown sugar
- 1/4 tsp crushed pepper flakes
- 4 tbsp water, or more

DIRECTIONS

FOR THE DRESSING

1. In a bowl, food processor, or blender, mix all ingredients. Add more water if necessary to thin. The amount of water will depend on the consistency of your peanut butter. Set aside.

FOR THE SALAD

1. Steam or blanch edamame beans for 5 minutes or until tender. Drain and run under cold water to cool after cooking.

2. Chop peanuts and set aside for garnish.

3. Slice all the vegetables using a sharp knife or mandolin. Chop cilantro. Toss everything together in a large bowl.

4. Add dressing and toss to combine.

5. Serve garnished with copped peanuts and lime wedges.

NOTES:

STORAGE: Store, covered, in the refrigerator for up to one week. The salad will wilt as it sits but remains crunch and delicious!

SUBSTITUTIONS: Substitute green cabbage with savoy or red cabbage, or a combination. Substitute peanut butter for almond or cashew butter. For a completely nut-free alternative try using Sunbutter which is made from sunflower seeds.

HAVE IT FOR DINNER: Serve as a side to your favourite protein!

DINNER RECIPES

TEX-MEX CHICKEN BAKE

A quick and easy one pot meal that will soon become a family favourite! Colourful vegetables and fresh flavours will make your mouth water!

Servings: 4 to 6

Prep & Cook Time: 1 hour

INGREDIENTS:

- 6 chicken thighs, bone-in, skin on
- 1 large white onion, peeled and diced
- 1 large red bell pepper, or any colour, diced
- 1 large zucchini, diced
- 2 large cloves garlic, finely chopped, 1 tbsp.
- 1 tsp chili powder
- 1 cup fresh or frozen corn kernels
- 2 cups of your favourite salsa
- salt and pepper to taste
- fresh cilantro, one small bunch, washed and roughly chopped. Divide in two portions. One half is for garnish
- 150 g or about 2 cups old cheddar cheese, grated
- 2-3 green onions, sliced, for garnish

SUGGESTED TOPPINGS

- Sour cream
- guacamole or avocado
- pickled jalapenos

INSTRUCTIONS:

1. Preheat oven to 400 degrees F.
2. Season chicken thighs on both sides with salt and pepper.
3. Heat olive oil in large sauté pan over medium-high heat.
4. Add chicken thighs, skin side down and set sear, without moving them, for 4-5 minutes

or until golden brown. Flip over and sear the other side for 3-4 minutes more or until golden brown.

5.   Remove chicken to a large plate or dish and set aside.

6.   Add diced onion to the pan with the oil and fat from the chicken. Sauté, stirring occasionally, for about 5 minutes or until soft and glossy.

7.   Add diced zucchini, red pepper, garlic, cumin, and chili powder. Continue cooking and stirring occasionally for 3-4 minutes.

8.   Add corn and cook for 2 more minutes. Add salsa and half the chopped cilantro. Taste and add salt and pepper as needed.

9.   Bring to a boil and reduce heat to a simmer. Nestle chicken pieces into the vegetable mixture.

10.   Top with grated cheddar leaving the chicken skin exposed.

11.   Bake in preheated oven for 30 minutes or until a thermometer reads 165 degrees F.

12.   Top with remaining cilantro and sliced green onions.

13.   Serve on its own or with rice or quinoa. Top with sour cream and/or guacamole.

NOTES:

STORAGE: Keep covered in the fridge for 3 days or freeze for up to 3 months.

SUBSTITUTIONS: Black beans, tofu, or shrimp work well in place of chicken. Use any combination of vegetables you like. You can use boneless thighs or breasts. Cooking times may vary.

HAVE IT FOR LUNCH: Have a larger portion of vegetables than chicken/protein and serve on a bed of leafy greens.

ADD LEAFY GREENS: Serve with a side salad or add 3-4 cups chopped spinach, kale, collard greens, or Swiss chard in step #7.

MAKE IT VEGETARIAN: Omit the chicken and add 1-2 cans of black beans. Add the beans in step #9. Or slice a block of firm tofu and follow recipe as is, browning the tofu first.

TERIYAKI SALMON BAKE

Who doesn't love a one pan meal? This Teriyaki Salmon Bake is so easy, super nutritious, and lip-smacking good! The teriyaki sauce is delicious on any type of fish, seafood, meat, poultry, and tofu so make a big batch and keep it in the fridge for quick access.

Servings: 3 or more (you can add as many filets as you like)

Total Prep & Cook Time: 45 minutes

INGREDIENTS:

- 3 salmon filets or as many as you need
- 1/2 head Napa or savoy cabbage, Bok choy or other Asian greens, chopped or sliced in large pieces
- 1 red pepper, sliced
- 1 medium carrot, thinly sliced
- 1 handful green beans or asparagus, cut into 2-inch pieces
- 2 tbsp olive or avocado oil
- 1/2 tsp salt, or to taste

TERIYAKI SAUCE

- 1/2 cup soy sauce
- 3 tbsp brown sugar
- 1 tbsp garlic, minced
- 3 tbsp mirin
- 1 tsp sesame oil
- 1/4 cup water
- 2 1/2 tsp cornstarch

OPTIONAL TOPPINGS

- toasted sesame seeds
- sliced green onions

INSTRUCTIONS:

1.   Preheat oven to 400 degrees F. Place rack in center of oven.

2. In a small saucepan mix together all the ingredients for the Teriyaki sauce. Bring to a boil and stir until slightly thickened. Set aside to cool.

3. Prepare all the vegetables and place in a 9" x 13" baking dish or something similar that will fit vegetables in an even layer. Drizzle with olive oil, sprinkle with salt and toss to coat.

4. Bake vegetables for 15 minutes.

5. Meanwhile, rinse salmon filets and pat dry. After 15 minutes remove vegetables from the oven and lay salmon filets on top.

6. Using about half of the Teriyaki sauce, coat the salmon and drizzle over vegetables.

7. Bake for 10 minutes. Remove from oven and turn broil to low.

8. Brush or drizzle the remaining sauce over salmon.

9. Broil on middle rack for 5 minutes. Check salmon for doneness. Internal temperature should read 145 degrees F. It should separate easily and be semi-translucent in the center.

10. Serve immediately. Top with toasted sesame seeds and/or sliced green onions if desired.

NOTES:

STORAGE: Salmon bake will keep in the fridge for 3 days. Teriyaki sauce will keep in the fridge for up to one month.

SUBSTITUTIONS: Substitute any vegetable you like including broccoli, cauliflower, Brussels sprouts, snow peas, etc. Substitute Mirin with white wine or rice vinegar mixed with 3 tsp sugar.

HAVE IT FOR LUNCH: Make veggies the star of the show when having for lunch.

ADD LEAFY GREENS: If you are looking to bump up your leafy greens you can serve on a bed of your favourite leaves.

MAKE IT VEGETARIAN: Substitute the salmon with slices of tofu marinated for 30 mins in the teriyaki sauce.

ZUCCHINI LASAGNA WITH SPINACH RICOTTA

Servings: 6

Prep time: 15 min

Cooking time: 40 min

INGREDIENTS:

- 1 lb lean ground beef
- 500 gr ricotta cheese
- 2 medium zucchini
- 2 roma tomatoes
- 1 cup canned diced tomatoes
- 1 egg
- 2 shallots
- 2-3 garlic cloves
- 2 cups baby spinach, packed
- 1 tsp oregano
- 1 tsp thyme
- 1/2 tsp chili flakes
- S&P
- Olive oil
- 1/4 cup shredded mozzarella
- chopped basil for garnish

DIRECTIONS:

1. Preheat oven to 425°F

2. Chop shallots, tomatoes and spinach. Mince the garlic. Using a vegetable peeler, ribbon the zucchini. Alternately, use a knife to slice as thinly as you can. Set the ribbons aside.

3. In a large bowl combine ground beef, garlic powder, oregano, thyme, and chili flakes. S&P generously and mix well. Using your hands, form a few patties.

4. Over medium-high, heat a splash of olive oil in a cast iron or in a large pan. Add shallots & garlic, cook, stirring occasionally until fragrant, about 1-2 min. Push the onions and garlic to the sides of the pan and place the ground beef patties in the middle. Let them brown on

each side, about 1-2 min. Using a wooden spoon break down the beef patties into smaller chunks. Add fresh & canned tomatoes. S&P to taste. Mix well, reduce the heat to medium, and simmer, stirring occasionally until the tomatoes soften and sauce reduced in half, about 10 min. Fold in half of the chopped spinach and set aside.

5.   While the sauce simmers, in a bowl combine ricotta, half of the spinach, and one egg. S&P to taste, mix well.

6.   Once the sauce is done, remove from heat and set aside.

7.   Assemble the lasagna by layering sauce, zucchini strips and ricotta mixture evenly into a deep baking dish. Repeat until you get about three layers (adjust as needed depending on the size of the dish you use). Sprinkle with grated mozzarella and transfer into the oven. Roast until the cheese is beginning to brown, about 15 min.

8.   Remove from the oven and let it cool down slightly. Serve with some fresh chopped basil and enjoy!

TEMPEH AND ROASTED CHICKPEA CURRY

If you follow a plant-based diet or are looking to consume less meat, tempeh is a fantastic source of protein. Similar to tofu but with a firmer, meatier texture that has a nutty taste. It's made of fermented soybeans so is also great for gut health!

Servings: 4

Prep & Cook Time: 40 mins

INGREDIENTS:

- 1 (390 ml/14 oz) can chickpeas, drained and rinsed
- 1/2 tsp ground cumin
- 1/2 tsp smoked paprika
- 1/2 tsp salt
- 1 tbsp coconut or olive oil
- 1 (250g) package tempeh, original flavour
- 1 tbsp cornstarch
- 1/2 tsp salt
- 1/2 large red onion, sliced thinly
- 1 medium to large fresh tomato, chopped
- 3 cloves fresh garlic, chopped
- 3 + 1 tbsp coconut oil
- 2 tbsp curry paste
- 1 (398 ml/14 oz can) full fat coconut milk
- 1 tsp sugar
- 2 cups baby spinach leaves, packed

OPTIONAL GARNISHES

- Plain yogurt
- Sliced red onion
- chopped fresh cilantro
- fresh lemon wedges

INSTRUCTIONS:

1. Preheat oven to 400 degrees F.

2. Toss chickpeas with cumin, spoked paprika, and salt. Place on a parchment lined baking tray and bake for 10 minutes.

3. Cut tempeh into approximately 1 cm (1/2-inch) cubes. Toss with cornstarch and 1/2 tsp. salt.

4. Prepare the onion, garlic, and tomato.

5. Heat 2-3 tbsp coconut oil in a large sauté pan over medium-high heat. Add tempeh and fry to brown all sides. Lower heat if browning too quickly. Remove from pan to a bowl or plate.

6. Lower heat to medium-low. Add another tablespoon of coconut oil to the pan.

7. Add sliced onions and sauté until softened. 8-10 minutes.

8. Add garlic and tomatoes and stir for one minute.

9. Add tempeh, chickpeas, and curry paste. Stir to coat everything in the curry paste.

10. Add coconut milk and 1 tsp sugar. Mix everything together.

11. Increase heat and bring to a boil. Reduce heat to a simmer and continue simmering for 10 minutes or until it reaches your desired thickness.

12. Add spinach and stir until wilted.

13. Serve with your favourite rice, spaghetti squash, cauliflower rice or zucchini "noodles".

NOTES:

STORAGE: Store covered in refrigerator for 5 days. Freeze for 3 months.

SUBSTITUTIONS: Instead of tempeh you could use extra firm tofu, chicken, fish or shrimp. In place of spinach use any leafy green you like. Substitute curry paste with 2 tsp. curry powder.

HAVE IT FOR LUNCH: Serve with extra vegetables or a side salad for lunch. You can also add in your favourite brown or dark rice here.

SERVE WITH: Spaghetti squash, spiralized zucchini, cauliflower rice.

SCIENCE GUIDE

This section contains more in-depth information and science behind The Livy Method. It is not mandatory reading, but is for those of you who want to dive deeper into the science behind the Program. This is an evolving section and we will continue to add more resources and articles in the future.

THE SET-POINT THEORY

Welcome to the science posts which are designed to help provide some foundational information and understanding of how our bodies function, and how implementing The Livy Method optimises our health, wellness, and mindfulness, by providing an environment where our bodies no longer feel the need to store fat!

We will begin this journey by discussing the Set-Point Theory and other theories of weight loss that might help us explain how The Livy Method works, and why it is different from other diets that involve deprivation and calorie restriction. Let's dive into this!!

THE HISTORY OF DIETING

It may be assumed by some that obesity and dieting is a concern of more recent times. But upon delving deeper into this subject matter, it is interesting to note that the concept of dieting or "slimming" has been around for centuries. The Ancient Greeks and Romans already understood that food and physical exercise influence our health and our weight. The Greek word 'diatia' (from which the word 'diet' is derived) referred to a whole way of living focused on self-control and eating in moderation. Interestingly, the first best selling diet book was written in 1474 by the Italian humanist Bartolomeo Sacchi, aka Il Platina. Advances in printing techniques meant that his *De honesta voluptate e valetudine* was read throughout Europe, and high society became obsessed with his recommendations regarding the relationship between gastronomic pleasure (voluptate) and health (valetudine).

Throughout the ages, humans have been in pursuit of fitting the criteria of what was deemed beautiful or accepted by the society they lived in. For many cultures, and in different eras, being thin has been one of the main measures of beauty. Although this can be problematic for so many different reasons, there is a distinction that needs to be made between weight loss and overall health, as opposed to seeking it to fit societal norms.

Hippocrates, who is considered the founder of medicine born in 460 BC, was one of the first to document the association between weight and health with the statement, "Those by nature overweight, die earlier than the slim". Today we know that obesity-related conditions which include heart disease, stroke, type 2 diabetes, and certain types of cancer, are among the leading causes of preventable, premature death.

Many health issues can be preventable by some degree of weight loss. From the ancient Greeks to current day, many of us have had some struggle with our weight and have likely tried many different diets in order to lose and gain the same weight, many times. There needs to be options for those that are looking to lose weight in a healthy, sustainable way! This is why The Livy Method is designed with overall health in mind, which includes not only a physical focus, but includes the mental, emotional, and for some even their spiritual health. Let's talk more about the impact of obesity on health and why one might consider trying to lose weight.

WHAT ARE SOME HEALTH RISKS OF OVERWEIGHT AND OBESITY?

TYPE 2 DIABETES

Type 2 diabetes is a disease that occurs when your blood glucose (or blood sugar), is too high. Your body cannot make enough insulin (a hormone that helps control the amount of glucose or sugar in your blood), or does not properly use the insulin it makes. Diabetes Canada (2022) reports that Type 2 diabetes is caused by several different risk factors and accounts for 90% of diabetes cases in Canada! According to the NIDDK (National Institute of Diabetes and Digestive and Kidney Diseases, 2018) About 8 out of 10 people with type 2 diabetes are overweight or have obesity. Over time, high blood glucose can lead to issues such as heart disease, stroke, kidney disease, eye problems, nerve damage, and other health problems.

If you are at risk for type 2 diabetes, losing 5 to 7 percent of your body weight and participating in regular physical activity may prevent or delay the onset of type 2 diabetes. (NIDDK, 2018) There is more discussion regarding the precursor to diabetes in the science post Hormones Important to Weight Loss & Digestion Part 1-Insulin, so check it out for more details!

HIGH BLOOD PRESSURE

High blood pressure, also called hypertension, is a condition in which blood flows through your blood vessels with a force greater than normal. High blood pressure can strain your heart, damage blood vessels, and increase your risk of heart attack, stroke, kidney disease, and even death. Being overweight and obese may raise your risk for high blood pressure.

HEART DISEASE

Heart disease is a general term used to describe several problems that may affect your heart, such as those that have suffered a heart attack, heart failure, angina, an abnormal heart rhythm (also called arrhythmia), or sudden cardiac death.

High blood pressure, abnormal levels of blood fats (blood lipids), and high blood glucose levels may increase your risk for heart disease. Blood lipids include HDL cholesterol, LDL cholesterol, and triglycerides. See the science post on The Science of Fat and Fat Loss for a more detailed description of fats in the body!

According to the NIDDK (2018, February) losing 5 to 10 percent of your weight may lower your risk factors for developing heart disease. Weight loss may improve blood pressure, cholesterol levels, and blood flow in the body.

STROKE

Stroke is a condition in which a blockage or the bursting of a blood vessel in your brain or neck, prevents blood flow from getting to the brain. A stroke can damage brain tissue, affecting your ability to speak or move parts of your body. According to the NIDDK (2018, February) High blood pressure is the leading cause of strokes. As discussed above, even a 5-10% reduction in weight can improve blood pressure, which could decrease the risk of stroke.

SLEEP APNEA

Sleep apnea is a sleep disorder in which your breathing can be affected while sleeping. Sleep apnea may present as irregular breathing patterns, or where your breathing stops (apnea) altogether for short periods of time. According to Jonathan Jun, M.D., (Johns Hopkins Medicine, 2022) a pulmonary and sleep medicine specialist at the Johns Hopkins Sleep Disorders Centre, sleep apnea happens when upper airway muscles relax during sleep and pinch off the airway, which prevents you from getting enough air. Your breathing may pause for 10 seconds or more at a time, until your reflexes kick in and you start breathing again. This results in decreased oxygen to the body and vital organs. If left untreated, sleep apnea may raise your risk of other health problems, such as type 2 diabetes and heart disease.

Jun discusses that sleep apnea occurs in about 3 percent of normal weight individuals but affects over 20 percent of people with obesity. In general, sleep apnea affects men more than women. However, sleep apnea rates increase sharply in women after menopause.

There are two kinds of sleep apnea: obstructive sleep apnea and central sleep apnea. Obstructive sleep apnea happens when air can't flow into or out of the nose or mouth, although you're trying to breathe. Central sleep apnea happens when the brain fails to send the right signals to your muscles to make you start breathing. (This type is less common.)

Symptoms of sleep apnea can manifest in the following ways:

- Pauses in breathing, or snoring (both of which may be noticed by a partner). Snoring is the sound caused by the vibration created by airway resistance. Snoring can be caused by the relaxing of the airway as described above, so snoring as an isolated symptom does not mean you have sleep apnea. Also, you may have sleep apnea, without much snoring, so if you suspect sleep apnea may be an issue for you, further testing may be necessary.

- Unexplained fatigue and mood swings due to the prevention of settling into the deep stages of restorative sleep. This may lead to increased tiredness and grogginess resulting in decreased productivity, impacting focus and attention. This can also result in dire consequences if one participates in activities that require attention such as driving a car, or operating machinery.

- Waking up with a dry mouth, as those with sleep apnea tend to breathe with their mouths wide open. This leads to the saliva in their mouths drying out.

- Headaches upon waking, which may be caused by low circulating blood oxygen or high carbon dioxide levels during sleep due to inadequate breathing.

- Although one can have sleep apnea independent of being overweight, evidence suggests a link between sleep apnea and diabetes, as sleep apnea can cause an increase in blood sugar levels.

- For those who are overweight or obese, weight loss is key for treating or avoiding sleep apnea. People who accumulate fat in the neck, tongue and upper belly are especially vulnerable to getting sleep apnea. This weight reduces the diameter of the throat and pushes against the lungs, contributing to airway collapse during sleep.

METABOLIC SYNDROME

Metabolic syndrome is a group of conditions that put you at risk for heart disease, diabetes, and stroke, and is related to obesity. These conditions include high blood pressure, high blood glucose levels (pre-diabetes and type 2 diabetes), high triglyceride levels in your blood, low levels of HDL cholesterol (the "good" cholesterol) in your blood, and the accumulation of fat around the abdomen.

As discussed in the science post Hormones Important to Weight Loss & Digestion Part 1-Insulin, experts believe obesity, especially too much fat in the abdomen and around the organs (called visceral fat) is a main cause of insulin resistance. Insulin resistance may lead to pre-diabetes and type 2 diabetes. A lack of physical activity may also be a factor.

Insulin resistance is when cells in your muscles, fat, and liver don't respond well to insulin and are not able to easily take up glucose from your blood. As a result, your pancreas increases the production of insulin to help glucose enter your cells, a condition called **hyperinsulinemia**. However, as long as your pancreas can produce enough insulin to overcome your cells' weak response to insulin, your blood glucose levels should stay in the healthy range.

Having a waist measurement of 40 inches or more for men and 35 inches or more for women is linked to insulin resistance. This is true even if your body mass index (BMI) falls within the normal range. However, research has shown that Asian Americans may have an increased risk for insulin resistance even without a high BMI. (The discussion of BMI is used in reference to this study, although the concept of BMI is problematic as a measure of obesity).

Studies have also shown that belly fat produces hormones and other substances that can contribute to chronic, or long-lasting, inflammation in the body. Inflammation may play a role in insulin resistance, type 2 diabetes, and cardiovascular disease. Since excess weight may lead to insulin resistance, this also is a contributing factor in the development of fatty liver disease.

FATTY LIVER DISEASES

Fatty liver diseases are conditions in which fat accumulates in the liver that can, over time, affect liver function and cause liver injury. Fatty liver diseases include non-alcoholic fatty liver disease (NAFLD) and non-alcoholic steatohepatitis (NASH). Fatty liver diseases may lead to severe liver damage, cirrhosis (late-stage scarring or fibrosis of the liver), or even liver failure.

People who drink too much alcohol may also have fat in their liver, but that condition is different from fatty liver disease.

There are 2 types of fatty liver disease. If you just have fat accumulation but no damage to your liver, the disease is called non-alcoholic fatty liver disease (NAFLD). If you have fat accumulation in your liver plus signs of inflammation and liver cell damage, the disease is called non-alcoholic steatohepatitis (NASH). According to Johns Hopkins Medicine, about 10% to 20% of Americans have NAFLD and about 2% to 5% have NASH.

Fatty liver disease is sometimes called a silent liver disease because it can occur without causing any symptoms. Most people with NAFLD live with fat in their liver without ever developing liver damage, whereas a few people develop NASH. Symptoms of Nash may take years to develop, and can potentially cause cirrhosis. Symptoms from NASH may include severe tiredness, weakness, weight loss, yellowing of the skin or eyes (jaundice), spider-like blood vessels on the skin, and long-lasting itching.

NASH that turns into cirrhosis could cause symptoms like fluid retention, internal bleeding, muscle wasting, and confusion. People with cirrhosis over time may develop liver failure and need a liver transplant.

The exact cause of fatty liver disease is unknown, but it is thought that obesity is the most common cause. Obesity in the U.S. has doubled in the last decade, and health care providers are seeing a steady rise in fatty liver disease. Although children and young adults can get fatty liver disease, it is most common in middle age.

Risk factors include:

- Being overweight
- Having high blood fat levels, either triglycerides or LDL ("bad") cholesterol
- Having diabetes or prediabetes
- Having high blood pressure

Fatty liver disease can happen without causing any symptoms. It's usually diagnosed when you have routine blood tests to check your liver. Your health care provider may suspect fatty liver disease with abnormal test results, especially if you are obese.

If you have NAFLD without any other medical problems, making some lifestyle changes can control or reverse the fat buildup in your liver. However, you will want to work alongside your healthcare provider (HCP) as you work through this process.

This may include:

- Losing weight (losing just 3-5% of your weight can decrease the amount of fat in your liver)
- exercise
- Lowering your cholesterol and triglycerides
- Controlling your diabetes

- Avoiding alcohol
- Check out the Science Post on detox! It has many great suggestions on how to support your liver.

OSTEOARTHRITIS

Osteoarthritis is a common, long-lasting health problem that causes pain, swelling, and reduced motion in your joints. Being overweight or having obesity may raise your risk of getting osteoarthritis by putting extra pressure on your joints and cartilage.

According to the Arthritis Foundation in the US (2022, May), maintaining a healthy weight can ease the pain of arthritis and help your medicines work better. The CDC also reports that 31% of obese Americans have doctor-diagnosed arthritis.

The Arthritis Society of Canada (2022, November) discusses that excess weight can contribute to the onset and progression of knee and hip osteoarthritis. Furthermore, what we eat can be a key factor in the prevention/reduction of disease progression, as well as an identified risk factor for the development and management of gout.

Here are some reasons that the Arthritis Foundation suggest why reaching and maintaining a healthy weight can help ease your arthritis:

REDUCE PRESSURE ON YOUR JOINTS

A key study published in Arthritis & Rheumatism of overweight and obese adults with knee osteoarthritis (OA) found that **losing one pound of weight resulted in four pounds of pressure being removed from the knees**. In other words, losing just 10 pounds would relieve 40 pounds of pressure from your knees! This is so impactful when you really think about what weight loss means for the joints in your body. Even a small amount of weight loss can make a big difference on your joints.

EASE PAIN

Multiple studies show that losing weight results in arthritis pain relief. A 2018 study published in Arthritis Care and Research went further to find that losing more weight – to an extent -- results in more pain relief. The study of overweight and obese older adults with pain from knee OA, found that greater weight loss resulted in better outcomes than losing a smaller amount of weight. Losing 10–20 percent of starting body weight improved pain, function, and quality of life better than losing just five percent of body weight.

REDUCE INFLAMMATION

The tissue fat itself is an active tissue that creates and releases pro-inflammatory chemicals. By reducing fat stores in the body, your body's overall inflammation will go down. An article published in 2018 explained that obesity can activate and sustain body-wide low-grade inflammation. This inflammation can amplify and aggravate autoimmune disorders, such as rheumatoid arthritis, psoriatic arthritis, lupus and their associated comorbidities (like heart disease).

REDUCE DISEASE ACTIVITY

Losing weight can reduce the overall severity of your arthritis. A 2018 study reviewed the records of 171 RA (rheumatoid arthritis) patients and found that overweight or obese people who lost at least 5 kg (10.2 pounds) were three times as likely to have improved disease activity compared to those who did not lose weight. A smaller 2019 study found that short-term weight loss in obese people with psoriatic arthritis (PsA) yielded

"significant positive effects" on disease activity in joints, entheses (an enthesis is the site of attachment of tendon, ligament, fascia, or capsule to bone), and skin.

IMPROVE CHANCE OF REMISSION.

Several studies have shown that being obese reduces your chance of achieving minimal disease activity or remission if you have RA or PsA. A 2017 review article analyzed data from more than 3,000 people with RA and found that obese patients had lower odds of achieving and sustaining remission compared with non-obese people. A 2018 article analysed several studies totaling more than 3,800 patient records. The authors found that obesity "hampered the effects of anti-TNF agents" and showed that the odds of reaching a good response or achieving remission were lower in obese than non-obese patients taking anti-TNF medications. TNF or tumour necrosis factor is a protein that is produced by the body that causes inflammation. In healthy individuals TNF is blocked naturally, but is elevated in the blood of those with rheumatic conditions (rheumatology.org, 2022). These medications help inhibit TNF in order to reduce inflammation.

LOWER URIC ACID LEVELS AND CHANCE OF GOUT ATTACK.

Gout is a common form of inflammatory arthritis that is very painful. It usually affects one joint at a time (often the big toe joint). There are times when symptoms get worse, known as flares, and times when there are no symptoms, known as remission. Repeated bouts of gout can lead to gouty arthritis, a worsening form of arthritis. Gout is caused by a condition known as hyperuricemia, where there is too much uric acid in the body. The body makes uric acid when it breaks down purines, which are found in your body and the foods you eat. When there is too much uric acid in the body, uric acid crystals (monosodium urate) can build up in joints, fluids, and tissues within the body. Hyperuricemia does not always cause gout, and hyperuricemia without gout symptoms does not necessarily need to be treated.

A 2017 analysis of 10 studies found that weight loss was beneficial for obese or overweight people with gout. Overall, people who lost weight had lower serum uric acid levels and fewer gout attacks.

The following make it more likely that you will develop hyperuricemia, which can cause gout:

- Being male
- Being obese

- Having certain health conditions, including: Congestive heart failure, hypertension (high blood pressure), insulin resistance, metabolic syndrome, diabetes, poor kidney function

- Using certain medications, such as diuretics (water pills).

- Drinking alcohol. The risk of gout is greater as alcohol intake goes up.

- Eating or drinking food and drinks high in fructose (a type of sugar).

- Having a diet high in purines, which the body breaks down into uric acid. Purine-rich foods include red meat, organ meat, and some kinds of seafood, such as anchovies, sardines, mussels, scallops, trout, and tuna.

SLOWS CARTILAGE DEGENERATION IN OSTEOARTHRITIS

A 2017 study assessed magnetic resonance images (MRIs) of osteoarthritic knees in 640 overweight or obese people. Participants who lost weight over 4 years showed significantly lower cartilage deterioration. The more weight lost, the lower the rate of disease progression.

For those navigating arthritis living in Canada, the Arthritis Society Canada, has some great resources to help support you in your learning and managing your diagnosis. This can allow you to better focus on reducing certain risk factors, such as weight loss, in order to help alleviate symptoms and disease progression.

https://arthritis.ca/

GALLBLADDER DISEASES

According to the NIDDK (2017, November) being overweight or having obesity may make you more likely to develop gallstones, especially if you are a woman. Researchers have found that people who have obesity may have higher levels of cholesterol in their bile, which can cause gallstones.

People who have obesity may also have large gallbladders that do not work well. Some studies have shown that people who carry large amounts of fat around their waist may be more likely to develop gallstones than those who carry fat around their hips and thighs.

Losing weight very quickly may raise your chances of forming gallstones. When you don't eat for a long period of time (fasting) or you lose weight too quickly, your liver releases extra cholesterol into the bile. Fast weight loss (associated with very low-calorie diets) can also prevent the gallbladder from emptying properly. Weight-loss surgery may lead to fast weight loss and higher risk of gallstones.

Weight cycling, or losing and regaining weight repeatedly, may also lead to gallstones. The more weight you lose and regain during a cycle, the greater your chances of developing gallstones.

Your chances of developing gallstones may depend on the type of weight-loss treatment you choose. A program like The Livy Method that supports the body, and helps people lose weight in a healthy way, is a good option when trying to lose weight.

Regular physical activity, which will improve your overall health, may also lower your chances of developing gallstones.

To improve health or prevent weight gain, aim for at least 150 minutes a week of moderate-intensity physical activity, like brisk walking or fast dancing. Also, muscle-strengthening activity, like lifting weights or using your own body weight (callisthenics) can be beneficial. The science post Issues of Digestion, discusses the gallbladder in further detail and options for those that have had it removed. Check it out for further details!

SOME CANCERS

Cancer is a collection of related diseases. In all types of cancer, some of the body's cells begin to divide without stopping and spread into surrounding tissues. Overweight and obesity may raise your risk of developing certain types of cancers.

KIDNEY DISEASE

Kidney disease is a generic term that means there is damage to the kidneys and they are not able filter blood of wastes like they should. This is a vital process for the body. Obesity raises the risk of diabetes and high blood pressure, the most common causes of kidney disease. Even if you do not have diabetes or high blood pressure, obesity itself may promote kidney disease and quicken its progression.

PREGNANCY PROBLEMS

Overweight and obesity raise the risk of health issues that may occur during pregnancy. Pregnant women who are overweight or obese may have a greater chance of:

- Developing gestational diabetes.
- Having pre-eclampsia, which presents initially as high blood pressure during pregnancy and can cause severe health problems for the mother and baby if left untreated.
- The need for a Caesarean section (C-section) which can come with increased risks, and a longer recovery after giving birth.

Overweight and obesity are also associated with mental health problems such as depression. People who deal with overweight and obesity may also experience the stigma of weight bias from others, including health care providers. This can lead to feelings of rejection, shame, or guilt, further worsening mental health.

THE RISE OF OBESITY IN THE WORLD

According to the World Health Organization (WHO), being overweight or obese is defined as having "abnormal or excessive fat accumulation that presents a risk to health". Although the BMI can be a problematic assessment of obesity, it is still widely used in order to categorise a person's weight. As per the WHO, a body mass index (BMI) over 25 is considered overweight, and over 30 is obese. A report from the global burden of disease describes that this issue has grown to epidemic proportions, with over 4 million people dying each year as a result of being overweight or obese in 2017.

The estimated annual medical costs related to obesity in the United States was nearly $173 billion in 2019. The medical costs for adults who were diagnosed with obesity were $1,861 higher than medical costs for people with a healthy weight.

In the US, the CDC discussed in their most recent report from 2017-2020, that the prevalence of obesity was 41.9%. They also report that from 1999 –2000 through 2017 –March 2020, that the prevalence of obesity had increased from 30.5% to 41.9% and the prevalence of severe obesity increased from 4.7% to 9.2% in this same time frame.

According to the Government of Canada, statistics gathered from the Canadian Risk Factor Atlas (CRFA) using pooled data from the Canadian Community Health Survey, 2015-2018 determined that:

- About 1 in 4 Canadian adults (26.6%) are currently living with obesity.
- Obesity rates in Canadian adults are higher in men compared to women (28.0% versus 24.7%).

In Canada, a health report released on October 20, 2021 from Statistics Canada, found that chronic diseases account for 89% of all deaths and more than $80 billion in annual health care costs. Adopting healthy lifestyle behaviours, such as healthy eating, has the potential to prevent 80% of type 2 diabetes and cardiovascular disease, 40% of cancers, and other chronic diseases. Despite healthy eating recommendations issued by Health Canada, eating habits continue to deteriorate, and overweight prevalence rates continue to increase!

Rates of those that are overweight and obese continue to grow in adults and children. From 1975 to 2016, the prevalence of overweight or obese children and adolescents aged 5–19 years increased more than four times from 4% to 18% globally.

The WHO describes obesity as one side of the double burden of malnutrition and states that today more people are obese than underweight in every region except sub-Saharan Africa and Asia. Once considered a problem only in high-income countries, being overweight and obese is now dramatically on the rise in low- and middle-income countries, particularly in urban settings. The vast majority of overweight or obese children live in developing countries, where the rate of increase has been more than 30% higher than that of developed countries. This can be attributed to the lower cost of calorie dense, but nutrient poor foods that are widely available all over the world. Decreased physical activity is also a factor.

Interestingly in Canada though, the rate of obesity is higher for adults living in rural areas compared with those living in urban areas, regardless if one identifies with being male or female. Living in an urban setting is defined as living in areas with a high-density concentration of population (i.e. areas with a population of at least 1,000 and a population density of at least 400 persons per km²). Living in a rural setting is defined as all areas outside urban areas, or embedded in urban areas.

- In rural areas, about 1 in 3 Canadian adults are living with obesity (31.4%).

- In urban areas, about 1 in 4 Canadian adults are living with obesity (25.6%)

This means that there are on average 5.8 more cases of obesity per 100 adults living in rural areas compared with urban areas. *Note: Not all provinces or Territories show higher rates of obesity in rural compared to urban areas.

Check out https://health-infobase.canada.ca/datalab/canadian-risk-factor-atlas-obesity-blog.html?=undefined&wbdisable=true for more details on the Canadian demographics!

OBESITY AFFECTS SOME GROUPS MORE THAN OTHERS

According to the CDC, in the US Non-Hispanic Black adults (49.9%) had the highest age-adjusted prevalence of obesity, followed by Hispanic adults (45.6%), non-Hispanic White adults (41.4%) and non-Hispanic Asian adults (16.1%). The prevalence of obesity was noted to be 39.8% among adults aged 20 to 39 years, 44.3% among adults aged 40 to 59 years, and 41.5% among adults aged 60 and older.

In the *Morbidity and Mortality Weekly Report (MMWR)* it is discussed that the association between obesity and income or educational level is complex and differs by sex and race/ethnicity. It was found that:

- In the US overall, men and women with college degrees had lower obesity prevalence compared with those with less education.

- This same obesity and education pattern occurred among non-Hispanic White, non-Hispanic Black, and Hispanic women, and non-Hispanic White men. However, the differences were not all statistically significant. Although the difference was not statistically significant among non-Hispanic Black men, obesity prevalence increased with increased education.

- No differences in obesity prevalence by education level were noted among non-Hispanic Asian women and men and Hispanic men.

SOCIO-ECONOMIC IMPACTS ON OBESITY

In the MMWR report, it was noted that the prevalence of obesity was lower in the lowest and highest income groups compared with the middle-income group. Researchers observed this same pattern among non-Hispanic White and Hispanic men. However, the prevalence of obesity was higher in the highest income group than in the lowest income group among non-Hispanic Black men. This can be attributed to how socio-economic and culture influence food choices, and lifestyle. In many cases those with more education, tend to have access to healthier food choices, and tend to be more active. Although interestingly in some cultures, greater affluence leads to more indulgent choices and activities leading to obesity (PRB, 2013).

Historically, urbanisation was considered one of the most important drivers of the rise in obesity in industrialised countries. However, in Canada, it has been more recently shown that the urbanisation of rural life has contributed to a larger increase in rural obesity.

This change in the geographic distribution of obesity can be partly explained by the growing economic and social disadvantage that rural communities experience compared to urban cities. In particular, rural communities experience lower education and income, lower availability of healthy and fresh foods at a reasonable cost, less access to public transportation, and lack of supportive environments to promote walkability, sports and recreational activities.

In Canada overall, adult obesity is more prevalent among disadvantaged population groups such as those unemployed or with lower household income and education levels.

Recent global trends show that the prevalence of obesity is rising faster among people living in rural areas than those living in urban areas. When looking at cities in Canada

- The lowest rates of adult obesity were observed in the largest urban census metropolitan areas.

- In general, obesity rates in adults tend to be higher in smaller cities.

- Although adult obesity rates in the territories are among the highest in Canada, there were no urban-rural disparities.

- In Canada overall, adult obesity is more prevalent among disadvantaged population groups such as those unemployed or with lower household income and education levels.

Having access and understanding this data on how obesity rates in rural and urban populations is changing, as well as the socio-economic and cultural demographics, may assist policy-makers and local communities to target policies, programs and services aiming to promote healthy weight appropriately. This is where implementing a program like The Livy Method, and access to healthy food and activity could incite real change!!!

THE LIVY METHOD

To understand weight loss better, it's important to understand the problem of obesity and the impact it is having on society. After looking at these statistics, one thing is very clear, the way we approach our health at a global level needs to change. A big part of this would be having access to real nutritious food, clean water and sanitation, housing, fresh air, and feeling physically and psychologically safe amongst many other things. The other factor is understanding how the issue of obesity impacts our health, along with our food and lifestyle choices.

As you can now see The Livy Method is VERY different from many of the diets and weight loss methods that are out there or you may have experienced. The diet and food industry are a profit driven industry, with a focus on sales and retaining consumers. At WLBG, some of the core missions are to help people change their lives by improving their health, their relationship with food, the quality of food that they eat and the way in which they eat it, and to promote people prioritising and showing up for themselves. This all ultimately leads to weight loss.

However, many question, how does this program work? How can I be losing weight when I am eating more than I ever have? I have always been taught to count macros and/or calories!

These are all great questions and points, so let's dive into this deeper!

THE SET POINT THEORY

According to Ghoshal (2020, March), set point theory in relation to weight loss states that we have a pre-set weight baseline that is hardwired in our DNA, and specific for our individual bodies. Based on this theory, our weight and how much it changes from that set point might be limited. The theory states that some of us have higher weight set points than others and our bodies fight to stay within these ranges.

Recent studies point to body weight being affected by a combination of factors. Weight can be determined by inherited traits, the environment, and by hormonal, psychological, and genetic elements. Weight can also depend on energy expenditure compared to what kinds of foods and how much has been ingested.

The set point model relies on the concept of a genetic pre-set weight range that's controlled by biological and physiological signals in our bodies (NIDDK, 2011). The body has a regulatory system that keeps you at a steady-state level, or set point. You may have also heard this called homeostasis.

The hypothalamus, a small region of the brain located at the base of the brain, near the pituitary gland, is involved in the integration of signals directed to it from hormones like leptin (from adipose or fat cells), ghrelin (from the digestive system), insulin (the pancreas), along with many other hormones that regulate our hunger and satiety. Your metabolism also constantly adjusts up or down based on a variety of signals. The set point theory also suggests that your weight may go up or down temporarily but will ultimately return to its normal set range. The signalling system we have in place helps to maintain our weight.

The science post Hormones Important to Weight Loss & Digestion Part 2-Hormones of Hunger and Satiety and Timing of Digestion, takes a much deeper dive on how our hormones influence our hunger and satiety, and how The Livy Method helps to support these hormones, which can help influence weight loss and a drop in set point!

*Check out this video to see a detailed breakdown of the important role the hypothalamus plays in our body!

https://www.youtube.com/watch?v=xCXtcoUxJZc

This model is consistent with many of the biological aspects of energy balance, but struggles to explain the significance that environmental, economical and social influences play on obesity, food intake and physical activity. More on this later!

However, why does our weight climb beyond a few pounds if we have a set point?

Some researchers (Jung, C.H. & Kim, M.S., 2013) believe that the reactive signal system stops working efficiently over time and leptin and insulin resistance develop, causing us to gain weight. Although not a human study, Dalvi et al. (2017), found that when mice were fed a mostly high fat diet, it led to inflammation of the hypothalamus. However, a different study in mice that same year, concluded that a diet high in both fat *and* sugar, caused inflammation of the hypothalamus (Gao et al., 2017). The thought is that foods that are high in fat and sugar, like many processed foods available today, lead to not only inflammation in the body, but also in the brain. Because the hypothalamus is so important in regulating, and interpreting the signals involved in hunger, satiety, and metabolism, inflammation can lead to a disruption in the pathway of these signals and even in how fat is stored. This can lead to weight gain.

It is also important to note that adequate sleep is also important to keep our hypothalamus healthy. The anterior region has an important role in regulating our circadian rhythm (which are physical and behavioural changes that occur on a daily cycle). An example of a circadian rhythm is being awake during the day and sleeping at nighttime which is influenced by the presence or absence of light (Seladi-Schulman, J., 2022, Jan). Adequate good quality sleep, which has been discussed in most of the science posts, has a great positive impact on many aspects of our weight and health.

Other influences also contribute to weight gain over time. According to the NIDDK (2018, February) weight gain can be influenced by: Family history and genes, race or ethnicity, age, sex, eating and physical activity habits, where you live, work, play, and worship, stress, lack of sleep, medical conditions and medications.

Gradually, according to set point theory, the normal body set point keeps adjusting upward over time if there is any disruption in our signalling system. Many factors influence this system and can lead to weight gain if the balance is interrupted. Factors include: lack of good sleep, poor digestion, lack of nutrition and vitamin/mineral deficiencies, increased stress, inadequate hydration, the development of insulin resistance, lack of movement/exercise, or any health/medical issues.

When we try to lose weight, our body fights to maintain the higher set point weight by slowing down our metabolism. This can ultimately limit weight loss. This is also when strategies such as eating less and/or exercising more begin to backfire, by feeding into that negative feed-back loop that further affects our hormones, stresses our body, and an even further lack of nutrition/vitamins/minerals, causing our bodies to hold onto our fat stores even more. This can also lead to mental and emotional duress as by implementing what we thought would help us lose the weight, actually sets us up for further weight gain and a sense of failure.

THE SETTLING POINT MODEL

However, there is a secondary theory for weight called the "settling point" model that is an enhancement to the set point theory. This concept suggests our weight is influenced by more than just physiological factors. How we navigate our food choices together with our biological traits and our energy balance affects weight shifts over time. This model can help us further understand obesity, especially in its rise, as it incorporates the influence of family/social dynamics of food, how the food itself has changed (food science and big business), environmental (chemicals/obesogens), socio-economic (having access to healthy food or alternatively living a more indulgent lifestyle) and the kind lifestyle you lead (active or inactive).

Overall, there are an abundance of different theories out there as well as groups researching obesity that have widely different views. However, what seems clear is the evidence that our weight is influenced by a complex set of internal and external signals — a combination of environmental and biological factors. The good news? The Livy Method helps us address all of these influences, including giving us the tools to do so!

CAN WE CHANGE OUR SET POINT WEIGHT? ACCORDING TO SET POINT THEORY, YES!

In order to reset our set point to a lower level, set point theory proponents recommend going slowly with weight loss goals. A gradual 10% step-down weight loss approach with persistent maintenance at each stage can help prepare the body to accept the new lower set point! This further corroborates why it is so important to allow our bodies to settle into its new weight and set point and embrace plateaus or stabilising periods as part of successful weight loss. This is also why it is important to allow adequate time for the body to adjust to maintenance by "consolidating your weight in maintenance" as Gina says. This is achieved by continuing with the plan for a few months upon achieving your goal, before reintroducing foods back into your life. Then it's about living your life, eating the foods that make you feel good, and doing so mindfully!

WHAT ABOUT CALORIES IN VS. CALORIES OUT?

According to set point theory, the reason typical diets don't work is that after a time, your body will fight reduced calorie intake by influencing your hunger hormones to leave you in a constant state of hunger and feelings of deprivation. It will then proceed to slow down your metabolism in an attempt to bring you back to your normal set point.

This can lead to binge eating and cycling through various diet programs like so many of us have experienced in the past. Set point theory believes your body and brain are in a struggle to regain a set point weight. However, by following a plan like The Livy Method which focuses on eating and feeding into your hunger signals, and allowing your insulin levels to stabilise over time, your hormone feedback system will improve. The Livy Method also focuses on improving digestive health, hydration, sleep, stress

management, eating nutrition rich foods to satisfaction, rather than strict calorie restrictions with large energy burns from exercise. All of these factors will ultimately help lower your set point.

Finally, it is important to stop thinking about food as calories. According to Harvard Medicine (2016, November), looking only at calories, and comparing calorie to calorie, ignores the important fact that our body processes various foods differently. In fact, the calories in more nutrient dense foods with higher fibre and water content, actually changes in how you digest it and retrieve the energy from that food (metabolic effect). An example of this would be when comparing a chocolate bar, and comparing its caloric equivalent in spinach, or nuts. You would feel naturally full on less when eating the spinach and nuts. Also, your body would receive much more nutritional benefit in the form of vitamins, minerals, and hormone stability. The chocolate bar would increase your blood sugar more than the spinach or nuts would, causing your body to release insulin to store the excess glucose. Increased insulin eventually leads to more intake, and thus the negative feedback loop has been stimulated.

Another consideration is that different foods go through different metabolic pathways. Some of these pathways are more efficient than others. According to Healthline (2018, May), the more efficient a metabolic pathway is, the more of the food's energy is used for work and less is dissipated as heat. The metabolic pathways for protein are less efficient than the metabolic pathways for carbs and fat. Protein contains 4 calories per gram, but a large part of these protein calories is lost as heat when it is metabolised by the body.

The thermic effect of food is a measure of how much different foods increase energy expenditure, due to the energy required to digest, absorb and metabolise the nutrients. Sources vary on the exact numbers, but it's clear that protein requires much more energy to metabolise than fat and carbs.

Therefore, to illustrate this when ingesting 100 calories of food, with a thermic effect of 25% for protein and 2% for fat, this would mean that 100 calories of protein would end up as 75 calories available, whereas 100 calories of fat would end up as 98 calories available to be used as energy or to be stored by the body.

Another example of this principle would be in how the body utilises fibre. There are 2 different types of fibre, soluble and insoluble. Both are important for health, digestion, and preventing diseases.

- **Soluble fibre** attracts water and turns to gel during digestion. This slows digestion. Soluble fibre is found in oat bran, barley, nuts, seeds, beans, lentils, peas, and some fruits and vegetables. It is also found in psyllium, a common fibre supplement. Some types of soluble fibre may help lower risk of heart disease.
- **Insoluble fibre** is found in foods such as wheat bran, vegetables, and whole grains. It adds bulk to the stool and appears to help food pass more quickly through the stomach and intestines.

The higher the fibre in foods, not only the better for your health, but less caloric energy is actually extracted from it for storage in the body. An example of this would be corn. Corn on the cob is nutritious, delicious, and high in fibre. In fact, it is very difficult for the body to process, requiring lots of chewing and work for the body to break down to use what it needs. However, if you take this same amount of corn and crush it into a flour and make a tortilla, the body hardly has to work, as it is already ground down and processed. In fact, most of its caloric energy is made available to the body, as opposed to when eating it in its whole form. This means the body will utilise almost all of the calories from the processed form, whereas the body will only use some of the calories in its whole form. Furthermore, its processed form can also impact the hormones in the body very differently. This may lead to an increased release in insulin and other hunger and satiety hormones, that can impact our hunger and satisfaction levels, which may lead us to eating more of it than we need! Hopefully this makes sense when understanding why it is recommended to eat food in its most whole form as much as possible, and there is a much clearer understanding behind the premise and science behind how The Livy Method results in weight loss.

Next week, we will be discussing The Basics of Digestion. Having a healthy digestive system is fundamental in optimizing weight loss, and an important focus of The Livy Method. Join us as we embark on the journey of learning more about the process of digestion, and how The Livy Method supports it.

REFERENCES

A history of restriction. (n.d). Alimentarium. https://www.alimentarium.org/en/fact-sheet/history-restriction

American College of Rheumatology. (2022, February). *Tumor necrosis factor (TNF) inhibitors.* https://www.rheumatology.org/I-Am-A/Patient-Caregiver/Treatments/TNF-Inhibitors

Aristizabal, J.C., Freidenreich, D.J., Volk, B.M., Kupchak, B.R., Saenz, C., Maresh, C.M., Kraemer, W.J., & Volek, J.S. (2015). Effect of resistance training on resting metabolic rate and its estimation by a dual-energy X-ray absorptiometry metabolic map. *European Journal of Clinical Nutrition, 69,* 831-836. https://doi.org/10.1038/ejcn.2014.216

Beth Israel Deaconess Medical Center. (2017, October 12). *Week one: The science of set point.* https://www.bidmc.org/about-bidmc/wellness-insights/nutrition/week-one-the-science-of-set-point

Centers for Disease Control and Prevention. (2022, May 17). *Adult obesity facts.* https://www.cdc.gov/obesity/data/adult.html

Centers for Disease Control and Prevention. (2022, June 3). *Obesity basics.* https://www.cdc.gov/obesity/basics/index.html

Centers for Disease Control and Prevention. (2022, July 14). *Why it matters.* https://www.cdc.gov/obesity/about-obesity/why-it-matters.html

Centers for Disease Control and Prevention. (2022, July 15). *Consequences of obesity.* https://www.cdc.gov/obesity/basics/consequences.html

Centers for Disease Control and Prevention. (2020, July 27). *Gout.* https://www.cdc.gov/arthritis/basics/gout.html#:~:text=quality%20of%20life%3F-,What%20is%20gout%3F,no%20symptoms%2C%20known%20as%20remission.

Considine, R.V., Sinha, M.K., Heiman, M.L., Kriauciunas, A., Stephens, T.W., Nyce, M.R., Ohannesian, J.P., Marco, C.C., McKee, L.J., Bauer, T.L., & Caro, J.F. (1996). Serum immunoreactive-leptin concentrations in normal-weight and obese humans. *The New England Journal of Medicine, 334,* 292-295. DOI: 10.1056/NEJM199602013340503

Dalvi, P.S., Chalmers, J.A., Luo, V., Han, D.-YD., Wellhauser, L., Liu, Y., Tran, D.Q., Castel, J., Luquet, S., Wheeler, M.B., & Belsham, D.D. (2017). High fat induces acute and chronic inflammation in the hypothalamus: Effect of high-fat diet, palmitate and TNF-α on appetite-regulating NPY neurons. *International Journal of Obesity, 41,* 149-158. https://doi.org/10.1038/ijo.2016.183

Diabetes Canada. (n.d.). *Type 2 diabetes.* https://www.diabetes.ca/about-diabetes/type-2

Dr. Wendi. (2020, September 15). *Hypothalamus and pituitary gland* [Video]. Youtube. https://www.youtube.com/watch?v=xCXtcoUxJZc

Gao, Y., Bielohuby, M., Fleming, T., Grabner, G.F., Foppen, E., Bernhard, W., Guzmán-Ruiz, M., Layritz, C., Legutko, B., Zinser, E., García-Cáceres, C., Buijs, R.M., Woods, S.C., Kalsbeek, A., Seeley, R.J., Nawroth, P.P., Bidlingmaier, M., Tschöp, M.H., & Yi, C.-X. (2017). Dietary sugars, not lipids, drive hypothalamic inflammation. *Molecular Metabolism, 6*(8), 897-908. https://doi.org/10.1016/j.molmet.2017.06.008

Geary, N. (2020). Control-theory models of body-weight regulation and body-weight-regulatory appetite. *Appetite, 144,* 104440. https://doi.org/10.1016/j.appet.2019.104440

Ghoshal, M. (2020, March 19). *What you need to know about set point theory.* Healthline. https://www.healthline. com/health/set-point-theory#summary

Government of Canada. (2020, November 5). Public Health Infobase. *Differences in obesity rates between rural communities and urban cities in Canada.* https://health-infobase.canada.ca/datalab/canadian-risk-factor-at-las-obesity-blog.html?=undefined&wbdisable=true

Government of Western Australia. (2018, January 25). *Set point theory.* Centre for Clinical Interventions. https:// www.cci.health.wa.gov.au/~/media/CCI/Mental%20Health%20Professionals/Eating%20Disorders/Eat-ing%20Disorders%20-%20Information%20Sheets/Eating%20Disorders%20Information%20Sheet%20 -%2024%20-%20Set%20Point%20Theory.pdf

Hall, K.D., Ayuketah, A., Brychta, R., Cai, Hongyi., Cassimatis, T., Chen, K.Y., Chung, S.t., Costa, E., Courville, A., Darcey, V., Fletcher, L.A., Forde, C.G., Gharib, A.M., Guo, J., Howard, R., Joseph, P.V., McGehee, S., Ouwerkerk, R., Raisinger, K., … Zhou, M. (2019). Ultra-processed diets cause excess calorie intake and weight gain: An inpatient randomized controlled trial of ad libitum food intake. *Cell Metabolism, 30(*1),67-77.E3. https://doi.org/10.1016/j.cmet.2019.05.008

Harris R. B. (1990). Role of set-point theory in regulation of body weight. *FASEB Journal.* 4(15), 3310–3318. https://doi.org/10.1096/fasebj.4.15.2253845

Heart attack. (n.d). Johns Hopkins Medicine. https://www.hopkinsmedicine.org/health/conditions-and-diseases/ heart-attack

Hjorth, M.F., Roager, H.M., Larsen, T.M., Poulsenn, S.K., Licht, T.R., Bahl, M.I., Zohar, Y., & Astrup, A. (2018). Pre-treatment microbial prevotella-to-bacteroides ratio, determines body fat loss success during a 6-month randomized controlled diet intervention. *International Journal of Obesity, 42,* 580-583. https://doi. org/10.1038/ijo.2017.220

Houle, B. (2013, December 3). *How obesity relates to socioeconomic status.* Population Reference Bureau. https:// www.prb.org/resources/how-obesity-relates-to-socioeconomic-status/#:~:text=They%20found%20that%20 obesity%20rose,less%20likely%20to%20be%20obese.

Jung, C. H., & Kim, M. S. (2013). Molecular mechanisms of central leptin resistance in obesity. *Archives of Phar-macal Research*, *36*(2), 201–207. https://doi.org/10.1007/s12272-013-0020-y

Kearns, C.E., Schmidt, L.A., & Glantz, S.A. (2016). Sugar industry and coronary heart disease research: A histor-ical analysis of internal industry documents. *JAMA Internal Medicine, 176*(11), 1680–1685. doi:10.1001/ jamainternmed.2016.5394

Liu, S., Munasinghe, L.L., Ohinmaa, A., & Veugelers, P.J. (2020). Added, free and total sugar content and consumption of foods and beverages in Canada. *Health Reports, 31*(10), 14-24. https://www.doi. org/10.25318/82-003-x202001000002-eng

Mayo Clinic Staff. (2021, February 6). *Cirrhosis.* Mayo Clinic. https://www.mayoclinic.org/diseases-conditions/ cirrhosis/symptoms-causes/syc-20351487#:~:text=Cirrhosis%20is%20a%20late%20stage,it%20tries%20 to%20repair%20itself

Müller, M. J., Bosy-Westphal, A., & Heymsfield, S. B. (2010). Is there evidence for a set point that regulates human body weight?. *F1000 medicine reports, 2,* 59. https://doi.org/10.3410/M2-59

Müller, M.J., Geisler, C., Heymsfield, S.B., & Bosy-Westphal A. (2018). Recent advances in understanding body weight homeostasis in humans [version 1; peer review: 4 approved]. *F1000Research*, *7*[F1000 Faculty Rev]1025 https://doi.org/10.12688/f1000research.14151.1

National Institute of Diabetes and Digestive and Kidney Diseases. (2018, February). *Factors affecting weight & health.* https://www.niddk.nih.gov/health-information/weight-management/adult-overweight-obesity/factors-affecting-weight-health

National Institute of Diabetes and Digestive and Kidney Diseases. (2018, February). *Health risks of overweight & obesity.* https://www.niddk.nih.gov/health-information/weight-management/adult-overweight-obesity/health-risks?dkrd=/health-information/weight-management/health-risks-overweight

National Institute of Diabetes and Digestive and Kidney Diseases. (2021, September). *Overweight & obesity statistics.* https://www.niddk.nih.gov/health-information/health-statistics/overweight-obesity

Nonalcoholic fatty liver disease. (n.d). Johns Hopkins Medicine. https://www.hopkinsmedicine.org/health/conditions-and-diseases/nonalcoholic-fatty-liver-disease

Pesta, D.H., & Samuel, V.T. (2014). A high-protein diet for reducing body fat: Mechanisms and possible caveats. *Nutrition & Metabolism*, *11*(1), 53. https://doi.org/10.1186/1743-7075-11-53

Petty, R.E. (2016). Structure and function. In R.E. Petty, R.M. Laxer, C.B. Lindsley & L.R Wedderburn (Eds.), *Textbook of pediatric rheumatology (7th ed., pp.* 5-13.e2). W.B. Saunders. https://doi.org/10.1016/B978-0-323-24145-8.00002-8

Pugle, M. (2022, January 27). *How your body tries to prevent you from losing too much weight.* Healthline.https://www.healthline.com/health-news/how-your-body-tries-to-prevent-you-from-losing-too-much-weight

SANESolution bibliography table of contents. (n.d.). SANESolution. https://sanesolution.com/sanesolution-bibliography/

Sarwan, G., & Rehman, A. (2022, June 5). Management of weight loss plateau. In *StatPearls*. StatPearls Publishing. https://www.ncbi.nlm.nih.gov/books/NBK576400/

Schoeller, D.A., Cella, L.K, Sinha, M.K., & Caro, J.F. (1997). Entrainment of the diurnal rhythm of plasma leptin to meal timing. *The Journal of Clinical Investigation, 100*(7), 1882-1887. https://doi.org/10.1172/JCI119717

Seladi-Schulman, J. (2022, January 31). *Hypothalamus overview.* Healthline. https://www.healthline.com/human-body-maps/hypothalamus

Soluble vs. insoluble fiber. (n.d). MedlinePlus. https://medlineplus.gov/ency/article/002136.htm#:~:text=Insoluble%20fiber%20is%20found%20in,through%20the%20stomach%20and%20intestines.

Stunkard, A.J., Harris, J.R., Pedersen, N.L., & McClearn, G.E. (1990). The body-mass index of twins who have been reared apart. *The New England Journal of Medicine, 322*, 1483-1487. DOI: 10.1056/NEJM199005243222102

The dangers of uncontrolled sleep apnea. (n.d). Johns Hopkins Medicine. https://www.hopkinsmedicine.org/health/wellness-and-prevention/the-dangers-of-uncontrolled-sleep-apnea

Wdowik, M. (2017, November 6). The long, strange history of dieting fads. *The Conversation.* https://theconversation.com/the-long-strange-history-of-dieting-fads-82294

World Health Organization. (n.d). *Obesity.* https://www.who.int/health-topics/obesity#tab=tab_1

THE BASICS OF DIGESTION

Our plan is to take a deeper dive into many topics, but we are going to start by building onto some of the fundamental concepts that are important to our overall health and subsequently weight loss. One of the most important topics that we are going to start with is the basics of digestion.

Many of you reported coming into this program with digestive issues, or wanting to know more about how your body may respond to the plan with issues like IBS, Crohn's disease, GERD (Gastric-Esophageal Reflux), missing your gallbladder, gastric bypass or other modifications. So, we are going to break this all down for you in our series about the digestive system!

WHY IS DIGESTION SO IMPORTANT?

Digestion is the complex process where our body breaks down the food and liquids that we eat in the form of carbohydrates, proteins and fats, into smaller components and nutrients, which the body uses for energy, growth, and cell repair. If there are any impairments in this process, there can be an impact in how our body is able to absorb and utilize the nutrients, vitamins, and minerals that we need to maintain optimal health! This is why with The Livy Method, there is a huge emphasis on improving digestive health, eating nutritious food, and making all meals and snacks as nutrient dense as possible.

THE CEPHALIC PHASE:

Many of us don't realize this, but digestion actually starts in our brain! When we think about, see, smell, touch, or taste food, our hormones become activated. We begin to secrete **saliva** in our mouths and our stomachs begin to secrete gastric juices. In fact, this phase is responsible for the secretion of up to 50% of our gastric and digestive hormone secretions, in order to aid in the processing of what we eat (Zafra, M.A., Molina, F., & Puerto, A., 2006)!

This is where our mindfulness should really start, in order to take full advantage of the optimal digestion of our foods. We can do this by checking in with ourselves to see what ingredients appeal to us most, taking the time to prepare our foods thoughtfully, and using all our senses in the food preparation process. Be in the moment and enjoy it!

Thus, the cephalic phase is a perfect time to really dive into the first two mindfulness questions of eating: Are you feeling hungry? How is this portion for me?

THE EATING PHASE:

The next phase of digestion continues to the mouth with the ingestion of food. This is where we begin to chew our foods and saliva continues to flood into our mouths. The action of chewing with our teeth helps to break down the foods we are eating into smaller bits for our body to process, mixing with enzymes contained in our saliva. **"Enzymes" are special proteins we have in our body that help speed up certain chemical reactions, and are involved in helping to build certain substances or break them down (like in the case of digestion).**

Although we have multiple glands that produce saliva and enzymes, the **parotid gland** is most responsible for producing **amylase (the enzymes that help break down carbohydrates into glucose).** Our saliva also provides lubrication to help our food to travel down our digestive tract. The most important part of this phase is the act of chewing, as it allows for good mixing of the broken-down food with the saliva and enzymes. It also does some good work of breaking down the food before it enters our stomach. The big takeaway here is, the better we are able to chew our food, the better our bodies are able to process it!

This is where we can really tune into the third set of mindfulness questions; Are you getting full? Is this food satisfying you? How would you feel if you took a few more bites? How would you feel if you stop eating now? Do you feel any physical effects of eating? Doing this allows us to chew our foods from our meals and snacks as they were meant to be chewed, instead of rushing through the process.

This is really important when we are eating those 4-5 token bites when we aren't hungry, in order to get the digestive process going. Which is why it is recommended to chew, chew, chew, chew, chew, chew, chew, chew with every bite while having our token bites!

THE PROCESS OF DIGESTION

ESOPHAGUS & STOMACH

When we swallow the food we have chewed (which is now called a "**bolus**"), it passes through our throat via the **pharynx** to the **esophagus**. The esophagus is a smooth muscular tube that is attached from our throat to our stomach that uses involuntary muscular contractions to propel the bolus to our stomach. This process is called **peristalsis.**

Once the food enters into the stomach, the cells in the stomach lining begin to secrete gastric juices that are rich in **HCl (Hydro-Chloric Acid)**. This increases the acidic environment of the stomach and activates **pepsin, the enzyme responsible for breaking down protein into amino acids**. Amino acids are then able to be used by the body as building blocks for vital processes such as building proteins, hormones, and neurotransmitters.

This acidic environment is also important for our immunity/defense system, as it creates an inhospitable environment for bacteria and other pathogens to grow, thus keeping us healthy!

The stomach begins to churn and contract, and that food we worked so hard to break down by chewing, forms a semi-liquid form of partially digested food called "**chyme**".

The small intestine, the liver, the gallbladder, and the pancreas

The stomach stores the contents of the chyme, and it is slowly emptied into the small intestine. The small intestine is divided into three different segments, known as the **duodenum, the jejunum** and the **ileum**.

The chyme first enters our **duodenum (the first part of our small intestine)** at a rate of about two teaspoons per minute. The duodenum receives enzymes from a variety of organs also involved in the digestive process; **the liver, the gallbladder, and the pancreas.**

The liver is a large organ located above the stomach in the upper abdomen. The liver produces bile which is stored in the gallbladder, stores nutrients, and helps remove toxins from the body.

When we eat fatty foods, the gallbladder (a small pouch) is stimulated to secrete **bile** via the **bile ducts** to the small intestine, which helps to emulsify the fats and makes it easier for **lipases (enzymes that break down fat)** to do their job!

The pancreas which is located in the upper part of the abdomen, behind the stomach, secretes what is known as "**pancreatic juice.**" This juice contains a substance called **bicarbonate (which helps to neutralize the high acidity of the incoming food)** and pancreatic enzymes. These pancreatic enzymes include **protease (which breaks down protein)** as well as amylase and lipase which have been discussed earlier. The pancreas also produces chemicals that help regulate blood sugar levels, which affect how much energy the body has available to use. One of these is the infamous **insulin**, which we will discuss in more detail in our series.

The small intestine also secretes its own enzymes for digestion known as **peptidases, sucrase, lactase** and **maltase.** These enzymes contribute mostly to the **hydrolysis of polysaccharides,** meaning they use water to break down these longer chain carbohydrate molecules into simpler sugars like glucose.

Once our food has been broken down into the basic building blocks of glucose, amino acids, vitamins, minerals, and fatty acids, they are ready to be absorbed into our bloodstream which carries the nutrients to cells throughout the body! The small Intestine is where most of digestion and absorption take place. The chyme moves in rhythmic movements along the intestines to allow for the mixing of fluids, and for a longer period of time for digestion to take place. The walls of the intestines are lined with finger-like projections called villi, which are then lined further with even tinier finger-like projections called microvilli. These allow for an incredibly expansive surface area for all of this absorption to take place, providing your body with those super important nutrients and energy!!!

THE LARGE INTESTINE

The last phase of digestion is the movement of the remaining undigested food into the large intestine (otherwise known as the **colon**) into the formation of stool or poop. The colon is primarily responsible for the reabsorption of water and the last bit of nutrients from this final stage of processing food, the content that remains forms stools which we poop out through our **rectum** via the **anus.**

The colon also contains our gut flora which is composed of trillions of microbes known as the **microbiome.** This is definitely a hot topic around here with our members, and a topic we will be looking further into down the road. These bacteria help to ferment the indigestible food and produce vitamins such as Vitamin K and B vitamins that are reabsorbed by the colon. But that's not all, an estimated 80% of our immune system is found in our gut (Wiertsema SP, Van Bergenhenegouwen J, Garssen J,

Knippels, 2021). Having a healthy digestive system, which includes a good balance of our healthy gut flora, ensures a healthier immune system and better nutrient absorption. This is why the Livy Method recommends taking a good quality probiotic, along with a prebiotic (if needed), to help feed those good microbes. Eating the high fibre, nutrient rich foods on plan not only gives our body what it needs, but is also vital in supporting our gut flora.

For a comprehensive video looking at digestion, check out this video:

https://www.youtube.com/watch?v=X3TAROotFfM

THE LAST QUESTION IN MINDFULNESS

This sums up the topic of the basics of digestion, and brings us to the fourth series of questions in mindfulness when eating. Do you feel full and if so, what is your definition of full? How do you know when you have eaten enough? How do you feel physically? Meaning, is it a physically full belly feeling, or is it more of an insulin rush or a tired feeling? Or is it that you just eat everything on your plate because it's there kind of thing? Or maybe you feel like you could eat more?

As you can see, establishing mindfulness around your eating not only helps you connect and become more in tune with your body, but additionally promotes optimal digestion! Hope this helps!

Now that we understand the basics of digestion, we will build upon this knowledge in the coming weeks. However, next week we will initiate the conversation regarding the concept of "effort", and how the psychology of effort can impact our weight loss journey and process.

REFERENCES

Anatomy of the digestive system. (2017). BarCharts, Inc.

Azzouz, L.L., & Sharma, S. (2021). *Physiology, large intestine.* StatPearls Publishing. https://www.ncbi.nlm.nih.gov/books/NBK507857/

Boland, M. (2016). Human digestion - a processing perspective. *Journal of the Science of Food and Agriculture, 96*(7), 2275–2283. https://doi.org/10.1002/jsfa.7601

Granger, N.D., Morris, J. D., Kvietys, P. R., & Granger, J. P. (2018). *Physiology and Pathophysiology of Digestion.* Morgan & Claypool Life Science Publishers.

McClements, D.J. (2019). *Future foods: How modern science is transforming the way we eat. Copernicus Publications.* https://doi.org/10.1007/978-3-030-12995-8

Morris, J.D., Granger, D. N., Granger, J. P., & Kvietys, P. R. (2018). *Physiology and Pathophysiology of Digestion: Part 2.* Biota Publishing.

Prados, A. (2022, February, 2). *Four science-backed ways of taking care of your gut microbiota.* Gut Microbiota for Health. https://www.gutmicrobiotaforhealth.com/four-science-backed-ways-of-taking-care-of-your-gut-microbiota

Schwenke, T. (2020, May 3). *Human digestive system - How it works!* [Video]. Youtube. https://www.youtube.com/watch?v=X3TAROotFfM

Sethi, S., & Jewell, T. (2019, February 1). *What causes dysbiosis and how is it treated?* Healthline. https://www.healthline.com/health/digestive-health/dysbiosis

Wiertsema, S. P., van Bergenhenegouwen, J., Garssen, J., & Knippels, L. M. J. (2021). The Interplay between the Gut Microbiome and the Immune System in the Context of Infectious Diseases throughout Life and the Role of Nutrition in Optimizing Treatment Strategies. *Nutrients, 13*(3), 886. MDPI AG. Retrieved from http://dx.doi.org/10.3390/nu13030886

Your digestive system & how it works. (2017, December). National Institute of Diabetes and Digestive and Kidney Diseases. Retrieved March 30, 2022, from https://www.niddk.nih.gov/health-information/digestive-diseases/digestive-system-how-it-works

Zafra, M.A., Molina, F., & Puerto, A. (2006). The neural/cephalic phase reflexes in the physiology of nutrition. *Neuroscience and Biobehavioral Reviews,* 30(7), 1032–1044. https://doi.org/10.1016/j.neubiorev.2006.03.005

THE PSYCHOLOGY OF EFFORT

In this post we are initiating the conversation about the concept of the psychology of "effort", and how effort can impact our weight loss journey and process. So, to better understand more about the psychological concept of effort and the kind of impact it has, let's take a deeper dive into effort! We will also discuss the concept of setting goals, the formation of habits (which will help in forming more positive ones in order to help with weight loss), and how to navigate through psychological roadblocks that may impact weight loss.

For so many of us, the journey behind weight loss can be a daunting and overwhelming process. Many of us have been on the hamster wheel of dieting and trying to lose weight for many years or have tried more diets than we can count. And yet here we are again, some of us at our wits end, unsure that The Livy Method will work. For many of us, this is our last attempt before giving up and accepting our current reality as our future.

HOW IS THE LIVY METHOD DIFFERENT?

With this method, there is a completely different emphasis on how we should be treating our bodies as well as our mindsets. We are changing our focus to supporting our bodies by giving our bodies what they need, establishing good nutrition, and on lifestyle changes that complement the weight loss process. We are also challenging ourselves in a more cerebral and emotional way, by purposefully implementing tweaks that address issues we may have consciously or subconsciously. The Livy Method post and video is an excellent resource, discussing how this process is different from the other diets that are out there or what we have experienced in the past!

However, this method is not a quick fix and may require some amount of effort in order to attain success! Although many members come into this process with gusto, ready to do all it takes, many can also be challenged as time evolves and their level of success may not be reflected by their perceived effort. Everybody is different, with different histories, physiologies and health issues they may be working through, varying mental/emotional experiences, stresses, financial situations, as well as life challenges. To be straight up, some people may need a lot of help and time before their body may be willing to make changes or start to drop weight on the scale. Some may really struggle with the time and energy it may take to work through this.

This raises the question, what happens when one's effort does not match their success on the scale? Many people use the scale to judge their level of achievement, yet discount any possible **NSVs (non-scale victories)** that they may have experienced or are experiencing. They may also not be realistic about the time that may be required to get their bodies healthy before they will begin to drop any weight.

Effort is a very interesting and complicated concept, as one may perceive they are exerting much more effort than they truly are, thus expecting a bigger return than they may be experiencing. In fact, they may be seeing themselves at their finish line in their minds, yet not putting in the actual level of effort required, thus feeling frustration with their current experience as reflected on the scale. Effort is subjective and irreflective of outcome. Let's delve deeper into the concept of Effort.

EFFORT DEFINED

Effort refers to the "subjective intensification of mental and/or physical activity in the service of meeting some goal" (Inzlicht, M., Shenhav, A., & Olivola, C. Y., 2018). Although related, effort is not the same as **motivation**, "which is a force that drives behavior by determining both a direction (e.g., goal) and the intensity or vigor with which this direction is pursued". Effort refers to the intensity of behavior but does not refer to any specific goal.

Effort is an "intentional process and application, therefore it corresponds with what a person is actively doing and not to what is passively happening to them. Effort is distinguishable from demand or difficulty, as effort corresponds to the intensity of mental or physical work that someone applies to achieve some outcome. Although effort typically involves demand (with people working harder when the task is more difficult), this relationship breaks down when incentives are too low or when demands are too high. Finally, it is important to distinguish effort from associated mental constructs, such as boredom." (Inzlicht, M., Shenhav, A., & Olivola, C. Y., 2018)

Effort can also be "visible to others and is difficult to fake, making it plain to observers whether someone is exerting themselves or not. The fact that effort is easily recognized in self and others gives it important signaling functions; for example, communicating dedication, intention, and commitment" (Inzlicht, M., Shenhav, A., & Olivola, C. Y., 2018).

THE PARADOX OF EFFORT

Effort, whether it is mental or physical, is a common occurrence in daily life and is encountered every time we need to push ourselves. We regularly face activities that require us to exert some level of energy to achieve a goal or task, whether it is forcing ourselves to get up for work, or exercise at the end of the day.

Effort is often associated with something that can feel difficult and averse and as a result, people tend to avoid effort, including the effort that comes from merely thinking things through. In fact, people often develop strategies that allow them to avoid situations that require more work or effort.

However, in contrast to this, while people will work hard to obtain something of value, working hard can also make those same things more valuable. In fact, effort can even be experienced as valuable or rewarding in its own right. People may readily apply more effort for better outcomes, and view those outcomes as more rewarding if more (not less) effort was used to attain them! In the example of weight loss, a person may see more value in the work they put in to achieve their weight loss goal, than in the actual weight loss itself!

COGNITIVE DISSONANCE THEORY AND EFFORT JUSTIFICATION

According to cognitive dissonance theory and its research, the more effort one exerts, the more valuable one perceives the reward associated with that effort (Harmon-Jones, E., Clark, D., Paul, K., & Harmon-Jones, C., 2020). This effect has been referred to as effort justification. Thus, cognitive dissonance theory would suggest that increasing the attractiveness of a reward would encourage greater effort, however we need to be clear on the effort we are really exerting. In the Livy Method members sometimes feel that the reward (e.g. weight loss) is not reflective of their effort. However, the Livy Method 20 questions assessment will help members to rate the effort they are truly exerting, and thus identify where they can level up. Basically, you may tell yourself that you are doing all the things, although in reality you may not be. While following the Livy Method may be challenging and unpleasant for some, being realistic about the effort you are applying (through the 20 questions) will help reduce the cognitive dissonance and stress when you think you are doing everything, but in reality there are ways we can always level up.

According to cognitive dissonance theory, when perceived effort does not match your results; "I should be at my goal" is in contradiction with the cognition, "I am not seeing the weight loss I had expected to see on the scale." The dissonance can be reduced by examining if "I am maximizing each aspect of the 20 questions and doing all the things." The variables of critical importance in dissonance theory are psychological (subjective) (e.g., the perception of effort). Because one may be perceiving themselves as exerting maximum effort, although they still have a long road ahead of them. They may be elevating the effort they are putting into the weight loss process, yet, in reality could be doing so much more.

Dissonance theory research suggests that people use effort justification when they perceive their goal cannot be predicted with certainty, and so they use how much effort they perceive they are exerting as a justification for obtaining the reward. This causes cognitive dissonance when the reward (in our case weight loss) is not immediately apparent.

Check out this video that explains the theory of cognitive dissonance in more detail!

https://www.youtube.com/watch?v=9Y17YaZRRvY

Check out this video that explains effort justification in more detail!

https://www.youtube.com/watch?v=PEGEJ21kASQ

WHAT IS BEING VALUED, EFFORT ITSELF OR THE PRODUCT OF EFFORT?

There is evidence that people hold greater value to goods and outcomes (e.g., group membership, furniture, coffee mugs, etc.) that they worked for and required effort, compared with identical goods and outcomes that they obtained without effort (e.g., by chance, as windfalls). Therefore, it can be assumed that those that achieved weight loss by following the plan and putting in a good effort to do so, will see the outcome of the process as more valuable.

People tend to associate effort with reward and will sometimes select objects or activities precisely because they require effort (e.g., mountain climbing, marathons). Effort adds value to the products achieved, but effort itself also has value. The value of effort is not only accessed concurrently with, or immediately following effort exertion, but is also in anticipation of such expenditure, suggesting that we already have an intuitive understanding of effort's potential positive value.

From examining the literature around effort, it can be seen that putting real effort into The Livy Method is putting in real effort into yourself. That effort alone may have value to you, even if it is difficult. Recognizing the scale and NSVs accomplished, will also increase the value you achieve from this process. However, it is important to see things from an accurate lens and to be real. Recognize where you could truly put in more effort. Be honest when answering the 20 questions so you can see where you can level up and maximize your efforts!

Now that we have discussed the importance of effort, let's talk about setting goals to put forth your effort into action!

SETTING GOALS REWIRES YOUR BRAIN'S EFFECTIVENESS

Goal setting can be very powerful and can motivate people to accomplish tasks they might not have thought they could.

A study in Behavioral and Cognitive Neuroscience Reviews showed that people that set goals are generally more "together" than everyone else (Top Stack, 2019, November). This is because goal setting rewires our brains to make the component parts work more effectively. This study showed that when you set a goal, multiple parts of the brain are suddenly engaged: The amygdala, which is the brain's emotional center, evaluates the goal for how important it is to you. The frontal lobe, which is the brain's logical problem-solving portion, defines the goal and digests it. Both the amygdala and the frontal lobe then work together to push you toward the completion of the goal. As the brain moves you into situations to help you achieve your goal, the organ changes to help you optimize behaviors and tasks.

Another study, in the Journal of Applied Psychology reports that people who established an ambitious goal usually achieved it. The study suggested that ambitious goals stimulate the brain more, motivating the person to accomplish the impossible. The study found that the higher the goal that was set, the more likely one would achieve it. The Psychological Bulletin said 90% of the studies showed that more challenging goals led to higher performance. More manageable goals, "do your best" goals, or no goals did not have the same effect on the brain, or the person's ability to achieve their goals. Researchers report that "goal setting is most likely to improve task performance when the goals are specific and sufficiently challenging" (Top Stack, 2019, November). Also, decades of research on achievement suggests that successful people reach their goals not simply because of who they are, but more often because of what they do.

Interestingly, these studies suggest brain rewiring occurs when the individual sets the goal themselves. However, the brain does not seem to change if the goal is set by someone else. When we apply this to the Livy Method it calls attention to the importance of regularly checking in on your "why" – it is only you who can decide your "why".

So, for those looking for success while following the Livy Method, let's talk more about the process of goal setting!

1. Get specific. When you set yourself a goal, try to be as specific as possible. "Lose 5 pounds" is a better goal than "lose some weight," because it gives you a clear idea of what success looks like. Knowing exactly what you want to achieve keeps you motivated until you get there. Also, think about the specific actions recommended by The Livy Method that need to be taken to reach your goal. Just stating you will "sleep more" is too vague, be clear and precise. "I'll be in bed by 10pm on weeknights, and sleep between 7-8 hours" is a specific goal.

2. Seize the moment to act on your goals. For example, increasing your activity or exercise is part of maximizing. Achieving your goal means organizing this activity into your calendar, especially as many of us live busy lives! Be as specific as possible (e.g., "on Monday, Wednesday, or Friday, I'll work out for 45 minutes before work."). Studies show that this kind of planning will help your brain to detect and seize the opportunity when it arises, increasing your chances of success by roughly 300% (Grant, H., 2011, February).

3. Know exactly how you are progressing. Achieving any goal also requires honest and regular monitoring of your progress. If you do not know how well you are doing, you are not able to adjust your behavior or strategies accordingly. While following The Livy Method, check your progress daily by using the APP to document your weight, water, activity, sleep, meals, snacks, and journal. This will keep your head in the game as you are maintaining accountability and seeing your daily weight progress will help keep you focused.

4. Be a realistic optimist. Believing in your ability to succeed is enormously helpful for creating and sustaining your motivation. However, do not underestimate how difficult it may be to reach your goal. Most goals worth achieving require time, planning, effort, and persistence. Studies show that people that assume that things will happen easily and with little effort, will have more difficulty achieving their goal as they may be unprepared for the journey ahead.

5. Have grit. Grit is a willingness to commit to long-term goals, and to persist in the face of difficulty. Grit is a good determiner of who will be successful in the long term. Everyone has the potential for grit!! By putting in the effort, planning, persistence, and strategies needed to succeed, will not only help you see yourself and your goals more accurately, but also do wonders for your grit.

6. Make sure your choices are in line with your goals. We make multiple choices and decisions every day. When you are choosing what to eat, take a minute to think through – is this in

line with my goals? Will this help advance my journey to finally and forever? Think through what choice you are making and be comfortable with the decision you make.

FOCUS ON WHAT YOU HAVE ACHIEVED

On the days when you feel frustrated with yourself for not meeting your goals, try taking a closer look at the things you have achieved. Revisiting what you have accomplished in the process so far can help you keep things in perspective. This is a good time to examine your "why" of wanting to lose weight or to get healthier by participating in the program. It is also important to look deeper at all the non-scale victories you have experienced!

KNOW YOUR LIMITS

Even with the best intentions and the willingness to put in maximum effort, you may not find it possible to improve every situation or meet every expectation. Although effort can get you closer to fulfilling your weight loss goal, you might need additional resources you just don't have access to, like the financial limitations of purchasing supplements, or may be overwhelmed with stress, or at capacity. You are a human being with normal physical and emotional limitations. If you find yourself not meeting an expectation you have set, acknowledge that you did your best and offer yourself compassion instead of blame. You will get there!

SHARE YOUR EXPECTATIONS

Discuss your goals and needs with the supporters in your life. By sharing your needs with those in your immediate circle, you are actively communicating what will help you be successful. This will help ensure your success in meeting your goals, but also allows those that care about you to support and be there for you!

KEEP A FLEXIBLE MINDSET

The more flexible you are with your goals, the better you will be able to accommodate life's unpredictability. The path to weight loss as we know is not a straight one. Just do the best you can and roll with the punches!

The last thing that will be discussed along with effort, goal setting, and expectations, is the formation of habits. Oftentimes it is certain habits that have led us to the path of weight gain or yo-yo dieting. However, The Livy Method is about real change, and implementing healthier life habits. Let's examine how long we may expect to incite real change into our lives.

HOW LONG DOES IT TAKE TO FORM A NEW HABIT?

According to a 2009 study published in the European Journal of Social Psychology, "it takes 18 to 254 days for a person to form a new habit" (Legg, T.J., & Frothingham, S., 2019, October). The study also concluded that, on average, it takes 66 days for a new behavior to become automatic, ultimately depending on the habit in question.

- Certain habits take longer to form. As demonstrated in the study, many participants found it easier to adopt the habit of drinking a glass of water at breakfast, than to do 50 sit-ups after their morning coffee.

- Some people are better suited to forming habits than others, as some gravitate towards a consistent routine, whereas others do not.

HOW THE MYTH OF "21 DAYS" CAME ABOUT

Many people subscribe to the belief that it takes 21 days to create a new habit. This concept can be traced back to "Psycho-Cybernetics," a book published in 1960 by Dr. Maxwell Maltz. Dr. Maltz identified this number as an observable metric in both himself and his patients and wrote, "these, and many other commonly observed phenomena, tend to show that it requires a minimum of about 21 days for an old mental image to dissolve and a new one to gel." As the book became more popular, this situational observation has become accepted as fact.

THE PSYCHOLOGY OF FORMING A HABIT

According to a 2012 study published in the British Journal of General Practice, habits are "actions that are triggered automatically in response to contextual cues that have been associated with their performance" (Legg, T.J., & Frothingham, S., 2019, October). For example, when you get into your car, you automatically put on the seat belt. You do not think about doing it or why you do it, you just do it. Your brain likes habits because they are efficient, and when you automate common actions, you free up mental resources for other tasks.

WHY IT CAN BE DIFFICULT TO BREAK A HABIT

According to the National Institutes of Health (NIH), pleasure-based habits are particularly difficult to break, because enjoyable behavior prompts your brain to release dopamine (Legg, T.J., & Frothingham, S., 2019, October). Dopamine is the reward that strengthens the habit and creates the craving to do it again. As discussed in the post on hormones, sugar also stimulates our dopamine response, eventually leading to a dulled response. We often seek more of these types of foods to stimulate the dopamine release. This may also account for snacking at night. You may enjoy some chips as you unwind for the night, while watching television. This will start to stimulate the dopamine reward center, reinforcing the habit of snacking while watching television. These types of habits may have a negative impact on the success of following The Livy Method.

HOW TO CHANGE A HABIT

Dr. Nora Volkow, director of the NIH's National Institute on Drug Abuse, suggests that the first step is to become more aware of your habits so you can develop strategies to change them. One strategy Volkow suggests is to identify the places, people, or activities that are connected in your mind to certain habits, and then adjust your behavior toward those things.

For example, if you like to eat chips, you can avoid buying chips until you feel more comfortable being around them without wanting to impulsively eat them. This can help you achieve your goal of avoiding them as you start your weight loss journey until your habit has changed.

Another strategy is to replace a bad habit with a good one. For example, instead of snacking on these same potato chips at night when watching TV, consider swapping them out for a nice warm cup of tea. Over time, you will change your association of watching tv with eating chips, creating a new routine with healthier habits when unwinding in the evenings.

In summation, it can take anywhere from 18 to 254 days for a person to form a new habit, and an average of 66 days for a new behavior to become automatic. Everyone is different, as well as their life circumstances, reinforcing why this time frame may be so different for everyone. Some habits are easier to form than others, and some people may find it easier to develop new behaviors than others. Just know that the only timeline that matters is the one that works best for you. If you maximize all your efforts, have the confidence that you WILL achieve your goals.

Now that we understand more about effort, setting goals, and the formation of habits that can influence our weight loss journey, stay tuned for the next post where we will be discussing DETOX!

REFERENCES

Axsom, D., & Cooper, J. (1985). Cognitive dissonance and psychotherapy: The role of effort justification in inducing weight loss. *Journal of Experimental Psychology, 21*(2), 149-160. https://doi.org/10.1016/0022-1031(85)90012-5

Berkman, E. T. (2018). The neuroscience of goals and behavior change. *Consulting Psychology Journal, 70*(1), 28–44. https://doi.org/10.1037/cpb0000094

Cherry, K., & Morin, A. (2020, July 22). *Self efficacy and why believing in yourself matters.* Verywell Mind. https://www.verywellmind.com/what-is-self-efficacy-2795954

Frey, M., & Goldman, R. (2021, June 28). *How to overcome 5 psychological blocks to weight loss.* Verywell Fit. https://www.verywellfit.com/overcome-emotional-stress-to-lose-weight-3495947

Grant, H. (2011, February 25). *Nine things successful people do differently.* Harvard Business Review. https://hbr.org/2011/02/nine-things-successful-people

Harmon-Jones, E., Clark, D., Paul, K., & Harmon-Jones, C. (2020). The effect of perceived effort on reward valuation: Taking the reward positivity (RewP) to dissonance theory. *Frontiers in Human Neuroscience, 14*(157). https://doi.org/10.3389/fnhum.2020.00157

Inzlicht, M., Shenhav, A., & Olivola, C. Y. (2018). The effort paradox: Effort is both costly and valued. *Trends in Cognitive Sciences, 22*(4), 337–349. https://doi.org/10.1016/j.tics.2018.01.007

Knight, R. (2014, December 29). *Make your work resolutions stick.* Harvard Business Review. https://hbr.org/2014/12/make-your-work-resolutions-stick

Krueger, J., & Perina, K. (2021, May 15). *Effort and value: Is the hard work worth it?* Psychology Today. https://www.psychologytoday.com/ca/blog/one-among-many/202105/effort-and-value

Legg, T.J., & Frothingham, S. (2019, October 24). *How long does it take for a new behavior to become automatic?* Healthline. https://www.healthline.com/health/how-long-does-it-take-to-form-a-habit

Legg, T.J., & Raypole, C. (2020, November 30). *Dreaming too big? 12 tips for understanding and reframing unrealistic expectations.* Healthline. https://www.healthline.com/health/mental-health/unrealistic-expectations

Maich, K.H. (2013). Reducing cognitive dissonance through effort justification: Evidence from past studies and daily experience. *Western Undergraduate Psychology Journal, 1* (1). https://ojs.lib.uwo.ca/index.php/wupj/article/download/1659/1038

Teixeira, P.J., Silva, M.N., Mata, J., Palmeir, A.L., & Markland, D. (2012). Motivation, self-determination, and long-term weight control. *International Journal of Behavioral Nutrition and Physical Activity, 9*, 22. https://doi.org/10.1186/1479-5868-9-22

Top Stack. (2019, November 29). *Learn how goal setting affects your brain.* https://topstackgroup.com/learn-how-goal-setting-affects-your-brain/

DETOX

In this post we are initiating the conversation about the concept of detoxification, otherwise known as detox, and how it relates to The Livy Method. To better understand what detoxification is and the relevance of how it impacts the weight loss process, let's take a deeper dive into the concept of detoxification, and what that actually means!

WHAT IS DETOXIFICATION?

Detoxification, or detox, has become pretty popular in the discussion of health in mainstream media over the years. However, this is not a new concept at all!! In fact, people have been trying to relieve their bodies of "toxins" for thousands of years. A toxin is defined "as a substance that is synthesized by a plant species, an animal, or by microorganisms, that is harmful to another organism". However, toxins can also include chemicals like pesticides, pollution, plastics, as well by consuming processed food which can include artificial ingredients, colours, and preservatives from the foods that we eat!

Some examples of traditional "detox" practices that have existed for centuries include bloodletting, enemas, sweat lodges, fasting, and drinking detoxification teas and tonics. Many of these practices were even used as medical treatments up until the early 20th century, however you still hear about many of these detox practices today. Those promoting these diets and products often imply and claim that by following their specific diet or by using their special products, your body will be rid of "toxins", thereby improving health and promoting weight loss.

A typical detox diet may involve a period of fasting, followed by a strict diet of fruit, vegetables, fruit and/or vegetable juices, and water. Sometimes a detox also includes herbs, laxatives, diuretics, teas, supplements, and colon cleanses or enemas.

These claim to:

- Rest your organs by fasting
- Stimulate your liver to help it rid of toxins
- Promote toxin elimination through stool, urine, and sweat
- Improve circulation
- Provide your body with healthy nutrients that it needs to help detox
- Change the PH of your body making it more alkaline in nature

These diets also claim to help with various health problems including obesity, digestive issues, autoimmune diseases, inflammation, allergies, bloating, and chronic fatigue.

However, human research on detox diets is lacking, and the handful of studies that exist are significantly flawed. In fact, popular detox diets rarely identify the specific toxins they aim to remove or the mechanism by which they supposedly eliminate them. There is also little evidence that supports the use of these diets for toxin elimination or sustainable weight loss.

The other concern is the potential for harm. Although some countries have strict regulations of supplements and products that are made available to consumers, many dietary supplements and detox products are not as strictly regulated in other countries. In fact, in the U.S, The FDA (The Food and Drug Administration) often finds "detoxifying" weight loss products contain dangerous drugs and chemicals not advertised on the packaging. These are listed on the FDA website. While some detox teas for example may contain natural tea ingredients like tea leaves, others could contain toxic or allergy-triggering substances, including drugs and medications! The other issue is that with today's technology, we are able to acquire these products for purchase online with just the click of a button. With the ease of online shopping, we are able to purchase pretty much any product from any country, so it can really be difficult to know what is in the products we buy.

Check out this link from the FDA showing the list for supplement advisories

https://www.fda.gov/food/dietary-supplement-products-ingredients/
dietary-supplement-ingredient-advisory-list#updates

Check out this list for Weight Loss and Detox tainted products

https://www.fda.gov/drugs/medication-health-fraud/tainted-weight-loss-products

For Canadians, check out the Natural Health Products Database

http://webprod.hc-sc.gc.ca/nhpid-bdipsn/atReq.do?atid=whats.quoi&lang=eng

This is the main page for Canadian consumers and those in the industry

https://www.canada.ca/en/health-canada/services/drugs-health-products/natural-non-prescription.html

IS THERE ANYTHING WE CAN DO TO FACILITATE DETOX?

Now it's time for the good news! Your body is very well-equipped to eliminate toxins on its own without the extra help from special diets or expensive supplements and products. Your body has a very self-sufficient and comprehensive way of eliminating toxins that involves the liver, kidneys, digestive system, skin, and lungs. However, it is only when these organs are healthy, that they can effectively eliminate unwanted substances.

Furthermore, you **can** enhance your body's natural detoxification system. In fact, by following The Livy Method, you are setting your body up for success in supporting your body's own detoxification pathways.

In order to understand the concept of detox, let's discuss some of the common misconceptions reviewed by Healthline, how our body naturally detoxifies itself, and how by following The Livy Method we can enhance and support our body's own detoxification system.

CAN WE TARGET THE ELIMINATION OF TOXINS?

As discussed above, detox diets rarely identify the specific toxins they aim to remove. According to Healthline, the mechanisms by which they work are also unclear. In fact, there is little to no evidence that detox diets can remove any toxins from your body.

Furthermore, your body is capable of cleansing itself by utilizing the liver as the primary detoxification organ, and through the elimination of stool, urine, breath, and sweat.

The liver initiates this process by transforming the toxic substances to a less harmful form, then ensures that the substance is eliminated from the body by way of the lungs, skin, kidneys and/or digestive system.

However, there are a few chemicals that may not be as easily removed by these processes, which can include persistent organic pollutants (POPs), phthalates, bisphenol A (BPA) found in plastics, and heavy metals.

These materials tend to accumulate in fat tissue or blood, and can take years for your body to eliminate. However, as we have gained an increased awareness about the harm that these compounds cause, many of these materials have been removed or limited in commercial products produced today. That being said, there is little evidence that detox diets help eliminate any of these compounds.

HOW EFFECTIVE ARE THESE DIETS?

Some people report feeling more focused and energetic during and after detox diets.

However, this improvement in well-being may simply be due to the elimination of processed foods, alcohol, and other unhealthy substances from their diets. They may also be receiving the nutrients, vitamins, and minerals that they were lacking before, thus resulting in feeling better.

EFFECTS ON WEIGHT LOSS

Very few scientific studies have investigated how detox diets impact weight loss. While some people may lose a lot of weight quickly, this effect is likely due the loss of fluid and carbohydrate stores rather than fat. This weight is usually regained fairly quickly once one resumes their previous lifestyle. If a detox diet involves severe calorie restriction, it may allow for weight loss, but will unlikely be sustainable in keeping the weight off in the long term. In fact, this is a major factor in creating an environment that promotes the body to store fat.

DETOX DIETS, SHORT-TERM FASTING, AND STRESS

According to Healthline (Bjarnadottir, A., 2019, January), several varieties of detox diets may have effects similar to those of short-term or intermittent fasting. Short-term fasting may improve various disease markers in some people, including improved leptin and insulin sensitivity.

However, these effects do not apply to everyone. Studies in women show that both a 48-hour fast and a 3-week period of reduced calorie intake may increase stress hormone levels. Crash diets can be a stressful experience, as they involve resisting temptations and feeling extreme hunger, ultimately affecting the hormones involved in hunger and satiety as discussed in the science post on hormones! These diets often lead to over indulgence from the deprivation involved, and stimulate/increase the hunger hormones and negative feedback loops that these diets perpetuate.

SEVERE CALORIE RESTRICTION

Several detox diets recommend fasting or severe calorie restriction. Short-term fasting and limited calorie intake can result in fatigue, irritability, and other physical symptoms.

Long-term fasting can result in energy, vitamin, and mineral deficiencies, as well as electrolyte imbalances and major health consequences, even death.

Furthermore, colon cleansing methods which are sometimes recommended during detoxes, can cause dehydration, cramping, bloating, nausea, vomiting, and the flushing out of the important bacterial microbiome that lives in the colon and is crucial to the digestive process.

OVERDOSING

Some detox diets may pose the risk of overdosing on supplements, laxatives, diuretics, and even water. There is a lack of regulation and monitoring in the detox industry, and many detox foods and supplements may not have any scientific basis on how their product is produced or manufactured.

In the worst and most insidious cases, the ingredient labels of detox products may be inaccurate. This can increase your risk of overdosing, potentially resulting in serious, and even fatal effects.

If you decide that you want to go down the path of a detox because it is something you choose to do, be sure to seek advice from a regulated health care professional, or Naturopathic Doctor that can oversee and monitor your health during the process!

SO, AFTER ALL THIS, HOW DOES THE BODY DETOX?

THE LIVER

The liver is such an amazing organ and does so much for our bodies! As discussed in the previous science posts, it has an important role in the digestive process and in storing and releasing energy in the form of glucose to the body! Let's discuss this amazing organ in more detail!

The liver is your body's largest solid organ. On average, it weighs around 3 pounds in adulthood and is roughly the size of a football. This organ is vital to the body's metabolic, detoxification, and immune system functions. Without a functioning liver, a person cannot survive.

The liver's position is held most prominently in the right upper region of the abdomen, just below the diaphragm. A portion of the liver is located in the left upper abdomen as well. The liver has two main segments, also called lobes. Each lobe is further divided into eight segments. Each segment has an estimated 1,000 lobules, also called small lobes. Each of the lobules has a small tube, a duct that flows into other ducts that join to become the common hepatic duct. This meets the cystic duct and then becomes the common bile duct.

Compared to the rest of the body, the liver has a significant amount of blood flowing through it, an estimated 13% of the body's blood is in the liver at any given time.

According to Johns Hopkins Medicine, the liver's major functions are in the metabolic processes of the body, but is also involved in many life-sustaining processes, which include:

- creating immune system factors that can help the body fight against infection or pathogens in the body

- producing proteins in conjunction with vitamin K (that is produced largely in the colon) that are important in the blood clotting process, and an important part of healing

- the liver is also one of the organs that help break down old or damaged blood cells and eliminate them from the body

From a digestive and metabolic standpoint, the liver produces an estimated 800 to 1,000 milliliters (ml) of bile each day. This yellow, brownish, or olive green liquid, is collected in small ducts and then passed on to the main bile duct which carries the bile to a part of the small intestine called the duodenum. The small intestine uses the bile to further help with the breakdown and absorption of fats. Any extra bile is stored in the gallbladder to be used later.

In the metabolism of carbohydrates, the liver helps to ensure that the level of sugar in your blood (blood glucose) maintains stability. As discussed in the science post on insulin, if your blood sugar levels increase, for example after a meal, the liver removes sugar from blood supplied by the portal vein and stores it in the form of glycogen. If the blood sugar levels drop or are too low, the liver breaks down glycogen and releases sugar into the blood to be used by the body as needed.

In addition to glycogen, the liver also stores fat-soluble vitamins and minerals such as copper and iron, and releases them into the blood when needed.

The liver also plays an important role in the metabolism of proteins. The liver cells change the amino acids in the foods we eat so that they can be used to produce energy, or make carbohydrates or fats for the body. A substance called ammonia is a by-product of this process which can be toxic to the body in large amounts. In order to prevent the ammonia from increasing to "toxic" levels, the liver cells convert the ammonia to a much less toxic substance called urea which is released into the blood. Urea is then transported to the kidneys and passes out of the body through urine.

The liver also controls the synthesis and removal of cholesterol in the body, which has a crucial role in the production of hormones.

LET'S TALK ABOUT THE LIVER AND DETOXIFICATION

The liver has a primary role in storing and releasing energy, but let's break down the vital role it plays in helping us eliminate toxins from our body.

The liver begins the process of making toxins less harmful to the body and removing them from the bloodstream, by receiving blood with nutrients from the digestive organs via a vein known as the hepatic portal vein. The hepatocytes (cells of the liver), accept and filter this blood. They act as little sorting centers, determining which nutrients should be processed, what should be stored, what should be eliminated via the stool, and what should be diverted back to the blood. In fact, as a last resort, the liver will even store toxins itself to protect the rest of the body!!

The liver filters toxins that enter or are produced by the body through an area called the sinusoid channels, which are lined with immune cells called Kupffer cells. These Kupffer cells engulf the "toxin", digest, and excrete it. This process is called phagocytosis.

As many chemicals are relatively "new", it may take thousands of years from an evolutionary standpoint before our body properly adapts to them. The main takeaway here is, if the liver cannot figure out what to do with a substance, it may simply store the substance(s), often in fat tissue, in other organs, or in the liver itself. This is potentially damaging to any of the tissues or organs involved in this process.

Check out these following videos for more information on how the liver functions and the detoxification process works.

https://www.youtube.com/watch?app=desktop&v=wbh3SjzydnQ

https://www.khanacademy.org/science/in-in-class-11-biology-india/
x9d1157914247c627:digestion-and-absorption/x9d1157914247c627:digestive-glands/v/liver

For a deeper dive on the removal of xenobiotics (substances that are foreign to the body or to an ecological system), check out this informative video

https://www.youtube.com/watch?v=zkS7PZUE27g&t=425s

So now, let's break down detox even further. The detoxification of substances that require elimination or results in storage in the body is thought to take place in three phases.

PHASE I

Two of the key phases of detox, Phase I and II, occur in the liver.

The first phase of detoxification occurs mostly in the liver and helps to transform potentially harmful lipid soluble (substances that dissolve in fat) molecules, into less harmful substances that will be easier for the body to excrete. This must occur prior to proceeding to phase II of detoxification.

In Phase I, a group of enzymes called cytochrome p450 enables the transformation of dangerous substances into less harmful substances through the chemical processes of oxidation (oxidation is a process in which a chemical substance changes because of the addition of oxygen), reduction (when a chemical substance loses an oxygen), hydration (when a chemical substance mixes with water), dehalogenation (a process when harmful compounds known as halogens are removed and converted to a more stable product), and hydrolysis (a reaction where water is used to break down a substance further).

These chemical changes require the activity of cytochrome p450 enzymes, as well as a variety of nutrients, to both support the activity of enzymes, and neutralize harmful molecules known as free radicals formed as a result of these processes. If free radicals are not neutralized, they can result in inflammation in the body. Many nutrients play a key role in phase I and the neutralizing of free radicals, including a variety of B vitamins, amino acids, vitamin C, zinc, vitamin A, and flavonoids.

Genetic issues, liver damage, nutrient deficiencies, and certain toxins can all impair the activity of p450 enzymes, reducing the ability of the liver to detoxify. Exposure to certain chemicals increases phase I activity, leading to a high production of phase I end products. If these products are not converted by phase II, they can be harmful to cellular DNA and RNA, and may be linked to diseases such as Parkinson's and cancer.

PHASE II

In phase II, the focus is on a process called conjugation. In conjugation, there is the addition of a chemical group to the by-product that was produced in phase I, making it water soluble and subsequently less harmful. Once the substance becomes water soluble, it can be excreted through the kidneys and intestines in the form of urine and bile.

There are many processes of conjugation. These include glutathionylation, methylation, glucuronidation, sulfation, and acetylation. Each of these processes involves the addition of a different substance to a phase I end-product, requiring specific nutrients, mostly amino acids, which must be obtained from our diet. Without these specific nutrients, phase II detoxification can be impaired. If phase II detoxification becomes impaired, an accumulation of phase I products occurs, resulting in inflammation and tissue damage in the body.

However, if phase I and II occur effectively, toxins can be eliminated by the kidneys and bowels via urine and stool. Although the liver is thought of as our primary detoxification organ, it requires a large variety of nutrients that must first be absorbed via the digestive system, in order to function optimally. Ironically though, the digestive system is also the initial site of exposure to ingested toxins. Due to these factors, it is recognized that there is an additional third phase of detoxification which occurs primarily in the digestive system.

PHASE III

The third phase of detoxification refers to a highly concentrated anti-porter (transport) system of proteins in the body. There are many anti-porters being researched, particularly P-glycoprotein, an anti-porter in the small intestine that moves toxins from cells into the gut. Another important protein known as blood-brain protein, is located in the kidneys, the blood brain barrier, and the liver. This transport system ensures the movement of harmful compounds out of the cell and into the detoxification organs.

A healthy diet and microbiome are key to the success of phase III, whereas digestive inflammation leads to the impairment of it. If phase III is compromised, an accumulation of toxins within the cell occurs. Errors in P-glycoprotein expression have been linked to Alzheimer's disease, and suspected to play a role in stress management and inflammatory bowel disease.

Due to the importance of these three phases, inefficient detoxification in any of the three phases can be detrimental.

Because of the constant stress placed on our detoxification systems, following a plan like The Livy Method which consistently supports these three phases can greatly help to also support our detoxification system and help keep us healthy! Let's talk more about strategies to best support our body in detox.

LIMIT ALCOHOL

More than 90% of alcohol is metabolized in your liver. Liver enzymes convert alcohol to a substance called acetaldehyde, a known cancer-causing chemical. Recognizing acetaldehyde as a toxin, your liver converts it to a harmless substance called acetate, which is later eliminated from your body.

Excessive drinking can severely damage liver function by causing fat buildup, inflammation, and scarring. When this happens, your liver cannot function properly and perform its necessary tasks, including filtering waste and other toxins from your body. Therefore, limiting alcohol can keep the liver healthy, thus supporting the body in detox.

FOCUS ON SLEEP

Ensuring adequate and quality sleep each night can help to support your body's health and natural detoxification system.

Sleeping allows your brain to reorganize and recharge itself, as well as remove toxic waste byproducts that have accumulated throughout the day. A waste product that the body produces is a protein called beta-amyloid, which contributes to the development of Alzheimer's disease. With sleep deprivation, your body does not have time to perform these functions, thus toxins can build up, affecting several aspects of health.

Poor sleep has been linked to health issues such as stress, anxiety, high blood pressure, heart disease, type 2 diabetes, and obesity. It is suggested to get at least seven to nine hours of good quality sleep per night, on a regular basis to promote good health and a healthy detoxification system. This is a foundational recommendation of The Livy Method!

DRINK ENOUGH WATER

Water and adequate hydration have a huge impact on how the body functions. Water regulates your body temperature, lubricates joints, aids digestion and nutrient absorption, and detoxifies your body by removing waste products.

Your body's cells must continuously be repaired to function optimally and break down nutrients for your body to use as energy. However, these processes release waste in the form of urea and carbon dioxide, which cause harm if able to build up in your blood.

Water allows for transport of these waste products, efficiently removing them through urination, breathing, or sweating. By increasing your water intake, your body reduces the secretion of the antidiuretic hormone and increases urination, eliminating more water and waste products. Thus, proper hydration is very important for detoxification of the body and to keep us healthy!

REDUCE YOUR INTAKE OF SUGAR AND PROCESSED FOODS

Sugar and processed foods are thought to be one of the root causes of today's public health crises. The increased consumption of sugary and highly processed foods has been linked to obesity and other chronic diseases, such as heart disease, cancer, and diabetes.

These diseases hinder your body's ability to naturally detoxify itself by harming organs that play an important role in the process, such as your liver and kidneys. For example, the high consumption of sugary beverages can cause **fatty liver disease**, a condition that negatively impacts liver function as discussed in the science posts on digestion. By following a healthful plan like The Livy Method during the weight loss process and in maintenance, by focusing on the foods that make you feel good, you can keep your body's detoxification system healthy in the long term.

However, with the onset of a diet and lifestyle change when initiating a program like The Livy Method, many people can experience symptoms from these changes. These changes are described in the program as detox.

SYMPTOMS OF DETOX

One of the common reactions to a healthier lifestyle/diet change is the onset of headaches.

Detox headaches are often caused by your body's reaction to missing an item, such as sugar or caffeine, that was habitually present. This may result in:

- a reduction in circulating hormones
- toxins such as chemical food additives or drugs leaching into your circulation to be eliminated
- a release of energy from tension and stress

However, headaches may also be a result of low sodium. Be sure to be mindful of adding in good salts like pink Himalayan, Celtic, and Sea Salts to your diet throughout the day! The low sodium post is a great one to refer to if you have any questions about this.

Along with headaches, other symptoms of detox may include:

- fatigue
- irritability
- hunger pangs
- rashes/breakouts
- diarrhea

These symptoms may be called various names including healing reactions, cleansing reactions, detox symptoms, and healing crises.

EAT ANTIOXIDANT RICH FOODS

Antioxidants protect your cells against damage caused by molecules called free radicals. Oxidative stress is a condition caused by excessive production of free radicals. Your body naturally produces these molecules in everyday cellular processes, such as digestion. However, alcohol, tobacco smoke, a poor diet, and exposure to pollutants, can also produce excessive free radicals in the body. By causing damage to your body's cells, these molecules have been implicated in a number of conditions, such as dementia, heart disease, liver disease, asthma, and certain types of cancer.

However, eating a diet rich in antioxidants can help your body fight oxidative stress caused by excess free radicals and other toxins that increase your risk of disease. Examples of antioxidants include vitamin A, vitamin C, vitamin E, selenium, lycopene, lutein, and zeaxanthin. Foods like berries, fruits, nuts, cocoa, vegetables, spices, and beverages like coffee and green tea, have some of the highest amounts of antioxidants.

EAT MORE CRUCIFEROUS VEGETABLES, LEGUMES, NUTS/SEEDS, AND LEAFY GREENS

Cruciferous vegetables and leafy greens are not only high in fiber and dense with nutrients, vitamins and minerals, but help the body engage in and support each phase of the detoxification pathway. They also support the microbiome and organs involved in detoxification! A review in the Journal of Nutrition and Metabolism notes clinical evidence of the effects from cruciferous vegetables, allium vegetables (such as garlic, onions, leeks, chives, scallions, and shallots), apiaceous vegetables (such as carrots, parsnips, celery, parsley), grapefruit, fish oil, foods that contain daidzein (found in abundance in legumes, especially in soybeans, but are present in many other vegetables, fruits, nuts, peas, lentils, and seeds), and eating food high in antioxidants have a profoundly positive nutritional impact on the detoxification process (Hodges, R. E., & Minich, D. M., 2015). The Livy Method recommends eating lots of vegetables, many of which include cruciferous vegetables (there is even a post about them), leafy greens, legumes, nuts, and seeds which will all support your body in detox!

EAT FOODS HIGH IN PREBIOTICS AND CONSIDER PROBIOTICS

Gut health is important for keeping your detoxification system healthy. Your intestinal cells have a detoxification and excretion system that protects your gut and body from harmful toxins, such as chemicals. Good gut health starts with prebiotics, a type of fiber that feeds the good bacteria in your gut called probiotics. With prebiotics, your good bacteria are able to produce nutrients called short-chain fatty acids that are beneficial for health.

The "good" bacteria in your gut can become unbalanced with "bad" bacteria from the use of antibiotics, poor dental hygiene, and a diet of poor quality.

Consequently, this unhealthy shift in bacteria can weaken your immune and detoxification system, increasing your risk of disease and inflammation. Eating foods rich in prebiotics can keep your immune and detoxification systems healthy. Good food sources of prebiotics include tomatoes, artichokes, bananas, asparagus, onions, garlic, and oats.

Take a good prebiotic, as well as a probiotic, both of which are recommended supplements of The Livy Method.

GET ACTIVE

Regular exercise is associated with a longer life and a reduced risk of many conditions and diseases, including type 2 diabetes, heart disease, high blood pressure, and certain cancers which have been discussed in previous science posts.

While there are several mechanisms behind the health benefits of exercise, reduced inflammation is a key factor. While some inflammation is necessary for recovering from infection or healing wounds, too much of it weakens your body's systems and promotes disease.

By reducing inflammation, exercise can help your body's systems including its detoxification system, function properly and protect against disease.

When maximizing The Livy Method, incorporating exercise will help the body support the detoxification system.

CAN I SWEAT OUT TOXINS THAT ARE IN MY BODY?

With some forms of exercise your body works up a sweat that helps to cool your body down. You may have also heard that sitting in a sauna, hot tub, or going to a hot yoga class will help your body sweat out toxins. However, your sweat is 99% water, and the rest of the 1% is composed of: electrolytes and minerals like sodium, potassium, calcium, and magnesium (It is important to replace them after periods of heavy sweating!); small amounts of pheromones, which are chemicals that act like hormones outside of your body; bacteria that grow in the sweat that you release and can cause body odor; and tiny amounts of toxins. Trace amounts of metals and other chemicals can be present in your sweat, but your kidneys and liver do most of the work when it comes to getting rid of toxins in the body.

Therefore, what you eat has a bigger impact when it comes to eliminating toxins in the body. That being said, saunas, hot yoga, hot tubs, and warm baths can be very relaxing with other health benefits, so can still have a positive impact on your health. However, if you have health issues such as cardiovascular disease, issues with blood pressure, or are pregnant, consult with your health care provider before using these types of heat-based therapies.

OTHER HELPFUL DETOX TIPS

Although no current evidence supports the use of detox diets for removing toxins from your body, certain dietary changes and lifestyle practices may help reduce toxin load and support your body's detoxification system.

- **Eat sulfur-containing foods**

  Food high in sulfur, such as onions, broccoli, and garlic, enhance excretion of heavy metals like cadmium.

- **Try out chlorella**

  Chlorella is a type of algae that has many nutritional benefits, and may enhance the elimination of toxins like heavy metals, according to animal studies.

- **Flavor dishes with cilantro**

  Cilantro enhances excretion of certain toxins, such as heavy metals like lead, and chemicals, including phthalates and insecticides.

- **Support glutathione**

  Eating sulfur-rich foods like eggs, broccoli, and garlic helps enhance the function of glutathione, a major antioxidant produced by your body that is heavily involved in detoxification.

- **Avoid the use of plastic and aluminum for heating and storing food**

  Use stainless steel or glass containers over plastic ones for foods and beverages. Avoid heating foods in plastic containers, and if using plastic containers, opt for ones featuring the BPA-free and phthalate-free labels.

- **Switch to natural cleaning products**

  Choosing natural cleaning products like vinegar and baking soda over commercial cleaning agents can reduce your exposure to potentially toxic chemicals.

- **Choose natural body care**

  Using natural deodorants, makeups, moisturizers, shampoos, and other personal care products can also reduce your exposure to chemicals. While promising, many of these effects have only been shown in animal studies. Therefore, studies in humans are needed to confirm these findings.

Hopefully you learned a bit more about the detox process and how by focusing on better nutrition, sleeping well, exercise, and positive lifestyle changes, will not only limit your exposure to chemicals, but help your body process them out optimally!

Stay tuned for next week's science post where we will build upon our knowledge of digestion, and discuss the migrating motor complex (MMC) and hunger!

REFERENCES

https://www.sciencedirect.com/topics/earth-and-planetary-sciences/toxin

https://www.sciencedirect.com/topics/medicine-and-dentistry/detoxication

https://www.sciencedirect.com/topics/agricultural-and-biological-sciences/daidzein#:~:text=Daidzein%20and%20genistein%20are%20in,peas%2C%20lentils%2C%20and%20seeds.

Balingit, A., & Nall, R. (2022, January 24). *The liver.* Healthline. https://www.healthline.com/human-body-maps/liver#keep-liver-healthy

Bjarnadottir, A. (2019, January 10). *Do detox diets and cleanses really work?* Healthline. https://www.healthline.com/nutrition/detox-diets-101#methods

Collins. (n.d.). Oxidation. In *Collinsdictionary.com dictionary.* Retrieved March 30, 2022, from https://www.collinsdictionary.com/us/dictionary/english/oxidation#:~:text=(Pharmaceutical%3A%20Physiology)-,Oxidation%20is%20a%20process%20in%20which%20a%20chemical%20substance%20changes,involves%20the%20oxidation%20of%20magnesium.

Detoxification. (n.d.). The Hepatitis C Trust. Retrieved March 30, 2022, from http://hepctrust.org.uk/information/liver/detoxification#:~:text=The%20liver%20filters%20toxins%20through,body%20properly%20adapts%20to%20them.

Detoxes and cleanses: What you need to know. (2019, September). National Center for Complementary and Integrative Health. Retrieved March 30, 2022, from https://www.nccih.nih.gov/health/detoxes-and-cleanses-what-you-need-to-know

Dietary supplement ingredient advisory list. (2021, October 29). U.S. Food & Drug Administration. Retrieved March 30, 2022, from https://www.fda.gov/food/dietary-supplement-products-ingredients/dietary-supplement-ingredient-advisory-list#updates

Han, S., & Frothingham, S. (2018, July 17). *Dealing with a detox headache.* Healthline. https://www.healthline.com/health/detox-headache

Higdon, J., Drake, V. J., Delage, B., & Traka, M. (2017, April). *Cruciferous vegetables.* Oregon State University. https://lpi.oregonstate.edu/mic/food-beverages/cruciferous-vegetables

Higdon, J., Drake, V. J., & McCann, S. (2021, March). *Lignans.* Oregon State University. https://lpi.oregonstate.edu/mic/dietary-factors/phytochemicals/lignans

Hodges, R. E., & Minich, D. M. (2015). Modulation of metabolic detoxification pathways using foods and food-derived components: A scientific review with clinical application. *Journal of Nutrition and Metabolism, 2015,* 760689. https://doi.org/10.1155/2015/760689

Institute for Quality and Efficiency in Health Care (IQWiG). (2016, August 19). *How does the liver work?* https://www.ncbi.nlm.nih.gov/books/NBK279393/

Jackson, E., Shoemaker, R., Larian, N., & Cassis, L. (2017). Adipose tissue as a site of toxin accumulation. *Comprehensive Physiology, 7*(4), 1085–1135. https://doi.org/10.1002/cphy.c160038

Jung, J.S., Kim, W.L., Park, B.H., Lee, S.O., & Chae, S.W. (2020). Effect of toxic trace element detoxification, body fat reduction following four-week intake of the wellnessup diet: a three-arm, randomized clinical trial. *Nutrition & Metabolism, 17, 47.* https://doi.org/10.1155/2015/760689

Kuczma, M. (n.d.). *Understanding the 3 phases of detoxification. Integrative Naturopathic Medical Centre.* https://integrative.ca/blog/3-phases-detoxification

Lang, A., & Rose-Francis, K. (2022, February 11). *What are obesogens, and should we be concerned? Healthline.* https://www.healthline.com/nutrition/what-are-obesogens

Liver: Anatomy and functions. (n.d.). Johns Hopkins Medicine. Retrieved March 30, 2022, from https://www.hopkinsmedicine.org/health/conditions-and-diseases/liver-anatomy-and-functions

Loconti, C., & Begum, J. (2021, December 1). *What to know about sweating.* WebMD. https://www.webmd.com/skin-problems-and-treatments/what-to-know-about-sweating

Narayan, R. [Khanacademymedicine]. (2014, May 15). *Liver | Gastrointestinal system physiology | NCLEX-RN* [Video]. Youtube. https://www.youtube.com/watch?v=rDjWrNRKfvg

Natural health products. (2022, March 22). Government of Canada. Retrieved March 30, 2022, from https://www.canada.ca/en/health-canada/services/drugs-health-products/natural-non-prescription.html

Natural health products ingredients database. (2022, March 25). Health Canada. Retrieved March 30, 2022, from http://webprod.hc-sc.gc.ca/nhpid-bdipsn/atReq.do?atid=whats.quoi&lang=eng

Ninja Nerd. (2018, June 11). *Gastrointestinal | Biotransformation of drugs and toxins* [Video]. Youtube. https://www.youtube.com/watch?v=zkS7PZUE27g&t=425s

Organ systems: Detoxification. (n.d.). Texas A&M College of Veterinary Medicine & Biomedical Sciences. Retrieved March 30, 2022, from https://vetmed.tamu.edu/peer/detoxification/

Peterson, S., Lampe, J. W., Bammler, T. K., Gross-Steinmeyer, K., & Eaton, D. L. (2006). Apiaceous vegetable constituents inhibit human cytochrome P-450 1A2 (hCYP1A2) activity and hCYP1A2-mediated mutagenicity of aflatoxin B1. *Food and Chemical Toxicology, 44*(9), 1474–1484. https://doi.org/10.1016/j.fct.2006.04.010

Petre, A. (2018, October 3). *Lycopene: health benefits and top food sources.* Healthline. https://www.healthline.com/nutrition/lycopene#cancer

Salehi, B., Mishra, A. P., Nigam, M., Sener, B., Kilic, M., Sharifi-Rad, M., Fokou, P., Martins, N., & Sharifi-Rad, J. (2018). Resveratrol: A double-edged sword in health benefits. *Biomedicines, 6*(3), 91. https://doi.org/10.3390/biomedicines6030091

Seitz, A., & Seitz, D. (2021, June 14). *The truth about the lemon water detox.* Healthline. https://www.healthline.com/health/lemon-water-detox-the-truth

Tainted weight loss products. (2022, March 22). U.S. Food & Drug Administration. Retrieved March 30, 2022, from https://www.fda.gov/drugs/medication-health-fraud/tainted-weight-loss-products

TED. (2021, July 8). *A cleanse won't detox your body but here's what will | Body stuff with dr. jen gunter* [Video]. Youtube. https://www.youtube.com/watch?v=DESCcjSQSKY

TED-Ed. (2014, November 25). *What does the liver do? - Emma bryce* [Video]. Youtube. https://www.youtube.com/watch?app=desktop&v=wbh3SjzydnQ

U.S. Food and Drug Administration. (2013, January 29). *Being fooled by empty diet promises* [Video]. Youtube. https://www.youtube.com/watch?v=wcdO6dDnUKE

Van De Wall, G. (2019, March 10). *Full body detox: 9 ways to rejuvenate your body.* Healthline. https://www.healthline.com/nutrition/how-to-detox-your-body

Woreta, T. (n.d.). *Detoxing your liver: Fact versus fiction.* Johns Hopkins Medicine. https://www.hopkinsmedicine.org/health/wellness-and-prevention/detoxing-your-liver-fact-versus-fiction

Zeratsky, K. (2020, April 18). *Do detox diets offer any health benefits?* Mayo Clinic. https://www.mayoclinic.org/healthy-lifestyle/nutrition-and-healthy-eating/expert-answers/detox-diets/faq-20058040

THE MIGRATING MOTOR COMPLEX (MMC) AND HUNGER

In this science post we are continuing the conversation on digestion (who knew there was so much to discuss?!?!) and will be exploring the fascinating function of our migrating motor complex or MMC, and the concept of hunger.

YOUR STOMACH IS "GROWLING", IS THIS A SIGN THAT YOU ARE HUNGRY AND NEED TO EAT?

Many of us growing up have learned to associate our stomach "growling" or noises coming from our abdomen, with hunger and the need to eat! In fact, many of us feel the immediate need to take action and eat as soon as we receive these signals from our bodies. But does this mean we are hungry and we should eat? This is one of the most common questions that our members have when they begin the journey of the Livy Method as they initiate the process of becoming more in tune with their bodies.

So, why do our stomachs and abdomens make these noises, and how do we distinguish some of the things that our body does (like our stomach churning, rumbling and growling) with the actual need to eat? Is it because we are hungry?

HUNGER

The feeling of "hunger" is fairly complex and can be affected by many things. Hunger can be influenced by physical/physiological, emotional, social, economic and mental factors, and can be a difficult thing to gauge at times.

In fact, many of us have lost touch with our hunger signals at a young age or never really become in tune with them in the first place. We may have become so detached from understanding or recognizing these cues because of the influence of our family, social/economic factors, years of dieting and cycles of deprivation, over training and exercise, and eating when we are not hungry because we are following a set number of calories or macros determined by others in the diet industry. It's no wonder that we do not even know where to start!

But not to worry!! These signals are still there, and an imperative part of The Livy Method process is reconnecting our members with these very important signals that their body provides to them!!

HOW CAN YOU GET BACK IN TOUCH WITH YOUR HUNGER SIGNALS?

JOURNALING AND SELF-REFLECTION

The Livy Method recommends journaling as a complementary process to the program as it can have a great benefit to the overall weight loss process. Also, as we mention in the science post Issues with Digestion (stay tuned for that post), can help identify any foods that have an impact on your digestion, as well as identify potential intolerances.

Journaling your feels/emotions and highlighting external factors such as stress, exercise/activity, and boredom can give you great insight into how your feelings, patterns, or behaviours, may influence your eating when not necessarily hungry. Using the traditional pen to paper process, or using the WLBG APP is a great way to do this!

If you are the type of person that needs a more **quantitative (quantitative data refers to any information that can be quantified, counted or measured, and given a numerical value)** way of understanding things, the use of a measurement tool such as a **hunger scale** may be of benefit to you!

A **hunger scale** is a tool that can help you learn how to identify the difference between actual physical hunger and the "feeling" of hunger that may be brought on by emotions like stress, boredom, sadness, or happiness.

Checking in and asking yourself the first two Mindfulness questions is a great way to assess this; but let's take this a step further by using a hunger scale.

Check out an example of a great hunger scale from Alberta Health Services! There are also additional questions and considerations that can help clarify the concept of eating to satisfaction.

https://www.albertahealthservices.ca/assets/info/nutrition/if-nfs-hunger-and-fullness-signals. pdf?fbclid=IwAR2m9j2uy8XsnUdcUQxAI6DX5T9fUMJDVErkWKVEhS-rsYw_E2h4WJ9KaVI

BEFORE YOU EAT, ASK YOURSELF IF YOU ARE HUNGRY?

WHEN SERVING OR PORTIONING OUT YOUR FOOD AND BEFORE YOU EAT ASK YOURSELF; HOW IS THIS PORTION FOR ME? HOW WOULD I FEEL IF I ATE ALL OF THIS?

When you start feeling like you want something to eat, rate your hunger on a scale of 1 to 10, with 1 being overwhelmingly hungry and 10 being so full you feel sick. A rating of 5 or 6 means you are comfortable, neither too hungry nor too full. When you feel hungry even though you recently ate, check to see if what you are feeling is really a craving brought on by something psychological or emotional. The goal is to bring awareness to your changing hunger levels. For example, sometimes you are really hungry but then when you eat, you feel full fast. Other times you are not hungry at all, but when you start to eat, you feel hungry. Both are completely normal to experience!

You may not get a really strong response or any answer from your body at first, but trust that once you begin this process of talking to yourself and taking the time to listen, your body will start to talk back!

WHILE EATING YOUR FOOD, PAY ATTENTION TO HOW YOU FEEL AND ASK YOURSELF:

Are you getting full, is this food satisfying you? How would you feel if you took a few more bites? How would you feel if you stop eating now? Do you feel any physical effects of eating? On the scale of 1-10 how are you feeling and where do you fall on that hunger scale?

WHEN YOU ARE DONE EATING, ASK YOURSELF HOW YOU FEEL:

Do you feel full and if so, what is your definition of full? How do you know when you have eaten enough? How do you feel physically; energetic, comfortable, tired? Are you just eating everything on your plate because it is there? Or maybe you feel like you could eat more? Again, you can rate how you feel on the scale from 1-10 to see where you fall with the goal being about a 5 or a 6!

In terms of journaling and using the scale as a tool to assess satisfaction, reflecting on when and what you eat, as well as what you were doing and feeling before you started eating can be really insightful in helping to identify psychological triggers for eating when you are not hungry. This may also help to identify habitual patterns of eating when you are not truly hungry. An example of this is wanting to eat a late-night snack while watching television, because this is a nightly ritual that you indulge in on evenings.

Here are a few more tips for assessing hunger devised by the University of Michigan Medicine (Healthwise Staff 2020, September), that very much align with the philosophy of The Livy Method:

- Try not to let your hunger drop to a 1 or 2 on the hunger scale. When you get that hungry, you are likely to eat faster, make poorer food choices, and keep eating past the "satisfied" point.

- On the other hand, let yourself feel **some** hunger between meals. Mild hunger is a good thing. After all, it›s a sign that you are not overeating. Teach yourself to appreciate hunger pangs as a natural part of life, and as a sign that you are a healthy eater.

- Give cravings 10 minutes. When you suddenly feel the need to eat, tell yourself that you will wait 10 minutes. If it was only a craving, you will have forgotten about it by then, and the urge will be gone. If 10 minutes goes by and you still have the urge to eat, you may be starting to get hungry. Also keep in mind, if you are craving something sweet, you may need more water, and if you are craving something salty, you may need more fat or salt!

- Don't eat more now because you think you might not have time to eat later. Eat what your body needs now, and worry about later, later.

- Does leaving food on your plate bother you? Take smaller servings. Save leftovers for another meal. Share plates with someone. Ask yourself what is more important—a few bites of "wasted" food, or your health? This aligns with the Ginaism, "your body is not a garbage can" so why would we treat it as such! This is truly a very impactful statement when framing leaving food on your plate!

- When you eat, make your food the main attraction. Sit down at the table with your family. Do not eat in front of the TV. Do not read while you eat. Give your attention to what you are putting in your mouth, how it tastes, and how your body reacts to what and how much you are eating.

Hopefully you found these tips helpful!

OK SO AFTER TUNING IN, YOU HAVE DETERMINED THAT YOU ARE NOT "FEELING" HUNGRY AND STILL HAVE TIME BEFORE YOU COULD EAT YOUR NEXT MEAL OR SNACK. HOWEVER, YOUR STOMACH IS RUMBLING…SHOULD YOU STILL EAT?

This is a great question, so let's take a deeper dive into answering this!

GASTRO INTESTINAL (GI) INNERVATION AND FUNCTION

As discussed in The Basics of Digestion, our digestive system, from our esophagus to our anus, is made up of a special type of muscle called smooth muscle. Smooth muscle, which like other muscles in our body, contracts and relaxes. However, this mostly occurs automatically in our bodies without our conscious thought, although we do have some control over some aspects of it, such as the act of eating or having a bowel movement.

See this video for more detail about smooth muscle!

https://www.youtube.com/watch?v=yh4bUdnU2MQ

Our digestive system is controlled by our **central nervous system (CNS),** and something called the **enteric nervous system (ENS).** These systems control our digestive processes primarily **motility (a term used to describe the contraction of the muscles that mix and propel [move forward] the contents in the GI tract)**, the secretion of hormones and enzymes important to hunger, satiety and digestion, the absorption of nutrients in digestion, and regulates blood flow to the digestive system. Our digestive system is often referred to as the "second brain" (containing as many neurons as the spinal cord!) because of the amazing capabilities it has to perform many of these functions without consulting the brain! However, that being said, our digestive system is still influenced by the **SNS (sympathetic nervous system) and the (PSNS) parasympathetic nervous system** as we discuss in the science post Issues With Digestion.

Check out this great short video about the ENS!

https://www.youtube.com/watch?v=lGdauJ9Fcdc

Normal gastrointestinal motility results from the coordinated contractions of the smooth muscle in the digestive system. There are 2 fundamental patterns of movement conducted by the digestive system, **propulsion** and **segmentation contractions.**

Propulsion is when the broken-down food (bolus) is propelled in a forward motion along the length of the digestive tube for the purposes of digestion and elimination (bowel movement). This movement is accomplished by **peristalsis**. In peristalsis, the smooth muscle contracts in a "ring" like form in front of the bolus (mouth side), propelling the bolus in the direction of the anus. The muscles on the opposite side of the bolus relax to allow the bolus to pass, and occur until the bolus is broken down, absorbed and eliminated from the body.

Check out this video to see what peristalsis looks like!

https://www.youtube.com/watch?v=kVjeNZA5pi4

As discussed in the last few posts, the majority of absorption occurs in the small intestine. For the purpose of optimal absorption, a movement involving **mixing** and a movement called **segmentation,** facilitates the combining of the ingested food with the secretions and enzymes needed for breaking down the carbohydrates, proteins and fats. These macronutrients are broken down into the smaller components needed to support body function, as well as allow for the extended time needed for absorption via the wall of the small intestine.

In segmentation**,** the muscular rings of the smooth muscle alternate between a state of contraction and relaxation of the muscles along the wall of the intestines, which promote the effective mixing of its contents. This movement is not meant to propel the contents forward. Segmentation's primary role is for mixing and allowing the time needed for optimal absorption of nutrients, vitamins, and minerals at the bowel wall.

Check out this video to see how segmentation facilitates absorption!

https://www.youtube.com/watch?v=ATXMxRPRPfU

SO, WHAT HAPPENS WHEN THE FOOD WE HAVE EATEN IS DIGESTED?

THE MIGRATING MOTOR COMPLEX (MMC) ALSO KNOWN AS THE MIGRATING MOTILITY COMPLEX

The MMC is a distinct pattern of muscular activity observed in gastrointestinal smooth muscle during the periods between eating, after most of the food that has been ingested has been digested.

The MMC is often referred to as the "housekeeper" of the digestive system. These muscular contractions facilitate the movement or "sweeping" of any residual undigested material through the digestive system.

Although the majority of our bacterial gut flora live in our colon or large intestine (which aid in digestion and promote the production of B vitamins and vitamin K), there is a small proportion of bacteria that do live in our small intestine. An important part of the MMC and its movement of undigested foods through our digestive tract is to prevent the proliferation or growth of these bacteria, which can lead to something called **SIBO or small intestine bacterial overgrowth.** So, the big takeaway here is that the MMC has a very important role in keeping us healthy and preventing the overgrowth of bacteria in our digestive system!

The MMC also stimulates peristalsis, which is important in moving food through our digestive system and out of our bodies (by the way of bowel movements) but interestingly, the MMC is stimulated and **only functions when we are not eating!**

The MMC is thought to be controlled by the CNS and elicited by the hormone **motilin.** The MMC is elicited when the body is in a "non-fed" state in a cycle that recurs every 1.5 to 2 hours, and consists of four distinct phases or stages. When the body is ready to stimulate the MMC to initiate its "housekeeping" of the digestive tract, motilin is released from the upper portion of the small intestine. However, all that one needs to do to halt this process, is to initiate eating again.

Stage 1 is initiated by a quiet period with minimal muscular activity. There is only the occasional contraction occurring in the digestive system, lasting approximately 45-60 minutes.

Stage 2 is about 30 minutes in duration. In this stage, peristalsis increases in intensity and occurrence. Peristalsis starts in the stomach and is directed towards the small intestine.

Stage 3 is about 5 to 15 minutes in duration and is initiated by the occurrence of rapid evenly spaced peristaltic contractions. The **pylorus** (lower part of the stomach connecting to the duodenum of the small intestine) remains open during these peristaltic contractions, allowing indigestible materials to pass into the small intestine. This is in contrast to what occurs during the ingestion of food.

After the completion of stage 3, there is a short period of time that elapses before these stages all begin again. This transition period is stage 4!

Interestingly, while the MMC is activated, there is an increase in gastric, biliary, and pancreatic secretions seen with this contractile activity, which also likely assists in controlling the bacterial population in the upper segments of the digestive system.

MYTH BUSTER- A GROWLING STOMACH DOES NOT NECESSARILY MEAN HUNGER IT IS LIKELY THE MMC IN ACTION.

As you can see, a "growling" stomach, even after a meal, does not mean you are hungry! This is the stimulation of your very important MMC doing its very important job of cleaning out your digestive tract and keeping you healthy!

THE LIVY METHOD AND HOW IT PROMOTES AN OPTIMAL FUNCTIONING MMC

1. A healthy digestive system promotes a healthy MMC! The focus of The Livy Method is to improve and optimize digestion and absorption, and although the MMC is engaged in the periods we are not eating, they both go hand in hand.

2. Although we are eating fairly frequently at least 6 times a day, we still have up to 3.5 hours in between meals and snacks that allows for the MMC to engage. Because we are not eating to the point of being over-full, and likely eating smaller amounts when eating to satisfaction, we are more likely to stimulate the MMC earlier than we might have in the past! Also, this is a means to an end in the pursuit of weight loss and change. Eventually, as we complete maintenance, we will not necessarily be eating this often unless it's what our body needs!

3. The recommendation of eating our dinner earlier in the evening and to minimize late night snacking is also in line with optimizing the role of the MMC. The body can focus on rest and repair, and allow the MMC a good period of time overnight to do its thing!

4. The Livy Method promotes prioritizing restful sleep, selfcare and stress management techniques that reduce cortisol levels and helps keep hormones in homeostasis, preventing us from "stressing" our digestive system or impairing the function of the MMC!

The following are a couple of videos that discuss digestion and the MMC in greater detail if you are interested!

https://www.youtube.com/watch?v=3Bl1wknR1lc

This is a great video on motility. Discussion of the MMC starts at about 10:35 min of the video if you choose to skip ahead.

https://www.coursera.org/lecture/physiology/helpUrl-nUnNY

Hopefully, this post has given you more insight into the amazing MMC, the importance of digestion and how the foods we choose impact our health, the concept of hunger, and how using the tools and strategies discussed may help in assessing your hunger better!

Stay tuned for our next science post where we will initiate the conversation regarding hormones important to digestion and weight loss. We will be focusing our discussion on INSULIN, its role in our bodies, and how following The Livy Method impacts it!

REFERENCES

https://www.sciencedirect.com/.../migrating-motor-complex

Al-Missri, M., & Jialal, I. (2021, September 28). *Physiology, motilin*. StatPearls Publishing. https://www.ncbi.nlm.nih.gov/books/NBK545309/...

Betts, G.J., Young, K.A., Wise, J.A., Johnson, E., Poe, B., Kruse, D.H., Korol, O., Johnson, J.E., Womble, M., & DeSaix, P. (2019, May 29). *Anatomy and physiology*. Openstax. https://opentextbc.ca/anatomyandph.../chapter/smooth-muscle/

Cabrey, J., & Jakoi, E. (n.d.). *Motility* [Video]. Coursera. https://www.coursera.org/lecture/physiology/helpUrl-nUnNY

Costa, M., Brookes, S.J.H., & Henning, G.W. (2000). Anatomy and physiology of the enteric nervous system. *Gut, 47*(4), iv15-iv19. http://dx.doi.org/10.1136/gut.47.suppl_4.iv15

Deloose, E., & Tack, J. (2016). Redefining the functional roles of the gastrointestinal migrating motor complex and motilin in small bacterial overgrowth and hunger signaling. *American Journal of Physiology, 310*(4), 228-233. https://doi.org/10.1152/ajpgi.00212.2015

Deloose, E., Janssen, P., Depoortere, I., & Tack, J. (2012). The migrating motor complex: control mechanisms and its role in health and disease. *Nature Reviews:Gastroenterology & Hepatology*, 9(5), 271–285. https://doi.org/10.1038/nrgastro.2012.57

Electrophysiology of gastrointestinal smooth muscle. (n.d.). Vivo Pathophysiology. Retrieved March 30, 2022, from http://www.vivo.colostate.edu/.../basics/slowwaves.html

Gastrointestinal motility and smooth muscle. (n.d.). Vivo Pathophysiology. Retrieved March 30, 2022, from http://www.vivo.colostate.edu/.../basics/gi_motility.html

Gastrointestinal transit: How long does it take? (n.d.). Vivo Pathophysiology. Retrieved March 30, 2022, from http://www.vivo.colostate.edu/.../dig.../basics/transit.html

Gorard, D.A., Vesselinova-Jenkins, C.K., Libby, G.W., & Farthing, M. (1995). Migrating motor complex and sleep in health and irritable bowel syndrome. *Digestive Diseases and Sciences*, 40(11), 2383–2389. https://doi.org/10.1007/BF02063242

Grundy, D., & Brookes, S. (2011). Neural control of gastrointestinal function. *Colloquium Series on Integrated Systems Physiology: From Molecule to Function, 3*(9), 1-134. (https://doi.org/10.4199/C00048ED1V01Y201111ISP030)

Healthwise Staff. (2020, September 23). *Healthy eating: Recognizing your hunger signals.* University of Michigan Health: Michigan Medicine. https://www.uofmhealth.org/health-library/zx3292

How long does it take to digest food: Breaking down digestion speed. (2021, April 19). Cleveland Clinic. Retrieved March 30, 2022, from https://health.clevelandclinic.org/how-long-does-it-take.../

Hunger and fullness signals. (2021, March). Alberta Health Services. Retrieved March 30, 2022, from https://www.albertahealthservices.ca/.../if-nfs-hunger...

Nao. (2017, March 21). Why does my tummy rumble? *Dr. How's Science Wows*. http://sciencewows.ie/blog/tag/migrating-motor-complex/

Takahashi, T. (2012). Mechanism of interdigestive migrating motor complex. *Journal of Neurogastroenterology and Motility, 18*(3), 246-257. https://doi.org/10.5056/jnm.2012.18.3.246

The migrating motor complex. (n.d.). Vivo Pathophysiology. Retrieved March 30, 2022, from http://www.vivo. colostate.edu/.../stomach/mmcomplex.html

Tomomasa, T., Morikawa, A., Sandler, R. H., Mansy, H. A., Koneko, H., Masahiko, T., Hyman, P. E., & Itoh, Z. (1999). Gastrointestinal sounds and migrating motor complex in fasted humans. *The American Journal of Gastroenterology*, *94*(2), 374–381. https://doi.org/10.1111/j.1572-0241.1999.00862.x

HORMONES IMPORTANT TO WEIGHT LOSS & DIGESTION PART 1 - INSULIN

Insulin, we have heard this word discussed throughout the program as an important part of The Livy Method process. We are encouraged to eat high quality foods, support our bodies with supplements if we can, approach eating to the point where we feel satisfied, incorporate some exercise or activity to move our bodies, manage our stress levels, and prioritize having good, restful sleep. All of these things will help not only improve our health, wellness, and promote weight loss, but will also help to naturally lower our insulin levels.

In this science post we will be taking a deeper dive in the exploration of this highly discussed hormone. So, what exactly is insulin, and what exactly is its role in the body?

INSULIN

Insulin is a very important hormone in digestion, and has a huge role in helping to process and store the energy provided from the food that we eat! It is composed of 51 amino acids and for this reason is called a **peptide hormone** (hormones that are composed of small chains of amino acids). It plays an important part in glucose regulation, cell growth, and metabolism.

Insulin was previously believed to be solely produced by special cells in the pancreas called beta cells; however, recent evidence has shown that low concentrations are also found in certain neurons of the central nervous system!

As we have discussed in previous articles, the pancreas plays a principal part in digestion by producing hormones and enzymes that are crucial to the digestive process. However, this amazing organ also has a critical role in using and storing the energy (in the form of **glucose**) that it had just helped to break down and process, from the foods that we just ate!

So, let's back up this conversation a bit further. Let's recap the basics of digestion and then discuss how the foods we eat are processed for their energy.

SHORT RECAP ON DIGESTION

All parts of our body need energy to work, and this energy comes from the food we eat. As discussed, our bodies begin the digestive process when we think about and use our senses when preparing our food. When we ingest it, it begins mixing in with the saliva and enzymes in our mouths through the process of chewing. Then, the food bolus enters the stomach by way of the esophagus, and begins mixing with fluids (containing acids and enzymes) in the stomach. As the stomach churns and mixes, the food is processed and broken down further, resulting in reducing the carbohydrates we eat (sugars and starches) to their simplest form, a sugar called glucose. Proteins are broken down into amino acids and fat is broken down into fatty acids to be used by the body.

Glucose is the main energy source for our body's cells, and what keeps us functioning at all times whether it is when we are active and moving, resting and sleeping, it keeps our heart beating and lungs breathing. It is what allows all the organs and cells in our bodies to do what they need to do to keep us alive!

So, let's break it down even further, let's take a deeper look at what glucose actually is.

WHAT IS GLUCOSE?

Glucose is the simplest form of carbohydrates and only has one sugar molecule, which is called a **monosaccharide**. Other monosaccharides that may sound familiar include fructose, galactose, and ribose, which the body also processes or may produce for energy. To understand the differences, let's look at all these in more detail!

GLUCOSE

Glucose comes from the Greek word for "sweet" (Watson, S., & DerSarkissian, C. 2020, June). As discussed, glucose is a type of sugar you get from the foods you eat, and is what your body uses for energy. You may have heard the terms **blood glucose** or **blood sugar**, which are often used to describe the amount of glucose measured in your blood as it travels through your bloodstream to your cells. This can be quantified in a lab blood test, and results can be measured in that moment in time as a blood sugar, as a "fasted" blood sugar (taking your blood sugar after not eating or drinking for 8-12 hours), and as an A1C [which measures the percentage of hemoglobin (a protein in your red blood cells) that are coated in sugar, and can analyze your average blood sugar for the last 3 months].

Glucose is the most common monosaccharide found in nature. Some plants store glucose in linked chains. These chains are called starch. Common starch-containing foods include corn, potatoes, rice, and wheat. Glucose monosaccharides are also found naturally in some foods. The most concentrated whole food source of glucose monosaccharides are honey, followed by dried fruits such as dates, apricots, raisins, currants, cranberries, prunes and figs.

Most of the cells in your body use glucose along with amino acids (the building blocks of protein) and fats for energy. However, glucose is the main source of fuel for your brain. Nerve cells and chemical messengers located there need it to help them process information, and having access to glucose is very important for overall brain function. Your brain uses about 60% of the glucose that our bodies use. However, glucose does not always have to come immediately from foods and beverages. Glucose is also generated by the body to ensure that we always have the amount that is needed. One way that this is achieved is by breaking down something called **glycogen**, in order to free up the glucose it contains.

Glycogen is released by an important hormone called **glucagon.** When the body does not need to use glucose for energy, it is stored in the liver and muscles by insulin. This stored form of glucose is made up of many connected glucose molecules and is the glycogen. When the body needs a quick boost of energy or is not getting glucose from food, glycogen is broken down to release glucose into the bloodstream to be used as fuel for the cells. **Your body can store enough glycogen in order to keep you fueled for about a day.**

The body can also produce glucose through a process called gluconeogenesis. This process occurs when the body (mainly the liver, followed by the kidneys, and to a lesser extent the small intestine) makes glucose from non-carbohydrate sources which include lactate (what our bodies produce during exercise), glycerol (is produced when fats are digested, can be used for energy or stored in adipose tissue) and amino acids. Gluconeogenesis occurs when glycogen stores become low and glucose consumption is too low or nonexistent, such as during periods of starvation or prolonged fasting. Although the body has enough glycogen stored in the muscles and liver to last about a day, after about 14 hours in a fasted state it will begin to increase its percentage of gluconeogenesis, generating energy in increased ratios as time goes on (Chourpiliadis, C., & Mohiuddin, 2021).

One very important consideration is that skeletal muscle (composed of amino acids) can be used as a source when generating glucose through this pathway. This can lead to muscle wasting and loss over time, which can have a major impact on the body!

An additional alternative form of energy that can be generated if needed, is the formation of **ketone bodies** from our fat reserves. Ketone bodies can serve as a fuel source if glucose levels are too low in the body. Ketones serve as fuel in times of prolonged starvation, carbohydrate deprivation, or when patients suffer from uncontrolled diabetes and cannot appropriately utilize the circulating glucose. In these scenarios, fat stores are liberated, generating ketone bodies that are sent to the body and brain for energy.

This brings us to the conversation about the famous Keto diet that has been popularized in recent years. There seems to be a lot of compelling research arguing the benefits of using Keto as a means for weight loss. However, a recent study out of George Washington University School of Medicine examined available literature looking at the Keto diet (Crosby, L., Davis, B., Joshi, S., Jardine, M., Paul, J., Neola, M., & Barnard, N.D., 2021). They found that the diet was especially unsafe for pregnant women, women who may become pregnant, and those with kidney disease. They concluded that keto could also lead to long-term health complications, such as cancer, heart disease, and Alzheimer's Disease for most people. The rationale behind this was that this diet includes foods like meats, fish, nuts, and fibrous vegetables while eliminating most fruits, grains, beans, and starchy vegetables resulting in low vitamins, minerals, micronutrients and fiber intake. As we know from our last few science posts, these are all very important components of improving our overall digestion, microbiome and health! This study further corroborates the evidence that the Livy Method, which includes the food listed above, while minimizing added sugar, sets up our bodies for the best success!

If you want to go even further down the rabbit hole of understanding glucose at the chemical level, check out this video that discusses the structure of glucose in a more simplified way!

https://www.khanacademy.org/science/biology/macromolecules/carbohydrates-and-sugars/v/molecular-structure-of-glucose

GALACTOSE

The main dietary source of galactose comes in the form of lactose. Lactose is derived from milk and yogurt, and then digested and processed by the body, and broken down into the simpler forms of galactose and glucose. Interestingly, foods containing small amounts of free galactose include low-lactose or lactose-free milk, certain yogurts, cheeses, creams, ice cream, and other foods artificially sweetened with galactose. Plain natural foods like fruits, vegetables, nuts, grains, fresh meats, eggs, and milk, usually contain less than 0.3 g galactose per serving.

Galactose is not an essential nutrient! This means that you do not need to get it from food to be healthy, as galactose can be synthesized from glucose in our bodies if we need it. This is why we are able function just fine if we need to limit dairy, such as with those that live a vegan lifestyle, those with lactose intolerance or issues processing galactose like the genetic issue **galactosemia.**

Galactose, like glucose, is absorbed in the small intestine and carried by special proteins called "transport proteins" in the lining of the small intestine. From here, most of the absorbed galactose enters the liver where it is mainly converted to glucose, which is then either incorporated into glycogen or used for energy. Interestingly galactose ingestion, like fructose ingestion (as you will see below), results in lower blood glucose and insulin levels than glucose ingestion.

A common question that many members have when learning about the food plan, is how come they can have something like milk as part of their fluid intake? The thought being, will it increase our blood sugars like juice? It is a liquid, do our bodies not have to work as hard to break it down like food? This is a great question, and one that can be answered in 2 ways!

Milk, although easier to digest, does not raise our insulin levels the way a sugary drink would because of its absorption pathway in the liver (as it contains lactose which is broken down into galactose and glucose). Glucose (which is found in that sugary drink) would more likely be transported directly from the small intestine to the bloodstream increasing blood sugar. Insulin would be released in order to process and store that sugar (do not worry, we are getting to the discussion of insulin in due time, but all this is vital to understanding the role of insulin)! Interestingly, glucose can be absorbed at the wall of the small intestine as well as the liver. The second reason that drinking milk may not increase blood sugar levels, is that it contains protein and fat, that helps slow down our gastric emptying time, which also slows the processing of the blood sugar by the body. However, all this being said, it is still important to remember that most of our fluid intake should still come in the form of water!!

RIBOSE

Ribose is a type of monosaccharide that is made by our bodies from glucose. It is an essential component of **adenosine triphosphate (ATP)** which supplies energy to our cells, **(RNA) ribose nucleic acids** and **(DNA) deoxyribose nucleic acids.** DNA is known as the information molecule and stores all the genetic material of a cell. It also contains instructions for the synthesis of other molecules, like proteins. While RNA's function is to carry out the instructions that are encoded in DNA.

Ribose can be found in both plants and animals, including: mushrooms, beef and poultry, cheddar cheese and cream cheese, milk, eggs, caviar, anchovies, herring, sardines, and yogurt. However, it is found in these foods in very small quantities.

FRUCTOSE

Fructose is a fairly sweet, naturally occurring sugar. It comes from most fruits, and even some vegetables.

Pure fructose is also much sweeter than other types of sugar. As a result, people can use less fructose than other sugars in cooking to achieve the same sweetness. The most significant sources of fructose in today's diet include: table sugar (which is called **sucrose**, made from sugar cane or beets, is composed of 50% glucose and 50% fructose), honey, agave nectar, fruit juices, palm sugar and **(HFCS)** high fructose corn syrup (HFCS is a highly processed, inexpensive substitute for cane sugar that was introduced in the 1970s, and is made from corn. It is used to sweeten a variety of processed foods, including soda, candy, baked goods, and cereals).

After we ingest food, the stomach and small intestine go right to work in breaking the food down into its simplest form of glucose, which is absorbed and then released into the bloodstream. Once in the bloodstream, glucose can be used immediately by the cells for energy, or stored in our bodies to be used later. However, glucose and fructose are metabolized very differently by the body. Before it can be used by the body, fructose needs to be converted into glucose, which is conducted by the liver. While every cell in the body can use glucose, the liver is the only organ that can metabolize fructose when ingested in significant amounts!

HOW HAS FRUCTOSE CHANGED?

Before the mass production of refined sugar, humans rarely consumed fructose in high amounts. But as food science has developed over the years, our food has greatly changed from its very simple former self (that is a whole other science article!!!)

While most whole fruits and some vegetables contain fructose, they provide relatively low amounts. Some examples of vegetables that include fructose are artichokes, asparagus, broccoli, leeks, mushrooms, okra, onions, peas, red peppers, shallots and tomatoes.

Unlike glucose, fructose causes a low rise in blood sugar levels. Therefore, some health professionals recommend fructose as a "safe" sweetener for people with type 2 diabetes.

However, here is the crux. Many others are worried that excessive fructose intake may in fact contribute to several metabolic disorders. There is quite the debate in the scientific community around this!

When people eat a diet that is high in calories and high in fructose, the liver is thought to become overloaded and starts turning the fructose into fat. Many scientists believe that excess fructose consumption may be a key driver in many of the most serious diseases today (Gunnnars, K., 2018, April). These include obesity, type 2 diabetes, insulin resistance, heart disease, and even cancer. However, more human evidence is needed. Although, researchers debate the extent to which fructose contributes to these disorders, there is a considerable mounting body of evidence justifying the concerns.

THE HARMFUL EFFECTS OF EXCESS FRUCTOSE

According to (Gunnars, K., 2018, April), eating a lot of fructose in the form of added sugars may:

Impair the composition of your blood lipids. Fructose may raise the levels of **VLDL (very-low-density lipoprotein)** cholesterol, leading to the accumulation of fat around the organs. It may potentially cause heart disease, as it may alter how the body breaks down fats and carbohydrates, and lead to **atherosclerosis** (the build-up of plaque in the arteries which can block blood flow to the heart and other vital organs).

Increase blood levels of **uric acid**, leading to **gout** (a common and complex form of arthritis, characterized by sudden and severe attacks of pain, swelling, redness, and tenderness in one or more joints, most often in the big toe) and high blood pressure. Uric acid is a chemical created when the body breaks down substances called purines. Purines are normally produced in the body and are also found in some foods and drinks. Foods with high content of purines include liver, anchovies, mackerel, dried beans, peas, and beer. Generally, uric acid dissolves in blood and travels to the kidneys. It is processed by the kidneys and is passed out in urine. If your body produces too much uric acid or does not remove enough of it, you can get sick. A high level of uric acid in the blood is called **hyperuricemia.**

Cause deposition of fat in the liver, potentially leading to non-alcoholic fatty liver disease as discussed above.

Cause **insulin resistance**, which can lead to obesity and type 2 diabetes. Some studies found that excess amounts of dietary fructose seemed to cause inflammation that could lead to insulin resistance. We will go into more detail about insulin resistance later!

Fructose does not appear to suppress appetite as much as glucose does. As a result, it might promote overeating. When a person consumes glucose, the chemical structure of that compound triggers the pancreas to release insulin, a hormone that allows cells to use glucose for energy. Fructose does not appear to trigger insulin release or the release of hormones such as **leptin** which tells the brain that a person is full. It also does not inhibit hormones that tell an individual's body that they are hungry. As a result, fructose may lead to weight gain because it may contribute to overeating. Look out for more information on leptin next week as we discuss the hormones involved in hunger and satiety!

Again, to clarify, not all of this can be proven in controlled studies. However, the evidence is still there, and over time with more human studies conducted, this will likely become more evident.

SO, DO I NEED TO GIVE UP ALL FOODS THAT CONTAIN FRUCTOSE?

The important takeaway here is to realize that all of this does not apply to foods that have naturally occurring fructose, like whole fruits, vegetables, some whole grains, and even having a little bit of good quality sugars like cane sugar, honey or maple syrup. Essentially all healthy carbohydrates that are recommended on The Livy Method food plan!

Fruits, veggies, and heavier carbohydrates like quinoa, darker rices, potatoes and squashes, although containing fructose, are real food packed with nutrition, water and lots of fiber. These foods give your body what it needs, and allow you to feel satisfied with less. This makes them hard to overeat and you would have to eat very large amounts to reach harmful levels of fructose.

Hopefully this helps with the understanding of how our bodies process carbohydrates in order to utilize them for energy! The old adage, you are what you eat really holds true and hopefully as we are progressing through the program, eating better quality carbohydrates, you can all feel the difference this is making.

Here is a good video that briefly describes the monosaccharides in more detail:

https://www.youtube.com/watch?v=q5q8NXSDV0s

For those that want to look at the chemical structures of these sugars in more detail, check out this video!

https://www.youtube.com/watch?v=p0soyMv8-Xo

WHAT ABOUT PROTEIN AND FAT? DOES OUR BODY ALSO CONVERT THESE INTO GLUCOSE FOR ENERGY IF WE NEED IT?

Great question, and the answer is yes it does! Fats are used for energy after they are broken into fatty acids and glycerol and protein can also be used for energy, but its primary role is to help with making hormones, muscle, and other proteins.

NOW WE ARE READY TO TALK ABOUT INSULIN!!!

Now that we have reviewed the basics of glucose and the various pathways that the body uses to utilize the different simple sugars, protein, and fat for energy, let's talk about how the body stores this energy.

When a person consumes glucose, the chemical structure of the compound triggers the pancreas to release **insulin**, a hormone that allows cells to use glucose for energy.

THE PANCREAS

To recap our discussion from the science post on The Basics of Digestion, the pancreas is an organ which is located behind your stomach in the upper left part (quadrant) of your abdomen, surrounded by other organs of digestion including the small intestine, liver, gallbladder and spleen. Although the pancreas has an important role in digestion by secreting pancreatic juice rich in digestive enzymes, it also has the critical role of regulating blood sugar!

The body is designed to keep the level of glucose in your blood constant. The human pancreas contains one to two million pancreatic **islets (also called endocrine pancreas cells and islet of Langerhans cells)** housing different endocrine cells, primarily insulin-secreting beta cells, glucagon-producing alpha cells, and somatostatin-secreting delta cells (which serve to block the secretion of both insulin and glucagon from adjacent cells). Interestingly, although islets compose only 1–2% of the human pancreas, they receive up to 10% of the total pancreatic blood supply (Rahman, M. S., Hossain, K. S., Das, S., Kundu, S., Adegoke, E. O., Rahman, M. A., Hannan, M. A., Uddin, M. J., & Pang, M. G., 2021).

The beta cells in your pancreas monitor your blood sugar level every few seconds. When your blood glucose rises after you eat, the beta cells release insulin into your bloodstream. Insulin acts like a key, unlocking muscle, fat, and liver cells, so that glucose can penetrate them. Once inside, the cells convert glucose into energy to use right then, or store it to use later.

As glucose moves from the bloodstream into the cells, blood sugar levels start to drop. The beta cells in the pancreas can tell this is happening, so they slow down the amount of insulin they are making. At the same time, the pancreas slows down the amount of insulin that it is releasing into the bloodstream. When this happens, the amount of glucose going into the cells also slows down. Interestingly, insulin also helps our bodies store fat and protein.

After you have not eaten for a few hours your blood glucose level drops, and your pancreas stops producing insulin. Alpha cells in the pancreas begin to produce glucagon, signaling the liver to break down stored glycogen and turn it back into glucose. This glucose then travels to your bloodstream to replenish your supply until you are able to eat again. Although, as discussed earlier, your liver can also make its own glucose using a combination of waste products, amino acids, and fats.

The big takeaway here is that by following The Livy Method as designed, you are providing your body with a steady supply of energy over the day from healthy nutrient rich sources. As you are eating to satisfaction, you are no longer overeating to the state of being full, which would stimulate your beta cells to secrete a larger amount of insulin to process and store all that glucose being digested! Smaller amounts of food over time means smaller amounts of insulin being produced, feeling more satisfied with less, decreasing stress on the body!

Here is a great video that discusses the role of the pancreas.

https://www.youtube.com/watch?v=NZ4zcrTzUjA

Here is a video that discusses glucagon and its role in glucose release.

https://www.youtube.com/watch?v=9dq3dtudQHM

Here is a great video that discusses the role of insulin in a little more detail.

https://www.youtube.com/watch?v=fPguYEDlQEQ

ISSUES WITH INSULIN

Without enough insulin, glucose cannot move into the cells and the blood glucose level remains elevated. This condition is called **hyperglycemia**. Prolonged hyperglycemia can damage the blood vessels that carry oxygen-rich blood to your organs, and can increase your risk for heart disease, heart attack, stroke, kidney disease, nerve damage, and an eye disease called retinopathy.

WHAT CAUSES HYPERGLYCEMIA?

Typically, hyperglycemia is a symptom and can be caused when there is an issue with the body's cells not responding to insulin (**insulin resistance**), or there is an issue with the beta cells not producing adequate insulin (**prediabetes and diabetes**).

Other hormones that can raise the blood sugar level include epinephrine (also called adrenaline)and cortisol which are released by the adrenal glands, and growth hormone which is released by the pituitary gland. This is again why it is vitally important to manage stress levels, as chronic stress can have an impact on blood sugar levels.

WHAT IS INSULIN RESISTANCE?

Insulin resistance is when cells in your muscles, fat, and liver do not respond well to insulin and are not able to easily take up glucose from your blood. As a result, your pancreas increases the production of insulin to help glucose enter your cells, a condition called **hyperinsulinemia**. However, as long as your pancreas can produce enough insulin to overcome your cells' weak response to insulin, your blood glucose levels should stay in the healthy range.

WHAT IS PREDIABETES?

Prediabetes means your blood glucose levels are elevated, but not elevated enough to be diagnosed as diabetes. Prediabetes usually occurs in people who already have some insulin resistance or whose beta cells in the pancreas are not making enough insulin to keep blood glucose in the normal range. Without enough insulin, extra glucose stays in your bloodstream rather than entering your cells. Over time, you are at increased risk for developing type 2 diabetes.

WHAT CAUSES INSULIN RESISTANCE AND PREDIABETES?

According to the National Institute of Diabetes and Digestive and Kidney Diseases, researchers do not fully understand what causes insulin resistance and prediabetes, but they speculate excess weight and lack of physical activity are major factors.

EXCESS WEIGHT

Many experts believe obesity, and especially visceral fat (the accumulation of fat in the abdomen and around the organs) are the main cause of insulin resistance. Having a waist measurement of 40 inches or more for men and 35 inches or more for women is linked to insulin resistance. This is true even if your body mass index (BMI) falls within the normal range. However, research has shown that Asian Americans may have an increased risk for insulin resistance even without a high BMI. (The discussion of BMI is used in reference to this study, although the concept of BMI is problematic as a measure of obesity).

Studies have also shown that belly fat produces hormones and other substances that can contribute to chronic or long-lasting inflammation in the body. Inflammation may play a role in insulin resistance, type 2 diabetes, and cardiovascular disease. Since excess weight may lead to insulin resistance, this also is a contributing factor in the development of fatty liver disease.

PHYSICAL INACTIVITY

Not getting enough physical activity is linked to insulin resistance and prediabetes. Regular physical activity causes changes in your body that help with glucose regulation. When you participate in moderate exercise that increases your heart rate and breathing, your muscles use more glucose from the body. Over time, this can lower your blood sugar levels and also allows the insulin in your body to work better. You will also receive these benefits for hours after your activity or workout.

However, very intense or strenuous exercise can cause the body to produce more stress hormones, which can lead to an increase in blood sugar as well as stress on the body. This can also help explain one of the reasons why overexercise is not a good weight loss tool!

As you can see by following The Livy Method, and incorporating the food plan and eating nutrient rich foods, including heavier carbs when needed, eating to satisfaction, incorporating stress management strategies, with a focus on getting quality sleep, you can greatly improve your state of health and wellness. By losing weight and following The Livy Method which can decrease abdominal visceral fat over time, health issues can be reversed! Many of our Livy Losers have shared their amazing health related NSVs, and are great reads to tap into motivation if you need to! Finally, incorporating exercise will also help with blood sugar regulation and can be a great stress reliever too! So, if you are feeling it, move that body!!!

Now that we understand more about the role of insulin in the body and some of the hormones involved in digestion and weight loss, join us for our next science post where we discuss some of the issues with digestion!

REFERENCES

https://www.sciencedirect.com/topics/agricultural-and-biological-sciences/galactose

All about your A1C. (2021, August 10). Centers for Disease Control and Prevention. Retrieved March 30, 2022, from https://www.cdc.gov/diabetes/managing/managing-blood-sugar/a1c.html

Betts, G.J., Young, K.A., Wise, J.A., Johnson, E., Poe, B., Kruse, D.H., Korol, O., Johnson, J.E., Womble, M., & DeSaix, P. (2019, May 29). *Anatomy and physiology.* Openstax. https://opentextbc.ca/anatomyandphysiologyopenstax/chapter/lipid-metabolism/

Biologydictionary.net Editors. (2021, January 09). *Dna vs rna.* Biology dictionary. https://biologydictionary.net/dna-vs-rna/

Brown, S. (2021, August 18). *Study: Keto diet may lead to long-term health risks.* Verywell Health. https://www.verywellhealth.com/keto-diet-long-term-risks-5197991

Bryant, E. (2020, September 15). *How high fructose intake may trigger fatty liver disease.* National Institutes of Health. https://www.nih.gov/news-events/nih-research-matters/how-high-fructose-intake-may-trigger-fatty-liver-disease#:~:text=Studies%20suggest%20that%20high%20fructose,%2Dalcoholic%20steatohepatitis%20(NASH).

Chourpiliadis, C., & Mohiuddin. (2021). *Biochemistry, gluconeogenesis.* StatPearls Publishing. https://www.ncbi.nlm.nih.gov/books/NBK544346/

Cleveland Clinic. (2021, March 1). *What is fructose intolerance? How to cope when your stomach says no to fruit.* Cleveland Clinic. https://health.clevelandclinic.org/what-is-fructose-intolerance/#:~:text=Common%20high%2Dfructose%20foods%20include,pepper%2C%20shallots%20and%20tomato%20products.

Crosby, L., Davis, B., Joshi, S., Jardine, M., Paul, J., Neola, M., & Barnard, N.D. (2021). Ketogenic diets and chronic disease: Weighing the benefits against the risks. *Frontiers in Nutrition, 8,* 702802.https://doi.org/10.3389/fnut.2021.702802

Diabetes tests. (2021, August 10). Centers for Disease Control and Prevention. Retrieved March 30, 2022, from https://www.cdc.gov/diabetes/basics/getting-tested.html#:~:text=Fasting%20Blood%20Sugar%20Test,higher%20indicates%20you%20have%20diabetes.

Frank, J. (2020, September 28). *What are purines?* Arthritis - health. https://www.arthritis-health.com/types/gout/what-are-purines

Greenlaw, E. & Martin, L. J. (2013, January 18). *Exercises to lower your blood sugar.* WebMD. https://www.webmd.com/healthy-aging/features/exercise-lower-blood-sugar#:~:text=When%20you%20do%20moderate%20exercise,in%20your%20body%20work%20better.

Gunnnars, K. (2018, April 23). *Is fructose bad for you? The surprising truth.* Healthline.

https://www.healthline.com/nutrition/why-is-fructose-bad-for-you

Healthwise Staff. (2020, August 31). *Carbohydrates, proteins, fats, and blood sugar.* University of Michigan Health: Michigan Medicine. https://www.uofmhealth.org/health-library/uq1238abc#:~:text=Protein%20can%20also%20be%20used,%2C%20muscle%2C%20and%20other%20proteins.&text=Broken%20down%20into%20glucose%2C%20used%20to%20supply%20energy%20to%20cells.

Higdon, J., Drake, V.J., Delage, B., & Liu, S. (2016, March). *Glycemic index and glycemic load.* Oregon State University. https://lpi.oregonstate.edu/mic/food-beverages/glycemic-index-glycemic-load

How our bodies turn food into energy. (n.d.). Kaiser Permanente. Retrieved Month Date, Year, from https://healthy.kaiser-permanente.org/colorado/health-wellness/healtharticle.how-our-bodies-turn-food-into-energy#:~:text=Our%20bodies%20digest%20the%20food,type%20of%20sugar%2C%20called%20glucose.

Islet cell. (n.d.). National Cancer Institute. Retrieved March 30, 2022, from https://www.cancer.gov/publications/dictionaries/cancer-terms/def/islet-cell

Khan Academy. (2015, July 10). *Molecular structure of glucose | Macromolecules | Biology.* [Video]. Youtube. https://www.youtube.com/watch?v=-Aj5BTnz-v0

Kitchin, B. (2009, July 24). *High fructose fracas.* The University of Alabama at Birmingham. https://www.uab.edu/shp/nutritiontrends/nutrition-know-how/consumer-concerns/high-fructose-fracas

Macrophage. (2013, May 31). *Insulin 2: What is glucagon?* [Video].Youtube. https://www.youtube.com/watch?v=9dq3dtudQHM

Macrophage. (2013, June 10). *Insulin 1: What does insulin do, and why do we need it?* [Video].Youtube. https://www.youtube.com/watch?v=fPguYEDlQEQ

Marengo, K., & Dix, M. (2021, April 1). *How is protein digested?* Healthline. https://www.healthline.com/health/protein-digestion

Mayo Clinic Staff. (2020, August 25). *Glycemic index diet: What's behind the claims.* Mayo Clinic.

https://www.mayoclinic.org/healthy-lifestyle/nutrition-and-healthy-eating/in-depth/glycemic-i dex-diet/art-20048478

McMillen, M., & Ratini, M. (2021, February 5). *Ribose.* WebMD. https://www.webmd.com/vitamins-and-supplements/ribose-uses-and-risks#:~:text= Ribose%20(d%2Dribose)%20is,supplies%20energy%20to%20our%20cells.

MedlinePlus. (2022, March 21). *Uric acid - blood.* https://medlineplus.gov/ency/article/003476.htm#:~:text=Uric%20acid%20is%20a%20chemical,beans%20and%20peas%2C%20and%20beer.

MedlinePlus. (2020, August 18). *Galactosemia.* https://medlineplus.gov/genetics/condition/galactosemia/

MedlinePlus. (2019, February 27). *Vldl cholesterol.* https://medlineplus.gov/vldlcholesterol.html

Nakrani, M.N., Wineland, R.H., & Anjum, F. (2021). *Physiology, glucose metabolism.* StatPearls Publishing. https://www.ncbi.nlm.nih.gov/books/NBK560599/

NutrientsReview. (n.d.). *Galactose.* https://www.nutrientsreview.com/carbs/monosaccharides-galactose.html

Pointer, K., & Luo, E.K. (2017, March 24). *Everything you need to know about glucose.* Healthline. https://www.healthline.com/health/glucose

Pereira, R. M., Botezelli, J. D., da Cruz Rodrigues, K. C., Mekary, R. A., Cintra, D. E., Pauli, J. R., da Silva, A., Ropelle, E. R., & de Moura, L. P. (2017). Fructose consumption in the development of obesity and the effects of different protocols of physical exercise on the hepatic metabolism. *Nutrients, 9*(4), 405. https://doi.org/10.3390/nu9040405

Rahman, M. S., Hossain, K. S., Das, S., Kundu, S., Adegoke, E. O., Rahman, M. A., Hannan, M. A., Uddin, M. J., & Pang, M. G. (2021). Role of insulin in health and disease: An update. *International Journal of Molecular Sciences, 22*(12), 6403. https://doi.org/10.3390/ijms22126403

Ribose. (2020, August 10). LibreTexts. Retrieved March 30, 2022, from https://chem.libretexts.org/@go/page/392

Richter, A., & Nall, R. (2021, December 16). *Is fructose bad for you?* Medical News Today. https://www.medical-newstoday.com/articles/323818#summary

Skrovan, S. (2017, August 14). *Manufacturers reformulate with sugar as consumers sour on corn syrup.* Food Dive. https://www.fooddive.com/news/manufacturers-reformulate-with-sugar-as-consumers-sour-on-corn-syrup/449233/

Sollid, K. (2021, May 24). *What is glucose?* Food Insight. https://foodinsight.org/what-is-glucose/

ThePancreasPatient. (2013, September 6). *The role and anatomy of the pancreas* [Video]. Youtube.https://www.youtube.com/watch?v=NZ4zcrTzUjA

The Organic Chemistry Tutor. (2019, October 14. *Monosaccharides - Glucose, fructose, galactose, & ribose - Carbohydrates.* [Video]. Youtube. https://www.youtube.com/watch?v=p0soyMv8-Xo

Utiger, R. D. (2011, February 7). *somatostatin.* Encyclopedia Britannica. https://www.britannica.com/science/somatostatin

Watson, S., & DerSarkissian, C. (2020, June 13). *What is glucose?* WebMD. https://www.webmd.com/diabetes/glucose-diabetes

Weatherspoon, D., & Whelan, C. (2018, September 17). *Everything you need to know about fasting before a blood test.* Healthline. https://www.healthline.com/health/fasting-before-blood-test

What is diabetes? (2021, December 16). Centers for Disease Control and Prevention. Retrieved March 30, 2022, from https://www.cdc.gov/diabetes/basics/diabetes.html#:~:text=Diabetes%20is%20a%20chronic%20(long,your%20pancreas%20to%20release%20insulin

Whats Up Dude. (2016, October 16). *What are simple carbohydrates - Monosaccharides - Glucose - Fructose - Disaccharides* [Video]. Youtube. https://www.youtube.com/watch?v=q5q8NXSDV0s

ISSUES WITH DIGESTION

In the post The Basics of Digestion, we discussed digestion fundamentals with a few important take-aways. To recap, we discussed the importance of:

1.   The cephalic phase of eating- In this phase, we engage with our brain-gut connection by creating a ritual around thoughtfully preparing our foods, using our senses and focusing on the first two mindfulness questions. We are allowing for adequate time for the stimulation of our saliva and gastric juices which contain digestive enzymes to flood our mouth and stomach, getting our bodies primed and ready for digestion. This sets us up for the optimal absorption of the nutrients we are eating!

2.   Chewing our food- In this phase we are ingesting our food and chewing it as best as we can, breaking it down into the smallest pieces possible. This allows for the best mixing of our food with saliva and enzymes which can facilitate optimal digestion. This is the perfect time to engage in the third set of mindfulness questions to see how we are feeling while eating as in the cephalic phase, we want to take our time with this process for it to be the most beneficial!

This brings us to this follow up science post that initiates the conversation about digestive issues. Now that we have a better understanding of how digestion works, let's take a deeper look at how The Livy Method can best support those who may have concerns or healing needed for their digestive issues.

Because there are so many possible digestive issues, this article will focus on the most common issues that most people have. These articles do not take the place of your doctor or health care provider (HCP). If you have more in-depth issues or concerns, it is very important to consult with your HCP and communicate any questions or concerns with them!

HYPOCHLORHYDRIA, OTHERWISE KNOWN AS THE LOW PRODUCTION OF THE STOMACH ACID HCL (HYDROCHLORIC ACID)

As we discussed in The Basics of Digestion, during the cephalic phase, once our chewed foods enter our stomach, **parietal cells** that are contained in the lining of our stomach begin to release hydrochloric acid. This occurs in order to create an acidic environment to activate the digestive enzyme called pepsin. This begins the process of converting proteins into amino acids to enable utilization by the body. This acidic environment also protects our bodies from bacteria and pathogens that may have been ingested. However, to do this effectively, the **PH ("Potential for Hydrogen" which is a scale from 1-14 that measures how acidic or alkaline a substance is)** must be extremely low or acidic, measuring between **1.5-2** on the PH scale. Now that is acidic!!!!

However, some people have issues producing enough stomach acid for a variety of reasons which can have a major impact on their digestion!

AGE

As we age our production of HCL decreases, becoming more common in those over 65. This can have an impact on how those who are aging digest their foods.

CHRONIC STRESS

Stressful events activate our brain and stimulate our **sympathetic nervous system (SNS)** which is also known as the "fight or flight" response in our bodies. This response is meant to be short-term and is activated to deal with whatever emergency has arisen. When the emergency is over, our bodies are meant to settle back down to our normal **parasympathetic nervous system (PSNS)** state, otherwise known as the "rest and digest" state. When our SNS is activated, we release cortisol which many of us know as the "stress hormone," in order to fight the emergency. From the perspective of digestion, the SNS decreases blood flow to the digestive system, including the stomach, so it can focus on providing good blood flow to the heart, lungs, and brain! This decreased blood flow ultimately leads to lower HCl levels and a decrease in mucous production (which lines and protects the stomach), which has the potential to injure the fragile lining of the gut. Damage to this lining may cause inflammation, ulcers, and impact nutrient absorption. As you can see, if our bodies are in a chronic or prolonged state of stress, there can be a great impact on our digestive system!

POOR DIET LOW IN NUTRIENTS & LIFESTYLE FACTORS

B vitamins and minerals, such as iron and zinc, are responsible for the production of HCL in our bodies. Having a diet low in these nutrients can affect our production of HCL. Lifestyle factors such as smoking and drinking can also decrease our absorption of these vitamins and minerals, impacting how much HCL we are producing.

HELICOBACTER PYLORI (H. PYLORI) INFECTION

H. Pylori is one of the most common bacterial infections in the world, being said to affect up to 67% of the global population (Bernstein, S., & Khatri, M., 2020, December). H. pylori colonizes and lives in the stomach lining of the stomach, and is thought to be transmitted by the ingestion of food, water, and/or shared food, water, and utensils. It can also be contracted through contact with saliva or other bodily fluids of infected people. H. pylori is more common in countries or communities that lack clean water or good sewage systems.

The stomach lining is responsible for producing HCL and mucous, but also protects the stomach itself from the HCL it produces. Any compromise in the tissue of the stomach can lead to something called **"gastritis" or inflammation of the stomach**, leading to the stomach becoming inflamed, ulcers (sores), and/or bleeding of the tissue. This affects the cells that secrete the HCL potentially causing a decreased production of this stomach acid, causing hypochlorhydria, as well as the potential for the decreased ability to digest the foods eaten.

Most cases of those colonized with H. pylori are **asymptomatic (show no symptoms)** but may lead to the emergence of symptoms showing later in life, develop into stomach or duodenal ulcers, or result in gastric cancer for 1-3% of those colonized. The good news is that with good hygiene, the likelihood of acquiring H. Pylori is greatly reduced, and is easily diagnosed and treatable with antibiotics and medications!

LONG TERM USE OF ANTACID MEDICATIONS AND OTHER MEDICATIONS

Sometimes those with hypochlorhydria, experience symptoms that are similar to acid reflux or **GERD (gastroesophageal reflux disease)** and take medications to suppress those symptoms. A specific kind of antacid that people take are called **proton pump inhibitors (PPIs).** PPIs target the production of stomach acid by suppressing the parietal cells in the stomach from producing HCL. However, these cells also produce something called **intrinsic factor (IF)** that helps the small intestine absorb vitamin B12. Long term use of these PPIs may potentially cause a deficiency in B12 absorption. Vitamin B12 is an important component in helping our body produce **red blood cells** and if deficient in this vitamin over time, can lead to a condition called **pernicious anemia**. These can also impact our absorption of minerals as well if taken for prolonged periods. The big takeaway here is that those who think they have acid reflux or GERD, may actually be affected by having low gastric acid. If there is not enough gastric acid in our stomach, the food is not able to be broken down in the way it was meant to and spends a prolonged amount of time there. This allows the food to ferment and begin to release gases which cause our stomachs to feel bloated, causes burping and creates an acidic feeling in our stomachs. However, if you have been on PPIs for a long time, it is very important to have a discussion and consult your HCP about your medications before discontinuing them, or if you have any questions or concerns about your symptoms! This is a very individualized process and can have different impacts for different individuals.

GASTRIC BYPASS AND OTHER GASTRIC SURGERIES

Finally, the last cause of hypochlorhydria is in the case of those that have a history of gastric bypass surgery or other surgeries of the stomach. In these cases, the stomach does not function in the way it had prior to the surgery. This can be a fairly large topic, but the big takeaway is that following The Livy Method as described in the summary can help support the digestive system as optimally as possible. You may have to be mindful of certain foods that can cause symptoms for you! This is very individual and is different for everyone!

SYMPTOMS OF HYPOCHLORHYDRIA

Here are some signs that you may not be producing enough stomach acid. They usually show up a few hours after you have eaten and may include:

Feeling like you want to eat even when you are not hungry, feeling too full after regular meals, indigestion, gas or flatulence, bloating, constipation, diarrhea, soreness or burning in your mouth, stomach upset and cramps, undigested food in stool, nausea, and heartburn.

ACID REFLUX AND GASTROESOPHAGEAL REFLUX DISEASE

In normal digestion, after chewing and swallowing your food, the food travels down the esophagus via muscular contractions called peristalsis. This "bolus" enters the stomach via the **LES** or **lower esophageal sphincter**, a muscular ring which opens to allow food into your stomach. Once the food or bolus enters, the LES closes to stop food and acidic stomach juices from flowing back into the esophagus.

WHAT IS GERD?

Gastroesophageal reflux disease or GERD, is a chronic digestive disorder that occurs when stomach contents, which includes the acidic digestive juices, backs up from the stomach via the LES into the esophagus resulting in heartburn or acid indigestion. This occurs when the LES is weak or relaxes when it should not. Interestingly, an acidic environment triggers the closure of the LES, so in some cases, acid reflux occurs when there is incidence of hypochlorhydria! While it is common for people to experience acid reflux and heartburn once in a while, having symptoms that affect your daily life or occur at least twice each week could be a sign of GERD.

RISK FACTORS FOR GERD

HAVING WEIGHT TO LOSE

Having extra weight and fat on our body, especially in the abdominal region, can increase the pressure on our stomach causing the LES to open and cause reflux. This can also make our bodies less efficient at emptying the stomach contents into our small intestine.

PREGNANCY

Heartburn is common in pregnancy and can get worse as the pregnancy progresses. Hormones that support pregnancy can cause the digestive system to slow down. Peristalsis decreases and as the baby grows, the pressure on the stomach increases and can cause reflux.

DELAYED EMPTYING OF THE STOMACH (GASTROPARESIS)

Some people have a medical condition called **gastroparesis** that causes a delay in gastric emptying time. To recap, our stomach and intestines have strong involuntary muscular contractions that propel food through the digestive tract. Gastroparesis is a condition that affects the normal spontaneous movement of these muscles, otherwise known as motility, in the stomach. The stomach's motility is slowed down or does not function, preventing the stomach from emptying properly. What this means is there can be a delay in the movement of the contents of the stomach to the small intestine, resulting in reflux. This can be an isolated issue, or precipitated by other medical conditions like diabetes.

LIFESTYLE FACTORS SUCH AS SMOKING, CERTAIN FOODS AND DRINKS INCLUDING CHOCOLATE, MINT, FRIED FOODS, COFFEE, AND ALCOHOL

The nicotine from tobacco, chocolate, mint and alcohol can actually relax the LES causing reflux. Some people find fried foods, coffee, acidic or spicy foods can make symptoms of GERD worse.

LARGE MEALS

Eating a large meal can cause an increase in abdominal pressure on the stomach resulting in reflux.

EATING TOO SOON BEFORE BED

After eating, wait 2 to 3 hours before lying down. When you are lying down, the contents of your stomach can push against the LES resulting in reflux, whereas sitting up allows gravity to promote the proper movement and flow of food down the digestive tract. Also, as we are preparing for bed, and the production and secretion of melatonin increases in our bodies as it gets darker, our bodies will want to focus on rest and repair as opposed to digestion. In fact, our digestion naturally slows due to the release of these hormones, and is an important part of something called our "**circadian rhythm**"! This is why it is recommended to finish our meals earlier in the evening, minimizing late evening snacking, as it promotes the optimal environment for digestion!

HYPERCHLORHYDRIA

Some people's bodies naturally have an overproduction of gastric HCL. It may not be an issue for some, but for others it may cause issues with reflux.

MEDICATIONS

Some prescription medications, over the counter medications, and supplements may cause GERD. Consult your HCP or pharmacist to discuss your medications if you have questions.

GERD SYMPTOMS

The most common symptom of GERD is heartburn (acid indigestion). It is described as a burning chest pain that starts behind your breastbone and moves upward to your neck and throat. Many people describe that it feels like food is coming back into the mouth, leaving an acid, sour or bitter taste, lasting as long as 2 hours. Besides pain you may also have nausea, bad breath, trouble breathing, difficulty swallowing, vomiting, the wearing away of tooth enamel, or the feeling of a lump in your throat. If you have acid reflux at night, you may also have a lingering cough, laryngitis that comes on suddenly or gets worse, or issues with sleep. If you have concerns with any of these symptoms, follow up with your HCP!

Check out this video for more details!

https://www.youtube.com/watch?v=TdK0jRFpWPQ

LIVING WITHOUT A GALLBLADDER

Many of our members are coming into this program without a gallbladder, and are concerned that they will have issues following the plan, or with weight loss because of this.

To recap from last week, the liver is a large organ located above the stomach in the upper abdomen. The liver produces bile which is stored in the gallbladder, stores glucose and nutrients and also helps remove toxins from the body.

When we eat fatty foods the gallbladder (a small pouch) is stimulated to secrete **bile** via the **bile ducts** to the small intestine, which helps to emulsify the fats making it easier for **lipases (enzymes that break down fat)** to do their job!

The good news is that your body can still function well without a gallbladder! Although it acts as a storage area for your bile, the liver amazingly adapts to this change in your body and will still produce bile! However, it does this by producing it in continuous drips delivering it directly into the small intestine. This means that your body is still capable of producing bile for the emulsification of fats.

Some people have no issues without having a gallbladder. However, others may have to monitor foods that may cause them digestive discomfort like gas, bloating and diarrhea, limit the ingestion of fried fatty foods, or limit large meals. But as discussed below, The Livy Method supports those without a gallbladder really well!!!

INFLAMMATORY BOWEL DISEASE (IBD) AND INFLAMMATORY BOWEL SYNDROME (IBS)

Inflammatory bowel disease (IBD) is a general term used to describe disorders that involve chronic inflammation of the digestive tract. The 2 major types of IBD include:

ULCERATIVE COLITIS

This condition involves inflammation and sores (ulcers) along the superficial (top layer) lining of the large intestine (colon) and rectum.

CROHN'S DISEASE

This type of IBD is characterized by inflammation of the lining of the digestive tract, which can involve the deeper layers of the digestive tract, involve any part of the small or large intestine, and may be continuous or involve multiple segments of the small or large intestine.

Those with ulcerative colitis and Crohn's disease have symptoms of diarrhea, rectal bleeding, abdominal pain, fatigue and weight loss.

IRRITABLE BOWEL SYNDROME (IBS)

Irritable bowel syndrome, or IBS, is a group of symptoms that affect your digestive system. It's a common but uncomfortable gastrointestinal disorder. Those with IBS have symptoms of excessive gas, abdominal pain, and cramps.

IBS is a type of **functional** gastrointestinal (GI) disorder. A functional disorder or issue is when a person has symptoms of a condition, but the condition itself is unable to be identified or diagnosed by medical testing methods. These conditions, also called disorders of the gut-brain interaction, can affect how the gut and brain work together. When one is affected by IBS, the IBS can cause the digestive tract to be easily stimulated, affecting peristalsis (contraction of the digestive smooth muscle). This overstimulation can result in abdominal pain, diarrhea and constipation. People with IBS may have a lower pain tolerance, and research has also suggested that people with IBS may have bacterial overgrowth in the GI tract which may also contribute to their symptoms (Cleveland Clinic, 2020, September).

Check out this video for more information!

https://www.webmd.com/ibd-crohns-disease/video/video-ibd-complications

HOW THE LIVY METHOD HELPS SUPPORT THE BODY

The Livy method by the very nature of its design helps to support the body in digestion and improve our overall health! Here is a summary of how the program best supports all aspects of your digestive health.

1. Chew, chew, chew, chew and take smaller bites when eating to stimulate your saliva and digestive enzymes, while focusing on your practise of mindfulness. This can eliminate symptoms associated with low stomach acid and can help maintain an appropriate level of HCL in your stomach.

2. The Livy Method recommends eating nutrient rich foods loaded with lots of veggies, leafy greens, some fruit, and grains, which are high in vitamins, minerals, and fiber. These recommended foods can help increase your stomach acid levels, heal the digestive system, promote vitamin absorption, and promote the growth of healthy gut flora. It is also recommended to decrease the ingestion of processed foods, deep fried foods, and foods high in sugars which can cause inflammation in the stomach, decrease acid activity, and trigger acid reflux symptoms. Adding in fermented vegetables and fluids such as kimchi, sauerkraut, kefir, and pickles can also naturally improve your stomach acid levels. These foods also have probiotic effects that can help improve digestion, fight harmful bacteria, and reduce inflammation caused by low stomach acid.

3. Raw apple cider vinegar with the mother is a fermented liquid made from crushed apples, bacteria, and yeast. ACV is rich in protein and enzymes and is bacterial in nature, which can help break down food and improve gut health. Like lemon juice, raw apple cider vinegar can help increase stomach acid levels because of its acidic properties, introducing more acid into the digestive tract when ingested. Both lemon juice and ACV are a 2 on the PH scale!

    There is definitely a rabbit hole one can enter when looking at the benefits of using ACV or lemon water! There is limited evidence on its use as something to help stimulate bile production and the diet industry's proclamation of it being a fat burner and insulin stabilizer. However, it can be a great way to start the day in a positive way, by cleansing our palate and setting us up for success!! It's much like a physical action led intention which is a great addition to our daily intentions!!

As a final note, to help protect your teeth and the more sensitive tissues of your mouth and esophagus, you may want to dilute your ACV or lemon juice in a good amount of water if you can, and/or brush your teeth after 30 minutes of drinking.

4. While following the Livy Method, we are aiming to consume at least six meals and snacks a day, with a good mix of carbs, protein, and healthy fat at each meal. The Livy Method also focuses on eating to satisfaction and not overeating during these meals. This ensures that the digestive system is not overloaded and can handle the amount of food we give it! This helps to prevent heartburn from the stomach acids going back from the stomach into the esophagus, and may also prevent any subsequent gas, nausea, or vomiting. This also maximizes nutrient absorption! Even though you will reach a point where you won't necessarily be eating this often, the principles will be the same, eating what makes you feel good, eating to satisfaction and nurturing your body!

5. The Livy Method also recommends eating earlier in the evening and not too late at night! As discussed, eating before dark or up to two hours after sunset promotes better digestion. This allows your body to focus on rest and repair as opposed to digestion when our natural levels of melatonin are at their highest! This also allows more time for our food to travel from our stomach to our small intestine, reducing the risk of reflux. Sleeping on our left side is the most optimal position for digestion as it applies the least amount of pressure on our LES, and promotes better flow in the digestion pathway. Lying on our right side causes increased pressure on our LES, and is the least favoured position for digestion.

6. Because many of us come into this process with digestive issues, we are less able to absorb and process nutrients, vitamins, and minerals from our food. This is why supplementation is recommended as a companion to the food plan. It can help our bodies function the most optimally and can also help heal our bodies, eventually allowing us to process our nutrients better on our own. As discussed in The Basics of Digestion: Part 1, adding in prebiotics and probiotics also aids in the production and absorption of B vitamins and vitamin K in the colon, and also improves the colonization of helpful bacteria in our digestive system, which is vital to the digestive process! Check out this video on the importance of the microbiome of our digestive system!

    https://www.youtube.com/watch?v=B9RruLkAUm8&t=329s

7. Canadian digestive bitters can also be very helpful for the digestive process as recommended in the supplements post. Digestive bitters are groups of herbs that have very bitter qualities and stimulate the bitter receptors that are found in the mouth, gut, and pancreas (contrary to popular belief that they are just found in the tongue). As a result, they stimulate the production of saliva and they can help to naturally stimulate gastric juices and bile flow, which results in enhanced digestion!

8. Maintaining a journal that includes a food diary is a great add when following The Livy

Method. Journaling how certain foods make you feel can really give insights into what foods cause digestive discomforts or issues, and help you identify potential intolerances!

9. Stress management is imperative to the weight loss process and also helps manage the brain-gut connection! Using stress management techniques and the other methods recommended on plan decreases external stimulation that can literally "stress" our digestive system, promoting the body to function as best it can!

10. Finally, following the Livy Method ensures that you are adequately hydrated! Water as we all know here is vital to life and can maximize our success! It is involved in almost every chemical reaction in the body, particularly in the processing of our nutrients and the absorption of vitamins and minerals in the body. It can be particularly helpful in preventing constipation because water helps soften your stools! So… sip, sip, sip that water and get in just enough!

Now that we have explored some of the issues with digestion, stay tuned for our next science post, where we will take a deeper dive into more of the hormones involved in regulating our hunger and feelings of satiety, eating breakfast and how making it high in protein sets up our day for success, and will conclude our discussion on digestion by looking at how long it takes our bodies to process and digest the foods that we eat.

REFERENCES

AllHealthGo. (2018, August 30). *Living without a gallbladder* [Video]. Youtube. https://www.youtube.com/watch?v=l2eb7mSIvuk

Bernstein, S., & Khatri, M. (2020, December 7). *What is H. pylori?* WebMD. https://www.webmd.com/digestive-disorders/h-pylori-helicobacter-pylori

Bhargava, H.D. (2020, September 11). *Gerd.* WebMD. https://www.webmd.com/heartburn-gerd/guide/reflux-disease-gerd-1#:~:text=Gastroesophageal%20reflux%20disease%2C%20or%20GERD,get%20heartburn%20or%20acid%20indigestion.

Bolen, B., & Hall, M. (2020, December 7). *Keep a food diary to identify food triggers.* Verywell Health. https://www.verywellhealth.com/how-to-keep-a-food-diary-1945006

Brennan, D. (2021, November 15). *What is hypochlorhydria?* WebMD. https://www.webmd.com/digestive-disorders/what-is-hypochlorhydria

Cuenca, L. (2013, May 30). The bittersweet truth of sweet and bitter taste receptors. *Harvard University: The Graduate School of Arts and Sciences.* https://sitn.hms.harvard.edu/flash/2013/the-bittersweet-truth-of-sweet-and-bitter-taste-receptors/

Dunne, C., Dolan, B., & Clyne, M. (2014). Factors that mediate colonization of the human stomach by helicobacter pylori. *World Journal of Gastroenterology, 20*(19), 5610–5624. https://doi.org/10.3748/wjg.v20.i19.5610

Granger, N.D., Morris, J. D., Kvietys, P. R., & Granger, J. P. (2018). *Physiology and Pathophysiology of Digestion.* Morgan & Claypool Life Science Publishers.

Guy-Evans, O., & McLeod, S. (2021, May 18). *Parasympathetic nervous system functions.* SimplyPsychology. https://www.simplypsychology.org/parasympathetic-nervous-system.html#:~:text=The%20parasympathetic%20nervous%20system%20is,voluntary%20control%2C%20therefore%20being%20automatic.&text=The%20parasympathetic%20nervous%20system%20leads%20to%20decreased%20arousal.

Healthwise Staff. (2020, April 25). *GERD: Controlling heartburn by changing your habits.* C.S. Mott Children's Hospital: University of Michigan Health. https://www.mottchildren.org/health-library/ut1339

Harvard Health Publishing. (2020, July 6). *Understanding the stress response: Chronic activation of this survival mechanism impairs health.* Harvard Medical School. https://www.health.harvard.edu/staying-healthy/understanding-the-stress-response

Heda, R., Toro, F., & Tombazzi, C.R. (2021, May 9). *Physiology, pepsin.* StatPearls Publishing. https://www.ncbi.nlm.nih.gov/books/NBK537005/#:~:text=Parietal%20cells%20within%20the%20stomach,hydrogen%20ions%20and%20decrease%20pH.

How to manage acid reflux after bariatric surgery. (n.d.). Southern Nevada Bariatrics. Retrieved March 30, 2022, from https://www.southernnevadabariatrics.com/blog/how-to-manage-acid-reflux-after-bariatric-surgery

Intrinsic factor. (2022, March 21). MedlinePlus. Retrieved March 30, 2022, from https://medlineplus.gov/ency/article/002381.htm#:~:text=Intrinsic%20factor%20is%20a%20protein,cells%20in%20the%20stomach%20lining.

Irritable bowel syndrome (IBS). (2020, September 24). Cleveland Clinic. Retrieved March 30, 2022, from https://my.clevelandclinic.org/health/diseases/4342-irritable-bowel-syndrome-ibs

Mayo Clinic Staff. (2021, July 8). *Chronic stress puts your health at risk: Chronic stress can wreak havoc on your mind and body. Take steps to control your stress.* Mayo Clinic. https://www.mayoclinic.org/healthy-lifestyle/stress-management/in-depth/stress/art-20046037#:~:text=Cortisol%20also%20curbs%20functions%20that,reproductive%20system%20and%20growth%20processes.

Mayo Clinic Staff. (2021, May 18). *Helicobacter pylori (H. pylori) infection.* Mayo Clinic. https://www.mayoclinic.org/diseases-conditions/h-pylori/symptoms-causes/syc-20356171

Mayo Clinic. (2010, April 22). *Heartburn, acid reflux, GERD* [Video]. Youtube. https://www.youtube.com/watch?v=TdK0jRFpWPQ

Mayo Clinic Staff. (2020, October 10). *Gastroparesis.* Mayo Clinic. https://www.mayoclinic.org/diseases-conditions/gastroparesis/symptoms-causes/syc-20355787#:~:text=Gastroparesis%20is%20a%20condition%20that,food%20through%20your%20digestive%20tract

Morris, J.D., Granger, D. N., Granger, J. P., & Kvietys, P. R. (2018). *Physiology and Pathophysiology of Digestion: Part 2.* Biota Publishing.

Nambudripad, R. (2021, February 28). *SIBO: A doctor's guide to the root cause of bloating and IBS* [Video]. Youtube. https://www.youtube.com/watch?v=1WPv2FijZ5s

Nelson, D. (2020, March 3). *What does pH stand for and mean?* Science Trends. https://sciencetrends.com/what-does-ph-stand-for-and-mean/

Overview: Gallbladder removal. (2021, December 8). NHS. Retrieved March 30, 2022, from https://www.nhs.uk/conditions/gallbladder-removal/#:~:text=Living%20without%20a%20gallbladder,continuously%20into%20your%20digestive%20system

Sethi, S., & Anthony, K. (2019, March 7). *How to increase stomach acid at home.* Healthline. https://www.healthline.com/health/how-to-increase-stomach-acid#outlook

Stomach. (n.d.). National Cancer Institute. https://training.seer.cancer.gov/anatomy/digestive/regions/stomach.html#:~:text=Four%20different%20types%20of%20cells,Chief%20cells

The brain-gut connection. (n.d). Johns Hopkins Medicine. Retrieved March 30, 2022, from https://www.hopkins-medicine.org/health/wellness-and-prevention/the-brain-gut-connection

Water Science School. (2019, June 19). *pH scale.* United States Geological Survey. https://www.usgs.gov/media/images/ph-scale-0#:~:text=pH%20is%20a%20measure%20of,hydroxyl%20ions%20in%20the%20water

Warwick, K.W., & Eske, J. (2020, July 29). *How can you naturally increase stomach acid?* Medical News Today. https://www.medicalnewstoday.com/articles/how-to-increase-stomach-acid

Your digestive system: 5 ways to support gut health. (n.d.). Johns Hopkins Medicine. Retrieved March 30, 2022, from https://www.hopkinsmedicine.org/health/wellness-and-prevention/your-digestive-system-5-ways-to-support-gut-health

HORMONES IMPORTANT TO WEIGHT LOSS & DIGESTION PART 2-HORMONES OF HUNGER AND SATIETY AND TIMING OF DIGESTION

In this science post we are continuing the conversation discussing the hormones that are involved in digestion and are important to weight loss.

We will be focusing on the hormones that are imperative to regulating our hunger and feelings of satiety, or what we at Weight Loss By Gina like to call, eating to satisfaction! We will also be looking at the concept of breakfast and how making it high in protein sets up our day for success. Finally, we will conclude our discussion on digestion by looking at how long it takes our bodies to process and digest the foods that we eat. All of these topics can give us more insight into the "rhyme and reason" behind the different tweaks and the organization of The Livy Method Food Plan, and how it promotes weight loss.

HUNGER

In the science post The Migrating Motor Complex (MMC) and Hunger, we discussed how the feeling of "hunger" is a fairly complex concept that can be influenced by many things including physical/physiological, emotional, social, economic, and mental factors. In fact, many of us have lost touch with gauging hunger signals, or never really become in tune with them in the first place.

We discussed strategies for reconnecting with these signals such as journaling, using a hunger scale, revisiting the four mindfulness questions at every meal and snack. We also discussed the importance of being in the moment when you are eating, minimizing distractions, to really tune into your food and how it is making you feel!

Let's dive in a bit deeper and look closer at the physiological processes that occur in our bodies that drive our feelings of hunger, but also lead to our feelings of satisfaction when we have eaten enough.

WHAT ARE HORMONES?

Hormones are defined as a special substance produced in the body that contains "chemical messengers" that control and regulate the activity of certain cells or organs (Davis, C.P., 2021, March). They are secreted into the blood or extracellular fluid by one cell and in turn, alter the functioning of other "targeted" cells. These target cells may be in glands, tissues, and other cells. The target cells recognize the hormone circulating that is specific to it, and become a "receptor" allowing the hormone to activate it! In fact, many hormones are active in more than one physical process and may have multiple functions!

Many hormones are secreted by special **glands** and are essential for every activity of life, including the processes of digestion, metabolism, growth, reproduction, and our mood.

There are two types of glands. **Endocrine glands**, which are ductless glands that release the hormones they make directly into the bloodstream. These glands form part of what we know as **the endocrine**

system. The other type of gland that is present in the body is called an **exocrine gland** (for example sweat glands and lymph nodes). These are not considered part of the endocrine system as they do not produce hormones, and they release their product through a duct.

Neurotransmitters, although not specifically hormones, are also special chemical messengers that help carry, promote, and balance signals between neurons (also known as nerve cells) and target cells throughout the body. Neurotransmitters are more specific to the central nervous system.

Neurotransmitters can also have strong influences on our hunger and satiety cues and signals!

Here is a great video that briefly talks about hormones and how they work in the body.

https://www.youtube.com/watch?v=-SPRPkLoKp8

This video explains the endocrine system for those that want to learn a little more about how it works!

https://www.youtube.com/watch?v=ER49EweKwW8

This video talks about how neurotransmitters travel across neurons in the body.

https://www.youtube.com/watch?v=WhowH0kb7n0&t=5s

Now that we understand a little more about how hormones and neurotransmitters work in our body, let's talk about how these chemical messengers influence our hunger, satiety, and can influence weight loss!

INSULIN

As we discussed in the science post Hormones Important to Weight Loss & Digestion Part 1-Insulin, the pancreas has a major role in digestion by producing and secreting digestive enzymes. However, it also produces the hormone insulin, which is responsible for regulating and storing glucose (a simple sugar that is broken down from food) in the muscles, liver, and fat cells, for later use when needed.

To recap, the beta cells in your pancreas monitor your blood sugar level every few seconds. When your blood glucose rises after you eat, the beta cells release insulin into your bloodstream. Insulin acts like a key, unlocking muscle, fat, and liver cells, so that glucose can penetrate them. Once inside, the cells convert glucose into energy to use right then, or store it to use later.

As glucose moves from the bloodstream into the cells, blood sugar levels start to drop. The beta cells in the pancreas can tell this is happening, so they slow down the amount of insulin they are making. At the same time, the pancreas slows down the amount of insulin that it's releasing into the bloodstream. When this happens, the amount of glucose going into the cells also slows down.

After you haven't eaten for a few hours, your blood glucose level drops, and your pancreas stops producing insulin. Alpha cells in the pancreas begin to produce glucagon, signaling the liver to break down stored glycogen and turn it back into glucose. This glucose then travels to your bloodstream to replenish your supply until you are able to eat again.

Insulin resistance has become an increasingly common condition in current society and causes the cells in the body to stop responding to insulin. This results in the body producing even more insulin, in an effort to increase the possibility of glucose absorption. This condition eventually may result in high blood sugar, because the insulin cannot move glucose into your cells, and is linked to obesity, inflammation, type 2 diabetes and heart disease. Although more research is needed, insulin resistance may be linked to carrying excess weight and to a lack of exercise.

Insulin sensitivity can be thought of as the opposite of insulin resistance. It means that your cells are having a healthy response to the insulin being produced in the body. By following The Livy Method, you are already actively focusing on habits that will help improve insulin sensitivity, such as:

REGULAR EXERCISE AND MOVING YOUR BODY

Research supports that exercise, at both high and moderate intensities, that increases your heart rate and breathing, results in your muscles using more glucose from the body (Landes, E., & Jones, J., 2022, January). Over time, this can lower your blood sugar levels and also makes the insulin in your body work better. You will also receive these benefits for hours after your activity or workout.

However, strenuous exercise can sometimes increase blood sugar temporarily after you stop exercising, and very intense exercise can cause the body to make more stress hormones which can lead to an increase in blood sugar, as well as stress on the body. This can also help explain one of the reasons why over exercise is not a good weight loss tool! We will be discussing this further down when we discuss the hormone cortisol.

IMPROVE YOUR SLEEP HABITS

Not getting enough sleep, or not getting quality sleep, is linked to obesity and insulin resistance.

According to the Sleep Foundation, sleep can both raise and lower glucose levels. Our bodies experience a cycle of changes every day, called a circadian rhythm, which naturally raises blood sugar levels at night and when a person sleeps. These natural blood sugar elevations are not a cause for concern.

Restorative sleep however, may lower elevated blood sugar levels by promoting healthy systems. Decreased sleep is a risk factor for increased blood sugar levels. Even partial sleep deprivation of only 1 to 2 hours in a night, increases risk of insulin resistance, which can in turn increase blood sugar levels. As a result, a lack of sleep has been associated with diabetes.

More research is needed to better understand the connection between sleep and blood sugar. However, the following factors have been found to influence the relationship between sleep and blood sugar levels (Sleep Foundation. Retrieved March 30, 2022):

- The amount of time a person sleeps (7-8 hours has been discussed as ideal).
- The stages of sleep a person experiences.

- The time of day of a person sleeps (considerations for shift workers).

- Age (as people age they often have more difficulty sleeping).

- Eating habits (for example eating before sleep and poor nutrition, which overlaps with nutrition and sleep).

Why Does Sleep Affect Blood Sugar? Researchers are beginning to uncover why sleep affects blood sugar and which underlying mechanisms are involved. So far, they've learned that the following physiological factors play a role in the relationship between sleep and blood sugar:

- **Cortisol** (the stress hormone) is increased by sleep deprivation and increases glucose.

- Insulin sensitivity is reduced by sleep deprivation and impacts glucose.

- The time of day a person sleeps impacts insulin and cortisol levels, both of which affect glucose.

- Increases in growth hormone accompany glucose increases during sleep.

- Oxidative stress and inflammation are increased by sleep deprivation and impact glucose.

- **C-reactive protein (CRP)** and other inflammatory markers are increased by sleep deprivation and can impact glucose.

FOLLOWING THE LIVY METHOD FOOD PLAN HELPS REGULATE INSULIN!

Eating a diet which includes protein, as well as healthy fats from nuts, avocados and good oils like extra-virgin olive oil, and eating a diet rich in carbohydrates that are known to keep blood sugars stable and are high in fiber, such as whole grains, fruits, legumes, and includes many vegetables, may help reduce insulin resistance. Decreasing your intake of saturated and trans fats may also help.

MAINTAIN A MODERATE WEIGHT

In people that are overweight, healthy weight loss and weight management may improve insulin sensitivity.

LEPTIN

Leptin is a hormone made by the fat cells that creates the feeling of "fullness" that works by telling your **hypothalamus**, the portion of your brain that regulates appetite, that you're full. It works in conjunction with the hormone **ghrelin** that increases appetite, and also plays a role in body weight.

Of the two hormones, leptin appears to have a greater influence in our body's energy balance. Some researchers even think that leptin helps regulate ghrelin.

In general, the more fat you have, the more leptin is in your blood. However, the level varies depending on many factors, including when you last ate and your sleep patterns.

However, people with obesity may experience **leptin resistance**. This means the message to stop eating doesn't reach your brain, eventually causing you to overeat. In turn, your body may produce even more leptin until your levels become elevated. The concept of this is very similar to that of insulin resistance.

The direct cause of leptin resistance is unclear, but it may be due to inflammation, gene mutations, and/or excessive leptin production, which can occur with obesity.

Inflammation is a big component of this phenomenon, according to endocrinologist Scott Isaacs, MD (McCulloch, M., 2015). Leptin resistance (as well as insulin resistance) is caused by fat cells, especially in visceral or belly fat, producing large numbers of inflammatory chemicals or cytokines, which block the effects of leptin. Eating healthful foods, including ones rich in anti-inflammatory antioxidants and omega-3 fats, can improve leptin resistance.

Although no known treatment exists for leptin resistance, a few lifestyle changes may help lower leptin levels. Here are a few tips that may help and all recommended by The Livy Method. As you will notice reading through the discussion of all the hormones and neurotransmitters, the tips will all come to be quite repetitive!

MAINTAIN A HEALTHY WEIGHT

Because leptin resistance is associated with obesity, it's important to maintain a healthy weight. Additionally, research suggests that a decrease in body fat may help reduce leptin levels. Like insulin resistance, and recommended above, reducing abdominal/visceral fat can greatly help reduce the inflammation that may contribute to leptin resistance.

IMPROVE YOUR SLEEP QUALITY

Leptin levels may be related to sleep quality in people with obesity. Although this association may not exist in people without obesity, there are numerous other reasons to get better sleep.

EXERCISE REGULARLY

Research links regular, consistent exercise to a decrease in leptin levels.

GHRELIN

The hormone ghrelin, is essentially the opposite of leptin. It's one of the primary and most powerful hunger-stimulating hormones involved in regulating hunger. It is produced and secreted from the stomach lining, that sends a message to your hypothalamus indicating that your body needs food. The main function of ghrelin appears to be to stimulate an increase in appetite. But some researchers believe that ghrelin is not as important in determining appetite as once thought (Magee, E., & Nazario, B., n.d.). They think that its role in regulating body weight may actually be a more complex process.

Normally, ghrelin levels are highest before eating and lowest after a meal, and appear to cycle through about every 4 hours. German researchers have suggested that ghrelin levels play a big role in determining how quickly hunger comes back after we eat. Normally, ghrelin levels go up dramatically before you eat, which signals hunger. They then go down for about three hours after the meal.

Eating at regular intervals is in sync with this cycle, but after overnight fasting, ghrelin levels are increased. Ghrelin levels rise approximately two times immediately before a meal, and then decrease to their lowest levels about one hour after a meal.

Ghrelin is a short-acting hormone, and it appears that there is not a limiting level, that just builds until you eat. Importantly, it doesn't seem to be affected by what you ate yesterday! Thus, it is important to eat when you are hungry, and not let these levels build too high, which may reinforce overeating as recommended by The Livy Method!

Although one might think that ghrelin levels are higher in an obese person, thus driving more hunger, the opposite is true. Human studies have found that ghrelin levels actually are lower in the obese, but they're more sensitive to its appetite-stimulating effects. This increased sensitivity may lead to overeating.

TIPS TO MANAGE GHRELIN LEVELS

One reason weight loss can be difficult is that restricting calories often leads to increased ghrelin levels, leaving you hungry. Additionally, metabolism tends to slow down and leptin levels decrease. The Livy Method reinforces feeding into these hunger cues thus preventing ghrelin levels from getting too high, and also giving your body what it needs! This is why it is important to eat when you are hungry!

MAINTAIN A MODERATE BODY WEIGHT

Obesity may increase your sensitivity to ghrelin, ultimately increasing your appetite.

TRY TO GET GOOD QUALITY SLEEP

Poor sleep may lead to increases in ghrelin, overeating, and weight gain.

EAT REGULARLY

Because ghrelin levels are highest before a meal, listen to your body and eat when you're hungry and then just eat to satisfaction! These are all fundamental principles of The Livy Method!

CORTISOL

Cortisol is known as the stress hormone and is produced by your adrenal glands, as discussed previously in the science post Issues With Digestion.

To recap, during times of stress, the release of cortisol, alongside the hormone epinephrine (also known as adrenaline) engages our sympathetic nervous system, which is commonly called the "fight or flight" response. This is so our bodies can fight the emergency!

While it's important for your body to release cortisol in dangerous situations, chronic high levels may lead to many health issues, including heart disease, diabetes, low energy levels, high blood pressure, sleep disturbances, and weight gain.

Certain lifestyle factors, which include inadequate or poor sleep habits, chronic stress, and an unhealthy diet, may contribute to high cortisol levels.

Importantly, obesity appears to raise cortisol levels, but high levels may also cause weight gain, creating a negative feedback loop, reinforcing the body's need to store fat!

Here are how strategies recommended by The Livy Method may help manage cortisol levels:

OPTIMIZE SLEEP

Chronic sleep issues, including insomnia, sleep apnea, and irregular sleep habits (like those of shift workers), may contribute to high cortisol levels. Focus on developing a regular bedtime and sleep schedule may help with lowering cortisol levels!

EXERCISE REGULARLY

Cortisol levels temporarily increase after high intensity exercise, but regular exercise generally helps decrease levels by improving overall health and lowering stress levels. However, stressing the body with strenuous exercise or over exercising may have the opposite effect, and in fact increase cortisol levels.

PRACTICE MINDFULNESS

Research suggests that regularly practicing mindfulness lowers cortisol levels (Landes, E., & Jones, J., 2022, January). Try adding meditation and other relaxation techniques to your daily routine. Epsom salt baths are also a great way to relax as the warmth and the magnesium in the Epsom salts, relaxes muscles, helping to decrease stress, and ultimately cortisol levels!

MAINTAIN A MODERATE BODY WEIGHT

Because obesity may increase cortisol levels and high cortisol levels can cause weight gain, maintaining a moderate weight may help keep levels in check.

EAT A BALANCED DIET

Research has shown that diets high in added sugars, refined grains, and saturated fat may lead to higher cortisol levels. Following a plan like The Livy Method may help lower cortisol levels.

ESTROGEN

Estrogen is a sex hormone responsible for regulating the female reproductive system, as well as the immune, skeletal, and vascular systems. Although estrogen is also present and is an important hormone for males as well!

Levels of this hormone change during life stages such as pregnancy, nursing, and menopause, as well as throughout the menstrual cycle. For men as testosterone declines with age, estrogen levels increase.

High levels of estrogen, which are often seen in people with obesity, are associated with an increased risk of certain cancers and other chronic diseases.

Conversely, low levels, typically seen in women with aging, perimenopause, and menopause, may affect body weight and body fat, therefore also increasing risk of chronic diseases.

Individuals with low estrogen levels often experience an accumulation of weight around the abdomen, which should now be a familiar concept. This metabolic visceral fat, can lead to other health problems which should also sound familiar, such as high blood sugar, high blood pressure, and heart disease.

By following The Livy Method, you will naturally keep estrogen levels stable by doing the following:

TRY TO MANAGE YOUR WEIGHT

Weight loss or maintenance may reduce the risk of heart disease due to low estrogen levels in women ages 55–75. Research also supports healthy weight maintenance for reducing chronic diseases in general.

EXERCISE REGULARLY

Low estrogen levels may decrease levels of energy that may affect your motivation for exercising. However, regular exercise is still an important aspect of maintaining health.

FOLLOW A HEALTHY DIET LIKE THE LIVY METHOD

Diets high in processed foods, sugar, and refined grains have been shown to increase estrogen levels, which may raise the risk of chronic disease. Limiting these foods increases the likelihood of reversing some of these health issues.

NEUROPEPTIDE Y

Neuropeptide Y (NPY) is a hormone produced by cells in your brain and nervous system that stimulates appetite and decreases energy expenditure in response to prolonged fasting or stress.

Because it may stimulate eating, NPY is associated with obesity and weight gain.

NPY production is activated in fat tissue and may increase fat storage and lead to abdominal/visceral weight gain and metabolic syndrome, a condition that can increase the risk of chronic diseases.

Research has shown that NPY's mechanisms that lead to obesity may also increase inflammation in the body, further worsening health conditions.

Here are some tips for maintaining healthy levels of NPY:

EXERCISE

Some studies suggest that regular exercise that increases your heart rate and rate of breathing may help decrease NPY levels, though research is mixed.

EAT A NUTRITIOUS DIET, LIKE THE LIVY METHOD

Although more research is needed, a diet high in fat, processed foods, and added sugars may increase NPY levels. Following a nutrition food plan like The Livy Method may help lower NPY levels!

GLUCAGON-LIKE PEPTIDE-1

Glucagon-like peptide-1 (GLP-1) is a hormone produced in the digestive system when nutrients enter the intestines. This hormone also plays a major role in keeping blood sugar levels stable and making you feel full.

Research suggests that people that struggle with obesity may have issues with GLP-1 signaling.

Here are some tips to help maintain healthy levels of GLP-1:

EAT PLENTY OF PROTEIN

Adding in protein rich foods have been shown to increase GLP-1 levels. The good news is that protein is an important part of The Livy Method, as it is highlighted in breakfast and dinner, but also an important component in almost all meals and snacks!

CONSIDER TAKING PROBIOTICS

Preliminary research suggests that probiotics may increase GLP-1 levels, though more human research is needed. These are recommended along with prebiotics (to feed these good gut bacteria!) as part of The Livy Method supplements list!

Cholecystokinin

Like GLP-1, cholecystokinin (CCK) is a satiety hormone produced by cells in your digestive system after a meal. It has an important role in energy production, protein synthesis, digestion, and other bodily functions. It also increases the release of the fullness hormone leptin which we discussed earlier.

People that struggle with obesity may have a reduced sensitivity to CCK's effects, which may lead to chronic overeating, similar to the hormone ghrelin. In turn, this may further reduce CCK sensitivity, creating a negative feedback loop, and a cycle of overeating, worsening the likelihood of increased weight gain.

Here are some tips for maintaining healthy levels of CCK:

EAT PLENTY OF PROTEIN

Some research suggests a diet high in protein may help increase CCK levels, and therefore help increase feelings of fullness.

EXERCISE

While research is limited, some evidence supports regular exercise for increasing CCK levels.

PEPTIDE YY

Peptide YY (PYY) is another gut hormone that has a role in decreasing the appetite, leading to increased feelings of satiety. PYY levels may be lower in those that struggle with obesity, and may lead to an increase in appetite and overeating. Maintaining sufficient levels are believed to play a major role in reducing food intake and decreasing the risk of obesity.

Here are some ways to promote healthy levels of PPY in your body:

FOLLOWING A WELL-BALANCED DIET LIKE THE LIVY METHOD

Eating a well-balanced diet that includes protein, fruits and vegetables may promote healthy PYY levels and fullness. Although more research is needed.

EXERCISE

While research on exercise and PYY levels is conflicting, staying active and moving your body is generally beneficial for health, well-being and stress management!

DOPAMINE

Interconnected with the hormones involved in satiety and hunger are neurotransmitters, one of which includes dopamine. Dopamine has a direct effect in activating the reward and pleasure centers in the brain, which can affect both mood and food intake.

Those that struggle with obesity often have a blunted dopamine pathway because of chronic exposure to highly palatable foods, such as foods that are high in added sugar and fats. This over-exposure, which leads to a blunted response when eating, has been suggested to contribute to increased reward-seeking behavior, including overeating.

EAT A BREAKFAST THAT IS HIGH IN PROTEIN

WHAT IS BREAKFAST?

Breakfast is unique because it breaks a time of fasting (after a night of sleep). You are considered a breakfast eater if you eat your first meal of the day following your longest period of sleep, within 2 to 3 hours of waking and if your meal contains food or beverage from at least one food group. This is why The Livy Method recommends eating within 2.5 hours of waking if you are active once awake.

Eating a breakfast that is high in protein has been shown to be one of the best methods of reducing post meal cravings and increasing dopamine levels, but also decreasing a blunted response to it. Protein contains amino acids, several of which are the building blocks of dopamine. Thus, increasing protein consumption has been suggested to increase the production of dopamine in the body!

In addition, getting enough of one amino acid, tyrosine, is an important component in the production of dopamine. Top tyrosine sources include meat, poultry, eggs, fish, cheese, soybeans, and peanuts.

There is also compelling data that shows improved satiety and reduced appetite with the consumption of a high-protein breakfast in normal-weight individuals!!!

SHOULD YOU EAT BREAKFAST?

In the past, skipping breakfast has been associated with weight gain.

However, there is evidence showing that recommendations to eat or skip breakfast have no effect on weight gain or loss (Bjarnadottir, A, 2017, June).

That being said, eating breakfast may be a good idea for other reasons. It may improve mental performance in school children, teenagers and certain patient groups. Although, this may also depend on the quality of the breakfast, and as discussed, a high protein breakfast can prove to be very beneficial!

Protein activates the body's signals that curb appetite, which reduces cravings and overeating, mostly due to a decrease in the hunger hormone ghrelin and a rise in the fullness hormones peptide YY, GLP-1 and cholecystokinin. Interestingly, several studies have now demonstrated that eating a high-protein breakfast changes these hormones throughout the day!

BREAKFAST EATERS TEND TO HAVE HEALTHIER HABITS

Many observational studies show that breakfast eaters tend to be healthier, and are less likely to be overweight/obese, and have a lower risk of several chronic diseases. This is mostly likely because those that put the time and energy into having breakfast, also tend to place importance on prioritizing their health in other ways.

A high protein breakfast has been shown to benefit muscle health and to support weight loss by increasing muscle mass, energy expenditure (calories burned), satiety hormones, glucose regulation and by decreasing the desire to snack at night .

Eating a high protein breakfast, has also been shown to improve the body's response to foods high in carbohydrate, up to 4-hours after the breakfast meal. A study looked at the effect of a high protein breakfast compared to a high fat or high carbohydrate breakfast on the body's ability to control glucose and insulin, following the consumption of white bread, four hours after the breakfast meal. Participants consuming a high protein breakfast had improved blood sugar control and insulin levels after consuming the white bread!

This all further reinforces that starting your day with a breakfast making protein the star of the show, not only helps to reduce cravings, improve the feelings of satiety, but also may help boost your mood and improve mental performance at the start of the day!

SEEK PLEASURE FROM OTHER ACTIVITIES

The classic approach of finding an alternate activity to get your mind off a craving has benefits beyond distraction. Activities such as listening to music and doing yoga also increase dopamine levels, and can also feed into feeling good!

CONSUME OMEGA-3 FATS

Omega-3 fats, by supplementation and included from foods rich in Omega 3 fats such as salmon and other fatty fishes, can increase the number of dopamine receptors and dopamine levels. Omega-3 fats also are anti-inflammatory and may help improve leptin sensitivity. Because of all the benefits they have, Omega 3 supplementation is also recommended as part of The Livy Method basic supplements list!

Now that we've discussed some of the important hormones and neurotransmitters involved in our hunger and feelings of satisfaction, let's complete our discussion of digestion with a short synopsis of how long it takes the average person to actually process, digest, and move food through their body.

BREAKING DOWN DIGESTION SPEED

Why is it that after eating certain foods, you can feel full for hours, but after others, you're looking for a snack within minutes?

HOW LONG DOES FOOD TAKE TO DIGEST?

The entire digestive process can take several hours. Food generally stays in your stomach between about 40 to 120-plus minutes. Then add another 40 to 120 minutes for time spent in the small bowel. The denser the food, composed with protein and/or fat, the longer it takes to digest. It can take about 24-36 hours for digested food to be eliminated from the body. Longer in those that have digestive issues.

Simple carbohydrates, such as plain rice, pasta or simple sugars, average between 30 and 60 minutes in the stomach, but with added proteins and fats, can take upwards of between two to four hours to leave your stomach.

HOW LONG DOES IT TAKE WATER TO DIGEST?

Liquids leave the stomach faster because there is less to break down:

Plain water: 10 to 20 minutes.

Simple liquids (clear juices, tea, sodas): 20 to 40 minutes.

Complex liquids (smoothies, protein shakes, bone broths): 40 to 60 minutes.

Please note that these times are estimates and how long it takes to digest food varies on factors depending on body type, metabolism, medications, the types of food you eat, level of physical activity overall exercise fitness, if you are living a sedentary versus physically active lifestyle, past surgeries you've endured, and stress level.

IS IT POSSIBLE TO TELL WHEN YOUR STOMACH IS EMPTY?

Just because you feel hungry doesn't mean your stomach is empty. Our hunger cues, as discussed, can be hormonally regulated, so if you have a high level of hunger hormones circulating, you may feel hungry, even if your stomach is full. Your perception of these sensations is also highly individual, but as discussed before, journaling, using a hunger scale, asking yourself the 4 questions, and following the Livy Method as designed, will help you become more in tune with your hunger and feelings of satisfaction when eating just enough.

Hopefully you all enjoyed this post as we continued to build upon our knowledge of hormones involved in digestion and weight loss! Stay tuned for our next science post where we will be discussing the science of fat and fat loss.

REFERENCES

About us. (n.d.). Sleep Foundation. Retrieved March 30, 2022, from https://www.sleepfoundation.org/about-us

Biggers, A., & Jewell, T. (2019, October 22). *Risk factors of having high or low estrogen levels in males.* Healthline. https://www.healthline.com/health/estrogen-in-men

Bjarnadottir, A. (2017, June 3). *Is Skipping Breakfast Bad for You? The Surprising Truth.* Healthline. https://www.healthline.com/nutrition/is-skipping-breakfast-bad

Brown, G. (2019, June 24). *Difference between hormones and neurotransmitters.* Difference Between. http://www.differencebetween.net/science/health/difference-between-hormones-and-neurotransmitters/#:~:text=Hormones%20are%20chemical%20signals%20secreted,the%20brain%20and%20the%20body.

Cherry, K., & Lakhan, S. (2021, July 8). *The role of neurotransmitters.* Verywell Mind. https://www.verywellmind.com/what-is-a-neurotransmitter-2795394

Davis, C.P. (2021, March 29). *Medical definition of hormone.* MedicineNet. https://www.medicinenet.com/hormone/definition.htm

Digestion and absorption of carbohydrates. (2018, October 12). Lane Community College. Retrieved March 30, 2022, from https://media.lanecc.edu/users/powellt/FN225OER/Carbohydrates/FN225Carbohydrates4.html

Gao, C., Liu, Y., Gan, Y., Bao, W., Peng, X., Xing, Q., Gao, H., Lai, J., Liu, L., Wang, Z., & Yang, Y. (2020). Effects of fish oil supplementation on glucose control and lipid levels among patients with type 2 diabetes mellitus: a meta-analysis of randomized controlled trials. *Lipids in Health and Disease, 19,* 87 (2020). https://doi.org/10.1186/s12944-020-01214-w

Glands. (n.d.). You and Your Hormones. Retrieved March 30, 2022, from https://www.yourhormones.info/glands/#:~:text=is%20a%20gland%3F-,A%20gland%20is%20an%20organ%20which%20produces%20and%20releases%20substances,hormones)%20directly%20into%20the%20bloodstream.

Hawley, A. (2018, December 17). *Protein, its what's for breakfast.* American Society for Nutrition. https://nutrition.org/protein-its-whats-for-breakfast/#:~:text=A%20high%20protein%20breakfast%20has,desire%20to%20snack%20at%20night%20.

Hjalmarsdottir, F. (2017, June 22). *How protein at breakfast can help you lose weight.* Healthline.https://www.healthline.com/nutrition/protein-at-breakfast-and-weight-loss#5-Healthy-Snacks-That-Can-Help-You-Lose-Weight

Hormones, receptors and target cells (n.d.). Vivo Pathophysiology. Retrieved March 30, 2022, from http://www.vivo.colostate.edu/hbooks/pathphys/endocrine/basics/hormones.html

How long does it take to digest food: Breaking down digestion speed. (2021, April 19). Cleveland Clinic. Retrieved March 30, 2022, from https://health.clevelandclinic.org/how-long-does-it-take-to-digest-food/

Hunger and fullness signals. (2021, March). Alberta Health Services. Retrieved March 30, 2022, from https://www.albertahealthservices.ca/assets/info/nutrition/if-nfs-hunger-and-fullness-signals.pd

Khanacademymedicine. (2015, April 16). *Hormone control of hunger* [Video]. Youtube. https://www.youtube.com/watch?v=EVkFPeP5sFI

Landes, E., & Jones, J. (2022, January 26). *9 hormones that affect your weight and how to improve them*. Healthline. https://www.healthline.com/nutrition/9-fixes-for-weight-hormones

Magee, E., & Nazario, B. (n.d.). *Your 'hunger hormones': How they affect your appetite and your weight*. WebMD. https://www.webmd.com/diet/features/your-hunger-hormones

Mawer, R., & Feller, M. (2021, October 8). *What is ghrelin? All you need to know about this hormone*. Healthline. https://www.healthline.com/nutrition/ghrelin

McCulloch, M. (2015). Appetite hormones. *Today's Dietitian, 17*(7), 26. https://www.todaysdietitian.com/newarchives/070115p26.shtml

Narayan, R. [Khanacademymedicine]. (2014, May 15). *Control of the GI tract: Gastrointestinal system physiology* [Video]. Youtube. https://www.youtube.com/watch?v=_kfB2qKjdgM

Pradhan, G., Samson, S. L., & Sun, Y. (2013). Ghrelin: much more than a hunger hormone. *Current Opinion In Clinical Nutrition and Metabolic Care, 16*(6), 619–624. https://doi.org/10.1097/MCO.0b013e328365b9be

Purves, D., Augustine, G.J., Fitzpatrick, D., Katz, L.C., LaMantina, A., McNamara, J.O., & Williams, S.M. (2001). Neuroscience (2nd Edition). Sinauer Associates. https://www.ncbi.nlm.nih.gov/books/NBK10957/

Shaikh, J., & Uttekar, P.S. (2021, September 1). *Does it take 30 minutes to digest food?* MedicineNet. https://www.medicinenet.com/does_it_take_30_minutes_to_digest_food/article.htm

van Galen, K.A., ter Horst, K.W., & Serlie, M.J. (2021). Serotonin, food intake, and obesity. *Obesity Reviews, 22*(7), e2210. https://doi.org/10.1111/obr.13210

Wurtman, J.J., & Schrader, J. (2010, August 5). *Serotonin: What it is and why it's important for weight loss: Serotonin is nature's own appetite suppressant*. Psychology Today. https://www.psychologytoday.com/us/blog/the-antidepressant-diet/201008/serotonin-what-it-is-and-why-its-important-weight-loss

Yeung, A.Y., & Tadi, P. (2021, November 14). *Physiology, obesity neurohormonal appetite and satiety control*. StatPearls Publishing. https://www.ncbi.nlm.nih.gov/books/NBK555906/

THE SCIENCE OF FAT AND FAT LOSS

In this science post, we are following up the conversation about the hormones and neurotransmitters involved with the regulation of our hunger and satiety cues, with how the body utilizes and releases fat in the weight loss process. So, to better understand what fat loss really is and what happens in the body to make this process happen, let's take a deeper dive into fat and fat metabolism!

WHAT ARE FATS?

Fats which are also called "fatty acids" or "lipids", are an essential component of the homeostatic function of the human body. They also contribute to some of the body's most vital processes.

Fats and oils are categorized in chemistry as a chemical compound called an ester, which is described as any class of organic compounds that react with water to produce alcohols, and organic or inorganic acids.

Fats are fatty, waxy, or oily compounds that are soluble in organic solvents (dissolve in a substance that contains carbon and nonpolar, for example paint thinner) and insoluble in polar solvents such as water.

These include:

- Fats and oils (triglycerides)
- Phospholipids
- Waxes
- Steroids

The human body is composed of two main types of fat tissue. **White fa**t is important in energy metabolism, heat insulation, and cushioning. **Brown fat**, also called brown adipose tissue, is a special type of body fat that is turned on (activated) when you get cold. Brown fat produces heat to help maintain your body temperature in cold conditions. Brown fat is found mostly in newborn babies, between the shoulders, and is important for thermogenesis (making heat without shivering). Scientists used to believe that only babies had brown fat. They also thought this fat disappeared by the time most people reached adulthood. However, researchers now know that even adults have small reserves of brown fat (Marcin, A., Hodgson, L. 2022, January). It's typically stored in small deposits around the shoulders and neck.

A third type of fat called **beige (or brite)** fat has been identified in humans, and is a relatively new area of research. These fat cells function along the spectrum between brown and white fat cells. Similar to brown fat, beige cells can help utilize fat rather than store it. It is thought that certain hormones and enzymes are released when you are stressed, cold, or during exercise, which can help convert white fat into beige fat. This is an exciting area of research to possibly help prevent obesity and maximize healthy body fat levels.

When you are first born, your body does not have much white fat to help insulate and retain body heat; although there are white fat cells, there is not much fat stored in them. Brown fat cells are somewhat smaller than white, are composed of several smaller fat droplets, are iron rich (hence the brown colour), and are loaded with mitochondria which can generate heat. A newborn baby produces heat primarily by breaking down fat molecules into fatty acids in brown fat cells. Instead of those fatty acids leaving the brown fat cell, as happens in white fat cells, they get further broken down in the mitochondria and their energy is released directly as heat. Brown fat contains more mitochondria than white fat, and has generated interest among researchers because it appears to be able to use regular body fat as fuel. In addition, exercise and the exposure to cold may stimulate hormones that activate brown fat.

All people have some "constitutive" brown fat, which is the kind you're born with. There's also another form that's "recruitable." This means it can change to brown fat under the right circumstances. This recruitable type is found in muscles and white fat throughout your body.

RECAP OF THE DIGESTION OF FAT

When you eat food that contains fat, mostly triglycerides, it is digested through the stomach and intestines.

In the intestines, the following happens: large fat droplets get mixed with bile salts from the gallbladder in a process called emulsification. The mixture breaks up the large droplets into several smaller droplets called micelles, increasing the fat's surface area. The pancreas secretes enzymes called lipases that attack the surface of each micelle and break the fats down into their components of glycerol and fatty acids. These components get absorbed into the cells lining the intestine. Once in the intestinal cell, the parts are reassembled into fat molecules (triglycerides) with a protein coating called chylomicrons. This protein coating makes the fat dissolve more easily in water. The chylomicrons are then released into the lymphatic system. They do not go directly into the bloodstream because they are too big to pass through the wall of the capillaries (which are a tiny network of blood vessels). The lymphatic system eventually merges with the veins, at which point the chylomicrons are able to pass into the bloodstream. Fat molecules get broken down into glycerol and fatty acids and are then reassembled because fat molecules are too big to easily cross cell membranes. So, when passing from the intestine through the intestinal cells into the lymph, or when crossing any cell barrier, the fats must first be broken down. However, when fats are being transported in the lymph or blood, it is better to have a few large fat molecules than many smaller fatty acids, because the larger fats do not "attract" as many excess water molecules by osmosis as many smaller molecules would.

The fat that we store in our body is also stored as triglycerides. When you eat, your body converts any energy it does not need to use right away into triglycerides. The triglycerides are then stored in your fat cells. Later, hormones release triglycerides for energy between meals if you need them. Triglycerides also provide insulation to cells, and aid in the absorption of fat-soluble vitamins.

A triglyceride is made up of glycerol (a 3-carbon sugar alcohol/polyol) and 3 fatty acids. Fatty acids are chains of hydrogen and carbon. They are composed of differing lengths and various degrees of saturation. The molecule ends with something called a carboxylic acid group. How they are "bonded" allows for the creation of many different types of fatty acids. Fatty acids in biological systems usually contain an even number of carbon atoms and are typically 14 carbons to 24 carbons long.

Check out this video for more information on the molecular structure of triglycerides!

https://www.khanacademy.org/science/ap-biology/chemistry-of-life/properties-structure-and-func-tion-of-biological-macromolecules/v/molecular-structure-of-triglycerides-fats

Fats are also an essential component of the cell membrane in our body's cells. In the cell membrane, phospholipids are arranged in a bilayer, providing cell protection and serving as a barrier to certain molecules. The structure is typically made of a glycerol backbone, 2 fatty acid tails (which are hydrophobic, meaning the structure tries to avoid water molecules), and a phosphate group (which are hydrophilic, meaning that group is attracted to water molecules). These molecules are called phospholipids, and are amphipathic (having parts that are both hydrophobic and hydrophilic). The hydrophilic part faces outward and the hydrophobic part faces inward. This physical arrangement of the cell membrane helps to monitor and act as a gatekeeper, as to which molecules can enter and exit the cell. For example, nonpolar molecules and small polar molecules, such as oxygen and water, can easily diffuse in and out of the cell. Large polar molecules, for example, glucose, cannot pass freely so they need the help of transport proteins.

Another type of lipid is wax. Waxes are esters made of a long-chain alcohol and a fatty acid. Waxes provide protection. Cerumen (also known as earwax) helps protect the skin of the ear canal.

Another class of lipids includes steroids, which have a structure of four fused rings. One important type of steroid is cholesterol. Cholesterol is produced in the liver and is the most common steroid. Cholesterol is the precursor to many steroid hormones such as estrogen, testosterone, and cortisol. It is also the precursor to Vitamin D as well as bile salts, which help in the emulsification of fats and their subsequent absorption by cells. Cholesterol is also an important part in the composition of the cell membrane. Cholesterol is inserted in the bilayer of the cell membrane and has a big influence on the fluidity of the membrane.

WHY IS DIETARY FAT IMPORTANT?

Most of the fat that we need can be made by our bodies, however, there are certain fats that our bodies cannot manufacture but are essential for our health and bodily functions.

These fats are called "essential" fats, essential fatty acids (EFAs), or polyunsaturated fats. Essential fats include Omega-3 fats (found in foods such as fish and flax seed) and Omega-6 fats (found in foods such as nuts, seeds, and corn oil).

Other components of omega-3 fatty acid that are found in fatty fish and shellfish are called eicosapentaenoic acid (EPA) and docosahexaenoic acid (DHA). Fish can contain the metal mercury which acts as a toxin in the body, so choosing a good quality Omega 3 supplement, or fish lower in mercury like salmon, anchovies, herring, sardines, Pacific oysters, trout, Atlantic mackerel, and Pacific mackerel will help provide the EPA and DHA that your body needs.

Fat is an important component in our diet because:

- Fat helps the body absorb and process fat soluble vitamins like vitamins A, D, E, and K

- Fat helps to keep our skin healthy

- Essential fats like Omega-3 are important for heart health and brain health. Omega-3 fatty acids may reduce inflammation throughout the body. Inflammation can cause damage to your blood vessels, leading to heart disease and stroke. Omega-3 fatty acids may benefit heart health by: decreasing triglycerides levels, slightly lowering blood pressure, reducing blood clotting that could lead to clots therefore decreasing your risk of stroke and heart attack, decreasing heart failure risk and reducing arrhythmias (Mayo Clinic 2019, September).

The omega-3 fatty acids EPA and DHA are critical for normal brain function and development throughout all stages of life. EPA and DHA seem to have important roles in the developing baby's brain, and are also vital for the maintenance of normal brain function throughout life. They are abundant in the cell membranes of brain cells, preserving cell membrane health and facilitating communication between brain cells. In older adults, lower levels of DHA in the blood have been associated with smaller brain size, which is a sign of accelerated brain aging. It is also thought that Omega-3 fatty acids also reduce inflammation in the brain.

- Healthy unsaturated fats, like monounsaturated fats and polyunsaturated fats, can help lower levels of LDL cholesterol. Monounsaturated fats are found in avocados, peanut butter, nuts like almonds, hazelnuts, cashews, and pecans, and seeds, such as pumpkin, sesame, and sunflower seeds. They are also found in plant oils such as olive, peanut, safflower, sesame, and canola oils. A study from Harvard researchers (Harvard Health Publishing 2021, April) found that consuming monounsaturated fats, especially from nuts and olive oil, can lower a person's risk of heart disease — especially if the healthy fat replaces saturated fat and refined carbs (which can also raise LDL low density lipoprotein levels, the type of cholesterol that causes plaque build-up in the arteries). Unsaturated fats help to raise the HDL high density lipoprotein (good) cholesterol levels. HDL picks up excess LDL in the blood and moves it to the liver, where it is broken down and discarded. The goal is to have a high HDL-to-LDL ratio for a healthy blood lipid profile. The researchers added that any benefit from consuming monounsaturated fats may be negated if a person continues to consume too much saturated fat.

- Fat adds flavour to food by making food taste better.

- Fat keeps you feeling satisfied longer after a meal as it helps to regulate blood sugar levels and the hormones involved in hunger and satiety. Fat also takes the digestive system longer to process and digest, thus also making you feel fuller longer.

Although fats are a healthy part of our diet, it is still important to acknowledge that only up to 10% of our fat intake should come from saturated fats. Saturated fat includes foods like meat, dairy and coconut oil. Those monitoring their cholesterol should be mindful of their saturated fat intake.

Fats are generally recommended to account for about 30% of our diet, with the majority of fat intake coming from the healthy unsaturated fats listed above. Trans fat (partially hydrogenated fats) found in processed food can be detrimental to our health, so avoid these as much as possible.

Check out this video for more details discussing the differences between these kinds of fats.

https://www.youtube.com/watch?v=mvvx2yQRbzQ

Now that we discussed the fundamentals of fat, let's talk about how our bodies use it for stored energy, and how it is released from the body!

RECAP ON THE PROCESS OF METABOLISM

When you are not eating, whether active or at rest, your body must draw on its internal energy stores of complex carbohydrates, fat, and proteins to provide your body with the energy it needs to do all the things it needs to do to keep you alive! Important activities like breathing, keep your heart pumping, digesting, or providing energy for that run you enjoy.

Most of the cells in your body use glucose along with amino acids (the building blocks of protein) and fats for energy. However, glucose is the main source of fuel for your brain. Nerve cells and chemical messengers located there need it to help them process information, and having access to glucose is very important for overall brain function. Your brain uses about 60% of the glucose that our bodies use. However, glucose does not always have to come immediately from foods and beverages. Glucose is also generated by the body to ensure that we always have the amount that is needed. One way that this is achieved, is by breaking down something called glycogen, in order to free up the glucose it contains.

Glycogen is released by an important hormone called glucagon. When the body doesn't need to use glucose for energy, it is stored in the liver and muscles by insulin. Glycogen is this stored form of connected glucose molecules. When the body needs a quick boost of energy or is not getting glucose from food, glycogen is broken down to release glucose into the bloodstream to be used as fuel by the cells. Your body can store enough glycogen in order to keep you fueled for about a day. This process is called glycogenolysis.

The body can also produce glucose through a process called gluconeogenesis. This process occurs when the body (mainly the liver, then kidneys and to a less extent the small intestine) makes glucose from non-carbohydrate sources which include lactate (what our bodies produce during exercise), glycerol (is produced when fats are digested, can be used for energy or stored in adipose tissue) and amino acids.

Gluconeogenesis occurs when glycogen stores become low and glucose consumption is too low or nonexistent, such as during periods of starvation or prolonged fasting. Although the body has enough glycogen stored in the muscles and liver to last about a day, after approximately 14 hours in a fasted state it will begin to increase its percentage of gluconeogenesis, generating energy in increased ratios as time goes on. In this stage, energy that is stored in adipose tissue all around your body in the form of triglycerides will be liberalized. In the fat cell, other types of lipases (enzymes that break down fats) work to break down fats into fatty acids and glycerol in a process called lipolysis. These lipases are activated by various hormones, such as glucagon, epinephrine, and growth hormone. The resulting glycerol and fatty acids are released into the blood and travel to the liver through the bloodstream. Once in the liver, the glycerol and fatty acids can be either further broken down directly to get energy, or used to make glucose.

One very important consideration though, is that skeletal muscle (composed of amino acids) can be used as a source when generating glucose through the pathway of gluconeogenesis. This can lead to muscle wasting and loss over time which can have a major impact on the body!

An additional alternative form of energy that can be generated if needed, is the formation of Ketone bodies from our fat reserves. Ketone bodies can serve as a fuel source if glucose levels are too low in the body. Ketones serve as fuel in times of prolonged starvation, carbohydrate deprivation, or when patients suffer from uncontrolled diabetes and cannot utilize most of the circulating glucose. In these scenarios, fat stores are liberated, generating ketone bodies to the body and brain for energy.

So, in losing weight, what happens to the fat we use for energy?

The body disposes of fat through a series of very complex metabolic pathways. For those of you that are interested in the biochemistry behind each of these processes, these videos are a great way to understand the different pathways of fat metabolism described simply above:

https://www.youtube.com/watch?v=9lElznAeI48

https://www.youtube.com/watch?v=Qep3wooEw5M

https://www.ninjanerd.org/lecture/mobilization-of-triglycerides

https://www.ninjanerd.org/lecture/fatty-acid-oxidation-part-1

https://www.ninjanerd.org/lecture/fatty-acid-oxidation-part-2

https://www.ninjanerd.org/lecture/the-metabolic-map-lipids

https://www.ninjanerd.org/lecture/lipoprotein-metabolism-chylomicrons-vldl-idl-ldl-hdl

This is where things become very interesting!!

As the body begins to draw on our fat stores for energy, although the number of fat cells remains the same, each fat cell simply gets smaller.

The byproducts of the metabolism of fat are processed by the body in the following ways:

As water, through your skin (when you sweat) and your kidneys (when you urinate), and as carbon dioxide (CO_2) through your lungs (when you breathe out). Exercise also increases your respiratory rate, so more CO_2 (and the by-products of fat) leaves your body when you work out. Being well hydrated is well documented in supporting the body in fat loss (also allowing for the release of fat by-products through urine). Fat breakdown also generates heat, which keeps body temperatures normal.

What happens to body fat when you exercise?

Your muscles first utilize stored glycogen for energy. After about 30 to 60 minutes of aerobic exercise, your body starts utilizing mainly fat stores depending on the intensity of the activity. If you are exercising moderately, this takes about an hour. Building your muscle mass will raise your basal metabolic rate, and the amount of energy your body uses at rest.

This leads us to the most interesting theory about how most of our fat leaves our body.

A study conducted by a team of Australian researchers Meerman and Brown (2014), calculated exactly what happens to our fat when we drop weight, and revealed that we don't convert our missing mass into heat or energy. We actually breathe it out.

Their results reveal that 22 pounds (10 kg) of fat turns into 18.5 pounds (8.4 kg) of carbon dioxide, which is exhaled when we breathe, and 3.5 pounds (1.6 kg) of water, which we then excrete through our urine, tears, sweat and other bodily fluids.

Lead author of the paper Ruben Meerman, a physicist, first became interested in the biochemistry of weight loss when he dropped 33 pounds (15 kg). However, when he asked his doctors where this weight went, he was surprised by the fact no one could tell him.

After surveying 150 doctors, dieticians, and personal trainers, he discovered that more than half thought that fat was converted into heat or energy as we break it down.

But, as a physicist, Meerman knew that this would violate the law of conservation of mass. This law states that in a closed or isolated system, matter cannot be created or destroyed. It can change forms but is conserved. This law also helped scientists understand that substances did not disappear as result of a reaction (as they may appear to do), rather they transform into another substance of equal mass.

We put on weight in the form of fat when excess stores of energy are converted into triglycerides (compounds made up of carbon, hydrogen, and oxygen), and are then stored in lipid droplets inside fat cells. To lose weight, you need to break down those triglycerides to access their carbon.

The results of this study showed that in order to completely break down 22 pounds (10 kg) of human fat, we need to inhale 64 pounds (29 kg) of oxygen (and somewhere along the way, burn 94,000 calories). This reaction produces 62 pounds (28 kg) of CO2 and 24 pounds (11 kg) of water. Their calculations show that the lungs are the primary excretory organ for fat!

However, they couldn't work out exactly what was happening to the fat cells in this reaction. After months of research, Meerman discovered a formula from a paper published in 1949 that solved the problem. It showed that oxygen atoms are shared between the carbon and hydrogen in fat at a ratio of 2:1 (forming carbon dioxide and water). This allowed them to come up with the final figure of 84 percent of a fat molecule's atoms being exhaled as carbon dioxide, and the remaining 16 percent ending up as water.

However, this doesn't mean that simply breathing deeply will help us lose weight, energy is still required to unlock the carbon and break down the fat in the first place.

Meerman stated that "You can only breathe so many times a day; on a day of rest, you breathe around 12 times a minute so 17,280 times you'll breathe in a day and each one takes 10 milligrams of carbon with it, roughly."

Check out this video for more details!

https://www.youtube.com/watch?v=C8ialLlcdcw

Hopefully you found that interesting! Stay tuned for the next science post, where we will be discussing added sugars and artificial sugars (otherwise known as non-nutritive sugars or NNS) and their impact on the brain and body.

REFERENCES

Ahmed, S., Shah, P. & Ahmed, O. (2021, May 9). *Biochemistry, lipids.* StatPearls Publishing. https://www.ncbi.nlm.nih.gov/books/NBK525952/

Betts, G.J., Young, K.A., Wise, J.A., Johnson, E., Poe, B., Kruse, D.H., Korol, O., Johnson, J.E., Womble, M., & DeSaix, P. (2019, May 29). *Anatomy and physiology.* Openstax. https://opentextbc.ca/anatomyandphysiologyopenstax/chapter/lipid-metabolism/

Cannon, B., Nedergaard, J. (2008). Neither fat nor flesh. *Nature, 454,* 947–948. https://doi.org/10.1038/454947a

Cleveland Clinic. (2019, January 17). *Where does body fat go when you lose weight?* https://health.clevelandclinic.org/where-does-body-fat-go-when-you-lose-weight/#:~:text=Your%20body%20must%20dispose%20of,(when%20you%20breathe%20out)

Constant, F., Popkin, B.M. & Gardner, C.D (2012). Drinking water is associated with weight loss in overweight dieting women independent of diet and activity. *Obesity, 16(11),* 2481-2488. https://doi.org/10.1038/oby.2008.409

El-Zayat, S.R., Sibaii, H. & El-Shamy, K.A. (2019). Physiological process of fat loss. *Bulletin of the National Research Centre*, 43. https://doi.org/10.1186/s42269-019-0238-z

Feingold, K. R. (2021). Introduction to lipids and lipoproteins. In K. R. Feingold (Eds.) et. al., Endotext. Mdtext.com, Inc. https://pubmed.ncbi.nlm.nih.gov/26247089/

Freudenrich, C. (n.d.). How fat cells work. How Stuff Works. https://science.howstuffworks.com/life/cellular-microscopic/fat-cell3.htm

Harvard Health Publishing. (2021, April 19). *Know the facts about fats.* Harvard Medical School. https://www.health.harvard.edu/staying-healthy/know-the-facts-about-fats#:~:text=%22Fat%20helps%20give%20your%20body,your%20body%20absorb%20vital%20nutrients.

Health e-University. (n.d.) *What are fats?* https://www.healtheuniversity.ca/EN/CardiacCollege/Eating/Fats/

Hensrud, D. (2020, November 5). *What is brown fat? How is it different from other body fat?* Mayo Clinic. https://www.mayoclinic.org/healthy-lifestyle/weight-loss/expert-answers/brown-fat/faq-20058388#:~:text=Brown%20fat%2C%20also%20called%20brown,mitochondria%20than%20does%20white%20fat.

Khan Academy. (2015, July 14). *Molecular structure of triglycerides (fats) | Biology* [Video]. Youtube. https://www.youtube.com/watch?v=OpyTJbzA7Fk

Laskowski, E. R. (2020, April 21). *When you lose weight, where does the lost body fat go?* Mayo Clinic. https://www.mayoclinic.org/healthy-lifestyle/weight-loss/expert-answers/body-fat/faq-20058251

LCR Staff Writer. (2019, November 6). *Weight loss info: What does fat in urine look like?* LCR Health. https://lcrhealth.com/fat-loss-urine-color/

Link, R., Chin, K. (2021, February 18). *Can peeing cause lasting weight loss?* Healthline. https://www.healthline.com/nutrition/do-you-lose-weight-when-you-pee

Marcin, A., Hodgson, L. (2022, January 24). *Brown fat: What you should know.* Healthline. https://www.healthline.com/health/brown-fat#purpose

Mayo Clinic Staff. (2020, September 29). *Triglycerides: Why do they matter?* Mayo Clinic. https://www.mayoclinic.org/diseases-conditions/high-blood-cholesterol/in-depth/triglycerides/

art-20048186#:~:text=Triglycerides%20are%20a%20type%20of,triglycerides%20for%20energy%20 between%20meals.

Mayo Clinic Staff. (2019, September 28). *Omega-3 in fish: How eating fish helps your heart.* Mayo Clinic. https://www.mayoclinic.org/diseases-conditions/heart-disease/in-depth/omega-3/ art-20045614#:~:text=Omega%2D3%20fatty%20acids%20are,Decreasing%20triglycerides

Meerman, R., Brown, A. J. (2014). When somebody loses weight, where does the fat go? *BMJ, 349(7257). https:// www.bmj.com/content/349/bmj.g7257*

Ninja Nerd. (2018, January 6). *Metabolism | Lipoprotein metabolism | Chylomicrons, vldl, idl, ldl, & hdl* [Video]. Youtube. https://www.youtube.com/watch?v=wQY0xpwqPfQ

Ninja Nerd. (2017, June 19). *Metabolism | Fatty acid oxidation: Part 2* [Video].Youtube. https://www.youtube.com/ watch?v=jxylGoJP9jY

Ninja Nerd. (2017, June 14). *Metabolism | The metabolic map: Lipids* [Video]. Youtube. https://www.youtube.com/ watch?v=Wm7UR0zCQzM

Ninja Nerd. (2017, June 7). *Metabolism | Mobilization of triglycerides* [Video]. Youtube. https://www.youtube.com/ watch?v=lD62q1hUae4&t=1s

Ninja Nerd. (2017, May 29). *Metabolism | Fatty acid synthesis: Part 1* [Video]. Youtube. https://www.youtube.com/ watch?v=nBFSz63T1c0

Oregon State University. (2019, June). *Essential fatty acids.* https://lpi.oregonstate.edu/mic/other-nutrients/ essential-fatty-acids

Pearson, K. (2017, December 5). *How omega-3 fish oil affects your brain and mental health.* Healthline. https://www. healthline.com/nutrition/omega-3-fish-oil-for-brain-health#TOC_TITLE_HDR_3

https://www.thoughtco.com/definition-of-conservation-of-mass-law-604412

SciShow. (2015, December 21). *The deal with fat* [Video]. Youtube. https://www.youtube.com/ watch?v=mvvx2yQRbzQ

SciShow. (2015, January 13). *When you burn fat, where does it go?* [Video]. Youtube. https://www.youtube.com/ watch?v=C8ialLlcdcw

The Editors of Encyclopedia Britannica. (2021, May 31.). *Ester.* Encyclopedia Britannica. https://www.britannica. com/science/ester-chemical-compound

Watson, H. (2015). Biological membranes. *Essays in Biochemistry, 59,* 43–69. https://doi.org/10.1042/bse0590043

Wondersofchemistry. (2019, March 4). *Fat metabolism introduction* [Video]. Youtube. https://www.youtube.com/ watch?v=Qep3wooEw5M

Wondersofchemistry. (2018, March 31). *Lipolysis* [Video]. Youtube. https://www.youtube.com/ watch?v=9lElznAeI48

https://www.cell.com/cell-reports/fulltext/S2211-1247(17)30751-9?_returnURL=https%3A%2F%2Flinkinghub. elsevier.com%2Fretrieve%2Fpii%2FS2211124717307519%3Fshowall%3Dtrue

https://www.healthline.com/health/types-of-body-fat

SUGARS AND THE BRAIN

In this science post, we are taking a closer look at sugar and non-nutritive sugars (NNS), alternatively known as artificial sweeteners. We already examined sugar quite closely, discussing all the reasons why it is beneficial to minimise the intake of it, especially if maximising the program. However, let's take a closer look at how sugar and NNS affect us, more specifically our brain, and how they may influence our bodies, and even the choices we make!

WHY DO WE LIKE SUGAR?

Sugar provides energy to our bodies in the form of calories, so humans, like most other creatures, have evolved to enjoy it. Our primitive ancestors were scavengers. Sugary foods are excellent sources of energy, so we have evolved to find sweet foods particularly palatable. Foods with unpleasant, bitter and sour tastes can be unripe, poisonous or rotting. These foods could cause sickness, so we are more likely to avoid those foods.

We need food to survive, and we need the amount that nature has provided for us in the perfect package, which is food in its whole form. This often includes fibre or other substances that allow for a slower digestion, and does not usually facilitate a fast rise in blood sugar, as well as it is more likely to create a feeling of satiety.

Therefore, to maximise our survival as a species, this innate brain system has us seeking out these foods.

Sugar comes in a variety of forms. To recap, glucose is the simplest form of carbohydrates and only has one sugar molecule, which is called a **monosaccharide**. Other monosaccharides that may sound familiar include fructose, galactose, and ribose, which the body also processes or may produce for energy.

We have discussed the importance of how our body breaks down our food into these simple sugars in order to provide energy to the body in the science post on Insulin. There was also discussion on how added sugar affects our bodies. But let's take a deeper dive into how added sugar affects our brain and nervous system, after a refresher on how our body processes these added sugars.

WHAT IS ADDED SUGAR OR FREE SUGARS?

The World Health Organization (WHO) has been cautioning people to reduce their intake of "free sugars" to less than 10 percent of daily calories since 1989. The WHO states that doing so can lower the risk of becoming obese or overweight, or experiencing tooth decay. Free sugars include both the sugars naturally found in honey and fruit juice, and sugar added to food and drinks. On food labels, added sugars include words such as glucose, fructose, corn syrup, brown sugar, dextrose, maltose, and sucrose, as well as many others.

As we had discussed in previous posts, the most significant sources of added sugar in today's diet consists primarily of the simple sugar fructose. Fructose is a fairly sweet, naturally occurring sugar. It comes from most fruits, and even some vegetables.

However, the majority of sources of fructose that people tend to consume are table sugar (which is called **sucrose**, made from sugar cane or beets, is composed of 50% glucose and 50% fructose), honey, agave nectar, fruit juices, palm sugar and (**HFCS**) high fructose corn syrup (HFCS is a highly processed and inexpensive substitute for cane sugar that was introduced in the 1970s, which is made from corn. It's used to sweeten a variety of processed foods, including soda, candy, baked goods, and cereals). Today's sugars are often refined and concentrated.

After we ingest food, the stomach and small intestine go right to work in breaking the food down into its simplest form of glucose, which is absorbed and then released into the bloodstream. Once in the bloodstream, glucose can be used immediately by the cells for energy, or stored in our bodies to be used later. However, glucose and fructose are metabolised very differently by the body. Before it can be used by the body, fructose needs to be converted into glucose, which is conducted by the liver. While every cell in the body can use glucose, the liver is the only organ that can metabolise fructose when ingested in significant amounts!

Before the mass production of refined sugar, humans rarely consumed fructose in high amounts. But as food science has developed over the years, our food has greatly changed from its very simple former self. When people eat a diet that is high in calories and high in fructose, the liver is thought to become overloaded and starts turning the fructose into fat. Many scientists believe that excess fructose consumption may be a key driver in many of the most serious diseases today. These include obesity, type 2 diabetes, insulin resistance, heart disease, and even cancer. However, more human evidence is needed. Although, researchers debate the extent to which fructose contributes to these disorders, there is a considerable mounting body of evidence justifying the concerns.

THE DATA BEHIND SUGAR

In 2015, the WHO further suggested reducing free sugar daily intake to less than 5 percent of calories, about 6 teaspoons, for optimising health. In the United States In 2017–2018, the average daily intake of added sugars was 17 teaspoons for children and young adults aged 2 to 19 years, as well as in adults over 20 years of age. Added sugar also accounts for 14 percent of the average person's daily calorie intake. Most of this comes from beverages, including energy drinks, alcoholic drinks, soda, fruit drinks, and sweetened coffee and teas.

Other common sources are snacks. These don't just include the obvious, like brownies, cookies, doughnuts, and ice cream. You can also find large quantities of added sugar in bread, salad dressing, granola bars, cereals, and even fat-free yoghurts to name a few.

In Canada, a health report released on October 20, 2021 from Statistics Canada, found that in a 2015 Canadian Community Health Survey (CCHS), the total sugar intake in Canada per person was estimated at 105.6 g/day. While this was down from the 110.0 g/day reported in a CCHS conducted in 2004, it was concluded that the apparent reduction between 2004 and 2015 may actually be caused by misreporting as a result of changes in survey methodology. They also reported that total sugar consumption from foods actually increased between 2004 and 2015, while total sugar intake from beverages decreased.

The Office of Disease Prevention and Health Promotion in the Dietary Guidelines for Americans 2020-2025, suggest cutting the consumption of added sugars to less than 10 percent of calories per day. This is actually in line with WHO's older recommendations, that were stated earlier back in 1989!

However, to help consumers, the Food and Drug Administration (FDA) has developed a new food label that lists added sugars separately, which manufacturers are required to use (though some smaller manufacturers had until 2021 to comply).

https://www.fda.gov/food/food-labeling-nutrition/changes-nutrition-facts-label

Canada has also updated their food labels, which now identifies the total percentage of sugars in a product. This change was imposed by the Canadian Food Inspection Agency (CFIA), with compliance to be enforced by Dec 15, 2022.

https://www.canada.ca/en/health-canada/services/food-labelling-changes.html

Check out the video to see how sugar can be hidden in the foods we buy!

https://www.ted.com/talks/robert_lustig_sugar_hiding_in_plain_sight?language=en

HOW DOES SUGAR AFFECT OUR BRAIN?

There is an increasing body of research that tells us excess sugar could be as addictive as some street drugs and have similar effects on the brain. The concept of food addiction is a very controversial subject among scientists and clinicians. While it is true that you can become physically dependent on certain drugs, it is debated whether you can be addicted to food when you need it for basic survival. There are also those that caution us in our language when using words like addiction when describing things like food. The drug crisis is very serious, and those with addiction are physiologically driven to get more drugs. This can also be said for those with other addictions such as alcohol and sex. They may resort to crime and violence to do so, whereas those seeking out food wouldn't necessarily go to those lengths. However, our environment today is abundant with sweet, energy dense, processed foods, which we have easy access to. Our portion sizes have also increased to a much greater degree. What is clear, is these foods are having some effects on us, and our drive to have more of it.

Given the rise of obesity, one could argue towards the theory that sugar can in fact be addictive to some sort of degree. However, despite the differing opinions regarding this, researchers and nutritionists can agree that sugar has addictive properties and we need to be having less of it. Furthermore, in certain individuals with certain predispositions, this could manifest as having a compulsion towards sugary foods.

Check out this video on the effects of sugar and the brain!

https://www.ted.com/talks/nicole_avena_how_sugar_affects_the_brain?language=en

DOPAMINE

Sugar increases activity in certain parts of our brains, which means that those parts become excited due to the incoming nutrition. When we eat sweet foods the brain's reward system, called the mesolimbic dopamine system, gets activated. Brain activation happens because of electrical activity that occurs within cells called neurons. A neuron is a nerve cell that sends and receives electrical and chemical signals.

All brain activity occurs in the form of electricity that is sent down small "wires" or "tunnels" in the neurons called axons. The electrical signal through the axons then results in the release of brain chemicals called neurotransmitters, which are a chemical substance released by neurons in the brain that send messages to our bodies and muscles.

Interconnected with the hormones involved in satiety and hunger are neurotransmitters, one of which includes dopamine. Eating sugar releases opioids and dopamine in our bodies. This is the link between added sugar and compulsive behaviour. Dopamine has a direct effect in activating the reward and pleasure centres in the brain, which can affect both mood and food intake.

Those that struggle with obesity often have a blunted dopamine pathway because of chronic exposure to highly palatable foods, such as foods that are high in added sugar and fats. This over-exposure, which leads to a blunted response when eating, has been suggested to contribute to increased reward-seeking behaviour, including overeating.

When a certain behaviour causes an excessive release of dopamine, you experience sensations of pleasure that you are inclined to re-experience, and so repeat the behaviour. As you repeat that behaviour more and more, your brain adjusts to release less dopamine. The only way to feel the same amount of pleasure as before, is to repeat the behaviour in increasing amounts and frequency. This then leads to the blunted response that was described above, subsequently leading one to seek out more sugar which ultimately leads to substance (sugar) abuse and weight gain. Also, every time we have sugar, we reinforce neuropathways, causing the brain to become increasingly hardwired to crave sugar, from a habit formation perspective.

Check out these videos to learn more about the dopamine reward system and the mesolimbic dopamine pathway system!

https://www.youtube.com/watch?v=YzCYuKX6zp8&t=10s

https://www.youtube.com/watch?v=f7E0mTJQ2KM&t=36s

Check out this video about the potentially addictive effects of sugar on the brain!

https://www.youtube.com/watch?v=ShQYz8AwKJE

HYPOTHALAMUS

As discussed in the science post The Set-Point Theory, the hypothalamus, a small region of the brain located at the base of the brain, near the pituitary gland, is involved in the integration of signals directed to it from hormones like leptin (from adipose or fat cells), ghrelin (from the digestive system), insulin (the pancreas), along with many other hormones that regulate our hunger and satiety. Your metabolism constantly adjusts up or down based on a variety of signals. The set-point theory also suggests that your weight may go up or down temporarily but will ultimately return to its normal set range. The signalling system we have in place helps to maintain our weight.

Some researchers (Jung & Kim, 2013) believe that the reactive signal system stops working efficiently over time and leptin and insulin resistance develop, causing us to gain weight. As discussed, the thought is that foods that are high in fat and sugar, like many processed foods available today, lead to not only inflammation in the body, but also in the brain. Because the hypothalamus is so important in regulating, and interpreting the signals involved in hunger, satiety, and metabolism, inflammation can lead to a disruption in the pathway of these signals and even in how fat is stored. This can lead to weight gain. This further corroborates the negative impact that sugar and processed high fat foods have on our brain!

MANAGING CRAVINGS

Many people experience food cravings. Cravings can occur particularly when one is stressed, hungry, or their gastronomic senses are inundated with the sight, sound, and aroma of their favourite foods being prepared.

To overcome cravings, we need to inhibit our natural response to indulge in these tasty foods. A network of inhibitory neurons is critical for adjusting our behaviour. These neurons are concentrated in the prefrontal cortex, a key area of the brain involved in decision-making, impulse regulation and delaying gratification.

https://www.youtube.com/watch?v=i47_jiCsBMs&t=2s

Inhibitory neurons are like the brain's brakes and release the neurotransmitter GABA or Gamma Aminobutyric Acid. GABA is considered an inhibitory neurotransmitter because it blocks, or inhibits, certain brain signals and decreases activity in your nervous system. When GABA attaches to a protein in your brain known as a GABA receptor, it produces a calming effect. This can help with feelings of anxiety, stress, and fear. It may also help to prevent seizures.

Research in rats has shown that eating high sugar diets can alter inhibitory neurons. Rats that were fed a high sugar diet were also less able to regulate their behaviour and make decisions.

This shows that there is the potential that what we eat can influence our ability to make choices that are beneficial to us, and may underlie why diet changes can be so difficult for people.

A 2017 study asked people to rate how much they wanted to eat a high calorie snack when they were hungry versus when they had recently eaten. The people who regularly ate a high-fat, high-sugar diet rated their cravings for snack foods higher even when they were not hungry. This suggests that regularly eating high-sugar foods could heighten cravings, creating a negative feedback loop of wanting more and more of these foods!

However, there is good news! Our taste buds can adapt to accept less sugar in a fairly short period of time. Following a plan like The Livy Method that promotes eating nutrient dense, whole foods, which are naturally lower in sugar, is a great way to support the body in addressing cravings. By reducing sugar, especially concentrated sugars (as recommended by The Livy Method), not only limits the amount of sugar ingested, but also makes foods that are less sweet seem sweeter. This is a common finding by members when participating in the plan. In fact, members often comment on how they start to really enjoy the natural taste and flavours of the food they eat. They also describe how when they indulge in eating sweet or processed food, it doesn't taste as good as they remember, or they can taste the chemicals and additives in the food which they never noticed before.

SUGAR AND MEMORY

Another brain area that can be affected by high sugar diets is the hippocampus. The hippocampus is a part of the brain found in the inner folds of the bottom middle section of the brain, known as the temporal lobe. Its main functions involve human learning and memory.

The hippocampus is part of the limbic system, which is associated with the functions of feeling and reacting. The limbic system is situated on the edge of the cortex, and it includes the hypothalamus and the amygdala. These structures help control different bodily functions, such as the endocrine system and what is commonly known as the "fight or flight" response.

The hippocampus helps humans process and retrieve two kinds of memory, declarative memories and spatial relationships.

Declarative memories are those related to facts and events. Examples include learning how to memorise speeches or lines in a play.

Spatial relationship memories involve pathways or routes. For example, when a cab driver learns a route through a city, they use spatial memory. Spatial relationship memories appear to be stored in the right hippocampus.

The hippocampus is also where short-term memories are turned into long-term memories. These are then stored elsewhere in the brain. Research has shown that nerve cells continue to develop throughout adulthood, and that the hippocampus is one of the few places in the brain where new nerve cells are generated.

Similar to animal research, there is emerging evidence that a Western-style (WS) diet – high in saturated fat and added sugar – impairs human hippocampal functioning. However, the conditions under which this occurs are not fully understood.

According to a scientific systematic review (Taylor et al., 2021), regular consumption of a Western-style diet places individuals at higher risk for mild cognitive impairment and dementia. With progressive memory loss and hippocampal damage being an early feature and neurological sign of dementia, diet-induced hippocampal impairment may have significant ramifications by initiating or speeding-up the disease process. Furthermore, the same physiological changes associated with a Western-style diet, including increased hippocampal inflammation and reduced hippocampal neurogenesis (the formation of new neurons), are associated with the pathology of dementia.

There are also further consequences in having an impaired hippocampus resulting from the western-style diet. The hippocampus has a role in appetite regulation, by its involvement in recalling previously consumed food to assist with conscious adjustment of intake – such as recalling what you recently ate, and so moderating your intake accordingly. When satiated, the hippocampus may automatically inhibit retrieval of pleasant food-related memories. Thus, when looking at food when satiated, it will no longer lead to the recollection of how pleasant it is to eat, thereby dulling desire. It is suggested that impaired hippocampal inhibition leads to an increase in the intake of the very foods (highly palatable sweet and fatty foods) that caused the hippocampal damage in the first place, creating a "vicious cycle". This model is actually called the vicious cycle model and is likely to lead to slow, long term weight gain.

Finally, the hippocampus seems to be involved in appetitive interoception. Interoception is the perception of sensations from inside the body. This includes the perception of physical sensations related to internal organ function such as a heart beat, respiration, satiety, as well as the autonomic nervous system activities that are related to emotions. Hippocampal impairment has been linked to interoceptive insensitivity which can result in a disconnection with hunger/satiety and thirst cues. This may lead to overconsumption, resulting in weight gain and obesity over the long term.

Check out this video on the hippocampus and limbic system!

https://www.youtube.com/watch?v=2K3GAaC2SEI

Check out this video on the effects of sugar on the brain and hippocampus

https://www.youtube.com/watch?v=Dacv_OoM62s

NON-NUTRITIVE SWEETENERS (NNS)

From reviewing this information, it can be seen that a diet high in sugar, especially when paired with poor quality fats (often seen in processed foods), has detrimental effects on not only our bodies, but our brain!

This is why there is a market for non-nutritive sweeteners. The purpose of these products is to satisfy the desire for a sweet taste, but has few or negligible calories. The thought is people can continue to enjoy the taste of "sweet", while being able to manage weight/weight loss and health issues such as diabetes.

NNS are made by chemical alternatives, altering existing sugars or amino acids, or are made from the derivatives of plants. Some examples of NNS are aspartame (Equal, NutraSweet), cyclamate (Sucaryl, Sugar Twin, Sweet 'N Low), saccharin, sucralose (Splenda), sugar alcohols (mannitol, sorbitol, and xylitol. Note: if you eat too much of them, sugar alcohols can cause diarrhea and bloating), polydextrose, stevia, steviol glycosides, and erythritol, amongst many others. The regulation of NNS varies in different countries, allowing for different product availability depending on where you live. NNS are found in many different products, and may even be listed as an ingredient that is not identified as a low sugar product, or used as an additive.

THE SCIENCE BEHIND THE USE OF NNS

When going down the rabbit hole of research into this area, it is honestly difficult to navigate how NNS truly affects us. There have been many studies that do report the safety of these products, which does allow for wide scale use of them through regulatory bodies such as the FDA and Health Canada. However, it is identified that there is still a need for both further primary research, and high quality comprehensive systematic reviews including meta-analyses, to inform future recommendations about the health benefits and risks of NNS, to advise and support health care practice and public health decision-making. There are noted controversies of the existing evidence between different artificial sweeteners surrounding their use.

Although NNS maintains a similar palatability as natural sugars, the way the body processes them is different. Interestingly, the gut microbiota may play a major role in the physiological effects of artificial sweeteners on body weight regulation and glucose homeostasis. According to Pang, Goossens, & Blaak (2021) there is mechanistic evidence that artificial sweeteners may induce gut microbiota dysbiosis, by altering the gut microbiota composition and function.

The gut microbiota appears to react differently to NNS than to real sugar. These organisms become less able to break down real sugars the more that they are exposed to artificial sweeteners. Not being able to break down sugars is a concern, because this change in the microbiota can affect the ability of our bodies to digest and process the nutrients from the food we eat. This can potentially lead to deficiencies in vitamins and minerals!

Although different physiological processes are involved in the effect of NNS on metabolic health, meta-analyses of Randomised Control Trials (RCTs) or RCTs and prospective cohort studies, suggest that artificial sweeteners may have a neutral effect on body weight and glycemic control, respectively, or may have a beneficial effect on long-term body weight regulation. Even though the majority of human studies report no significant effects of artificial sweeteners on body weight and glycemic control, it should be emphasised that the study duration of most studies is limited. Furthermore, unlike rodent studies, long-term studies investigating the underlying physiological effects of body weight control and metabolic health of humans and NNS use are scarce and therefore warranted. This is important to consider when interpreting the results.

Notably, artificial sweeteners are metabolised differently and may not all elicit the same metabolic effect. For instance, components of NNS may affect the gut microbiota composition directly and others are easily digested and absorbed. It is also important to note, most NNS provide little to no energy, so should not affect your blood sugar. However, this is not true in the case of sugar alcohols. They are a carbohydrate, and a hybrid form of sugar and alcohol. These products can affect your blood sugar, so those with diabetes should still be mindful of them.

Not all studies investigating the effects of artificial sweeteners on body weight control and glucose homeostasis, take into account the different metabolic pathways of distinct artificial sweeteners. Therefore, human data on the effects of distinct artificial sweeteners are limited or lacking. The difference in metabolic fate of artificial sweeteners may underlie conflicting findings that have been reported related to their effects on body weight control, glucose homeostasis, and underlying biological mechanisms. Thus, making conclusions of the metabolic effects of a single artificial sweetener to all artificial sweeteners is not appropriate.

An example of this is that there is growing evidence that indicates certain artificial sweeteners like sucralose reduce insulin sensitivity and affect the gut bacteria.

It is recommended that future studies should consider the metabolic pathways of different artificial sweeteners. Also, further (long-term) human research investigating the underlying physiological pathways of different artificial sweeteners on microbiota alterations and its related metabolic pathway is warranted to evaluate the potential impact of their use.

Finally, although Stevia in the purified form, called stevioside (known as stevia extract or *Stevia rebaudiana)*, is considered safe to use, whole stevia leaves or crude stevia extracts are not recommended, as there is not enough information about their potential impact on your health. There's concern that raw stevia herb may harm your kidneys, reproductive system, and cardiovascular system. It may also drop blood pressure too low or interact with medications that lower blood sugar.

The WHO has released this 2022 systematic review and meta-analysis of the health effects of the use of non-sugar sweeteners.

https://ewgagdyvsuu.exactdn.com/wp-content/uploads/2022/04/Health-effects-of-the-use-of-non-sugar-sweeteners-a-systematic-review-and-meta-analysis.pdf

Currently, project SWEET, a European Commission Horizon 2020 funded project and human multicenter study is being conducted over 5 years. It is supported by a consortium of 29 pan-European research, consumer and industry partners, who will develop and review evidence on long term benefits and potential risks involved in switching over to sweeteners and sweetness enhancers (S&SEs) in the context of public health and safety, obesity, and sustainability. Check out their website to follow their findings!

https://sweetproject.eu/

Check out this excellent video synopsis on the complexity of reviewing the literature related to NNS.

https://www.youtube.com/watch?v=L6pJrxmDYEI

Check out this video on the microbiome that includes some discussion on the effects of NNS on the microbiome.

https://www.youtube.com/watch?v=IDqMB6C1uys

The takeaway on sugar and NNS

After examining all the research on sugar and NNS, what is clear is that reducing both are beneficial to your health. The science is clear on the effect sugar has on the reward centre of the brain, and the impact of a diet high in sugar and fat, typical of today's processed diet, on the incidence of obesity and disease, also causing inflammation in the body and the brain.

An alternative has been presented to feed our sugar cravings in the form of NNS, which are presented as a safe alternative. However, the question is why do we need to feed into our need and want of sugar, with an alternative that is processed, chemically altered, made in a lab, and still needs more long term, rigorous human study? Other "sugar free" products often contain additives, dyes, colours, flavours and preservatives. These products are often marketed as "healthy"!

The Livy Method recommends eating whole, natural foods, that includes the option of adding in natural sugars on occasion if desired. This combined with proper hydration, and eating to satisfaction, allows one to experience and enjoy food as it was meant to be experienced.

Sweetness inundates our senses, dulling them over time. By reducing the amount of sweet we eat, our taste buds can actually "reset", and foods less sweet, actually taste sweeter. Therefore, we can actually enjoy eating foods in their natural state, while our bodies and brains reap all the nutritional benefits, becoming healthier because of it. Now that is truly sweet!

The microbiome has been a popular topic, which we have touched on with some of our science posts. Stay tuned next week for our last science post, when we will be looking deeper into the microbiome!

REFERENCES

Avena, N. (2017, September). *How sugar affects the brain* [Video]. TED. https://www.ted.com/talks/nicole_avena_how_sugar_affects_the_brain?language=en

Ahmed, S. H., Guillem, K., & Vandaele, Y. (2013). Sugar addiction: pushing the drug-sugar analogy to the limit. *Current opinion in clinical nutrition and metabolic care, 16*(4), 434–439. DOI: 10.1097/MCO.0b013e328361c8b8

BioBrainBuddies. (2020, May 8). *Memory and the hippocampus* [Video]. Youtube. https://www.youtube.com/watch?v=2K3GAaC2SEI

Changes to the nutrition facts label. (2022, March 7). U.S. Food and Drug Administration. https://www.fda.gov/food/food-labeling-nutrition/changes-nutrition-facts-label

Chong, C. P., Shahar, S., Haron, H., & Din, N. C. (2019). Habitual sugar intake and cognitive impairment among multi-ethnic Malaysian older adults. *Clinical Interventions in Aging, 14*, 1331–1342. https://doi.org/10.2147/CIA.S211534

Edwards, S. (2016). *Sugar and the brain.* Harvard Medical School. https://hms.harvard.edu/news-events/publications-archive/brain/sugar-brain

Government of Canada. (2008, April 30). *The safety of sugar substitutes.* https://www.canada.ca/en/health-canada/services/healthy-living/your-health/food-nutrition/safety-sugar-substitutes.html

Government of Canada. (2022, June 30). *Food labelling changes.* https://www.canada.ca/en/health-canada/services/food-labelling-changes.html

Guo, Y., Zhu, X., Zeng, M., Qi, L., Tang, X., Wang, D., Zhang, M., Xie, Y., Li, H., Yang, X., & Chen, D. (2021). A diet high in sugar and fat influences neurotransmitter metabolism and then affects brain function by altering the gut microbiota. *Translational Psychiatry, 11.* https://doi.org/10.1038/s41398-021-01443-2

Grech, A., Kam, C.O., Gemming, L., & Rangan, A. (2018). Diet-quality and socio-demographic factors associated with non-nutritive sweetener use in the Australian population. *Nutrients, 10*(7). doi: 10.3390/nu10070833

Healthline Medical Network. (2019, March 7). *What does gamma aminobutyric acid (GABA) do?* Healthline. https://www.healthline.com/health/gamma-aminobutyric-acid

How sweet it is: All about sugar substitutes. (2021, November 30). U.S. Food and Drug Administration. https://www.fda.gov/consumers/consumer-updates/how-sweet-it-all-about-sugar-substitutes

Hyman, M. (2018, January 15). *What's worse for you: Sugar or artificial sweetener?* Cleveland Clinic. https://health.clevelandclinic.org/whats-worse-sugar-or-artificial-sweetener/

Khanacademymedicine. (2014, June 25). *Reward pathway in the brain: Processing the environment* [Video]. Youtube. https://www.youtube.com/watch?v=YzCYuKX6zp8&t=10s

Kanwal, J.K. (2016, January 11). *Brain tricks to make food taste sweeter: How to transform taste perception and why it matters.* Science in the News. https://sitn.hms.harvard.edu/flash/2016/brain-tricks-to-make-food-taste-sweeter-how-to-transform-taste-perception-and-why-it-matters/

Jung, C. H., & Kim, M. S. (2013). Molecular mechanisms of central leptin resistance in obesity. Archives of Pharmacal Research, 36(2), 201–207. https://doi.org/10.1007/s12272-013-0020-y

Lee, A. A., & Owyang, C. (2017). Sugars, sweet taste receptors, and brain responses. *Nutrients, 9*(7). https://doi.org/10.3390/nu9070653

Leech, J., & Kubala, J. (2021, November 12). *What are sugar alcohols, and are they a healthy sugar swap?* Healthline. https://www.healthline.com/nutrition/sugar-alcohols-good-or-bad

Link, R. (2019, April 18). *Is stevia safe? Diabetes, pregnancy, kids, and more.* Healthline. https://www.healthline.com/nutrition/is-stevia-safe

Lohner, S., Toews, I. & Meerpohl, J.J. (2017). Health outcomes of non-nutritive sweeteners: Analysis of the research landscape. *Nutrition Journal, 16.* https://doi.org/10.1186/s12937-017-0278-x

Lustig, R. (2019, March.). *Sugar: Hiding in plain sight* [Video]. TED. https://www.ted.com/talks/robert_lustig_sugar_hiding_in_plain_sight?language=en

Mesolimbic pathway. (n.d.). Neuroscientifically Challenged. https://neuroscientificallychallenged.com/glossary/mesolimbic-pathway

Myüz, H., & Hout, M.C. (2019). Trick or treat? How artificial sweeteners affect the brain and body. *Frontiers for Young Minds, 7*(51). doi: 10.3389/frym.2019.00051

Neuroscientifically Challenged. (2015, February 13). *2-Minute neuroscience: Reward system* [Video]. Youtube. https://www.youtube.com/watch?v=f7E0mTJQ2KM&t=36s

Neuroscientifically Challenged. (2019, September 4). *2-Minute neuroscience: Prefrontal cortex* [Video]. Youtube. https://www.youtube.com/watch?v=i47_jiCsBMs&t=2s

Pang, M.D., Goossens, G.H., & Blaak, E.E. (2021). The impact of artificial sweeteners on body weight control and glucose homeostasis. *Frontiers in Nutrition, 7.* doi:10.3389/fnut.2020.598340

Petre, A. (2020, August 19). *Artificial sweeteners: Good or bad?* Healthline. https://www.healthline.com/nutrition/artificial-sweeteners-good-or-bad

Pugle, M. (2022, January 27). *How your body tries to prevent you from losing too much weight.* Healthline. https://www.healthline.com/health-news/how-your-body-tries-to-prevent-you-from-losing-too-much-weight

Price, C. J., & Hooven, C. (2018). Interoceptive awareness skills for emotion regulation: Theory and approach of mindful awareness in body-oriented therapy (MABT). *Frontiers in Psychology, 9.* https://doi.org/10.3389/fpsyg.2018.00798

Project overview. (n.d.). Sweet Project. https://sweetproject.eu/

REICHELT, A. (2019, December 26). *A neuroscientist explains what sugar really does to our brains.* Science Alert. https://www.sciencealert.com/research-shows-sugar-can-change-your-brain-here-s-how

Rios-Leyvraz, M., & Montez, J. (2022). *Health effects of the use of non-sugar sweeteners: A systematic review and meta-analysis.* Geneva: World Health Organization. https://ewgagdyvsuu.exactdn.com/wp-content/uploads/2022/04/Health-effects-of-the-use-of-non-sugar-sweeteners-a-systematic-review-and-meta-analysis.pdf

Rivera, L.S. (2020, January 15). *Effects of sugar on the brain: Cravings and inflammation.* UVAHealth. https://blog.uvahealth.com/2020/01/15/effects-sugar-brain/

Ruiz-Ojeda, F. J., Plaza-Díaz, J., Sáez-Lara, M. J., & Gil, A. (2019). Effects of sweeteners on the gut microbiota: A review of experimental studies and clinical trials. *Advances in Nutrition, 10*(Suppl.1), S31–S48. https://doi.org/10.1093/advances/nmy037

SciShow. (2019, January 14). *Are artificial sweeteners bad for you?* [Video]. Youtube. https://www.youtube.com/watch?v=L6pJrxmDYEI

Stevenson, R.J., Francis, H.M., Attuquayefio, T., & Ockert, C. (2017). Explicit wanting and liking for palatable snacks are differentially affected by change in physiological state, and differentially related to salivation and hunger. *Physiology & Behavior, 182,* 101-106. https://doi.org/10.1016/j.physbeh.2017.10.007

Taylor, Z.B., Stevenson, R.J., Ehrenfeld, L., Francis, H.M. (2021). The impact of saturated fat, added sugar and their combination on human hippocampal integrity and function: A systematic review and meta-analysis. *Neuroscience & Biobehavioral Reviews, 130,* 91-106. https://doi.org/10.1016/j.neubiorev.2021.08.008

TEDx Talks. (2016, June 27). *Microbiome: Gut bugs and you* [Video]. Youtube. https://www.youtube.com/watch?v=IDqMB6C1uys

TEDx Talks. (2016, June 29). *This is your brain on sugar* [Video]. Youtube. https://www.youtube.com/watch?v=xCXtcoUxJZc

TEDx Talks. (2017, March 1). *Society's sweet tooth... the brain's response to sugar* [Video]. Youtube. https://www.youtube.com/watch?v=ShQYz8AwKJE

TEDx Talks. (2018, September 25). *Misunderstanding dopamine: Why the language of addiction matters* [Video]. Youtube. https://www.youtube.com/watch?v=aqXmOb_fuN4

U.S. Department of Agriculture and U.S. Department of Health and Human Services. (2020, December). *Dietary guidelines for Americans 2020-2025 (9th ed).* https://www.dietaryguidelines.gov/sites/default/files/2020-12/Dietary_Guidelines_for_Americans_2020-2025.pdf

World Health Organization. (2015, March 4). *WHO calls on countries to reduce sugars intake among adults and children.* https://www.who.int/news/item/04-03-2015-who-calls-on-countries-to-reduce-sugars-intake-among-adults-and-children

Yang, Q. (2010). Gain weight by going diet? Artificial sweeteners and the neurobiology of sugar cravings: Neuroscience 2010. *The Yale Journal of Biology and Medicine, 83*(2), 101–108. https://www.ncbi.nlm.nih.gov/pmc/articles/PMC2892765/#!po=59.3750

Yeung, A.W.K., & Wong, N.S.M. (2020). How does our brain process sugars and non-nutritive sweeteners differently: A systematic review on functional magnetic resonance imaging studies. *Nutrients, 12.* https://doi.org/10.3390/nu12103010

MAINTENANCE AND THE MICROBIOME

We have talked about our microbiome in previous science posts, and how our health can be influenced by it. Just by following The Livy Method for these last 12 weeks, has had a major influence on our gut health and microbiome. In fact, as some of us head into maintenance, eating what makes us feel good, reinforces eating the foods that feed these good bacteria, continuing to keep us healthy. In this final science post, let's review all that we have discussed about the microbiome and then take a deeper dive into it.

THE MICROBIOME- A REVIEW

According to the National Institute of Environmental Health Science (NIEHS) in the United States, the microbiome is defined as the collection of all microbes, such as bacteria, fungi, viruses, and their genes, that naturally live on our bodies and inside us.

Bacteria, viruses, fungi and other microscopic living things are referred to as microorganisms, or microbes, for short. Although microbes are so small that they require a microscope to see them, they contribute in big ways to human health and wellness. They protect us against pathogens, help our immune system develop, help to produce vitamins that our body needs, and enable us to digest food to produce energy.

Because the microbiome is a key connection between the body and the environment, these microbes can affect health in many ways and can even affect how we respond to certain environmental substances. Some microbes alter environmental substances in ways that make them more toxic, while others act as a buffer and make environmental substances less harmful.

HOW CAN THE MICROBIOME AFFECT HEALTH?

More than 2,000 years ago, Hippocrates, the Greek physician who many attribute as the founder of modern medicine, suggested that all disease begins in the gut. It turns out he was onto something (Gunnars, K., 2019, February)!

Studies examining the diversity of the human microbiome started with Antonie van Leewenhoek, who, as early as the 1680s, had compared his oral and fecal microbiota (What is Biotechnology?). He noted the striking differences in microbes between these two habitats and also between samples from individuals in states of health and disease in both of these sites. Thus, studies of the profound differences in microbes at different body sites, and between health and disease, have existed since the science of microbiology itself. What is new today is the ability to use scientific techniques to gain insight into why these differences exist, and to understand how we can affect transformations from one state to another.

The human microbiome has a different community of microbes located in different areas in the body. Trillions of these microbes exist mainly inside your intestines and on your skin. Most of the microbes in your intestines are located in the large intestine in an area called the cecum, and they are referred to as the gut microbiome. They are also found in other areas of the body such as the oral and nasal cavities, and the conjunctiva of our eyes.

According to Gunners (2019, February), although many different types of microbes live inside you, bacteria are the most studied. In fact, there are more bacterial cells in your body than human cells. It is estimated that there are roughly 40 trillion bacterial cells in your body and only 30 trillion human cells. That means you are more bacterial than human!

Altogether, these microbes may weigh as much as 2–5 pounds (1–2 kg), which is roughly the weight of your brain. Together, they function and are considered as an extra organ in your body, playing a huge role in your health.

THE MICROBIOME AND DIGESTION

Humans have evolved to live with microbes for millions of years. During this time, microbes have learned to play very important roles in the human body. In fact, without the gut microbiome, it would be very difficult to survive. Interestingly, the food you eat affects the diversity of your gut bacteria.

There are up to 1,000 species of bacteria in the human gut microbiome, and each of them plays a different role in your body. Most of them are extremely important for your health, while others may cause disease. Interestingly, on average a person carries about 160 species in their gut.

As discussed in the science post The Basics of Digestion, the gut flora in our colon help to ferment the indigestible food and produce vitamins such as Vitamin K and B vitamins that are reabsorbed by the colon. But that's not all, an estimated 80% of our immune system is found in our gut. Having a healthy digestive system, which includes a good balance of our healthy gut flora, ensures a healthier immune system and better nutrient absorption. This is why the Livy Method recommends taking a good quality probiotic, along with a prebiotic (if needed), to help feed those good microbes. Eating the high fibre, nutrient rich foods on plan not only gives our body what it needs, but is also vital in supporting our gut flora!

A person's core microbiome begins to develop from birth and is formed in the first years of life, but can change over time in response to different factors including diet, medications, and environmental exposures. You are first exposed to microbes when you pass through your mother's vaginal canal. However, new evidence suggests that babies may come in contact with some microbes while inside the womb.

Breastfeeding introduces beneficial bacteria to a baby's gut which also contributes to their microbiome. As you grow, your gut microbiome begins to diversify, meaning it starts to contain many different types of microbial species. Higher microbiome diversity is considered good for your health.

Differences in the microbiome may lead to different health effects from environmental exposures and may also help determine individual susceptibility to certain illnesses. Environmental exposures can also disrupt a person's microbiome in ways that could increase the likelihood of developing conditions such as diabetes, obesity, cardiovascular and neurological diseases, allergies, and inflammatory bowel disease.

As your microbiome grows, it affects your body in a number of ways, including:

- **Digesting breast milk:** Some of the bacteria that first begin to grow inside babies' intestines are called ***Bifidobacteria***. They digest the healthy sugars in breast milk that are important for growth.

- **Influencing your immune system:** The gut microbiome also influences how your immune system works. By communicating with immune cells, the gut microbiome can influence how your body responds to infection.

- **Influencing your brain health:** Some research suggests that the gut microbiome may also affect the central nervous system, which controls brain function. See below for more details.

- **Digesting fibre:** Certain bacteria digest fibre, producing short-chain fatty acids in the gut, which are important for gut health. Fibre may help prevent weight gain, diabetes, heart disease and the risk of cancer.

Short-chain fatty acids are fatty acids with fewer than 6 carbon atoms. They are produced when the friendly gut bacteria ferment fibre in your colon and are the main source of energy for the cells lining it.

Excess short-chain fatty acids are used for other functions in the body. For example, they may provide roughly 10% of your daily energy needs. Short-chain fatty acids are also involved in the metabolism of important nutrients like carbohydrates and fat.

About 95% of the short-chain fatty acids in your body are: acetate (C2), propionate (C3), and butyrate (C4). Propionate is mainly involved in producing glucose in the liver and small intestine, acetate is important for energy production and synthesis of lipids, and butyrate is the preferred energy source for cells that line the colon (Brown, M.J., 2021, October).

Many factors affect the amount of short-chain fatty acids in your colon, including how many microorganisms are present, the food source, and the time it takes food to travel through your digestive system.

Eating a lot of fibre-rich foods, such as fruits, vegetables, and legumes, is linked to an increase in short-chain fatty acids. However, the amount and type of fibre you eat affects the composition of bacteria in your gut, which affects what short-chain fatty acids are produced.

For example, studies have shown that eating more fibre increases butyrate production, while decreasing your fibre intake reduces production.

The following types of fibre are best for the production of short-chain fatty acids in the colon:

- **Inulin.** You can get inulin from artichokes, garlic, leeks, onions, wheat, rye, and asparagus.
- **Fructo-oligosaccharides (FOS).** FOS are found in various fruits and vegetables, including bananas, onions, garlic, and asparagus.

- **Resistant starch.** You can get resistant starch from grains, barley, rice, beans, green bananas, legumes, and potatoes that have been cooked and then cooled.

- **Pectin.** Good sources of pectin include apples, apricots, carrots, oranges, and others.

- **Arabinoxylan.** Arabinoxylan is the most common fibre in wheat bran, making up about 70% of the total fibre content.

- **Guar gum.** Guar gum can be extracted from guar beans, which are legumes.

- Some types of cheese, butter, and cow's milk also contain small amounts of butyrate.

THE MICROBIOME AND WEIGHT GAIN

There are thousands of different types of bacteria in your intestines, most of which benefit your health. However, having too many unhealthy microbes can lead to disease. An imbalance of healthy and unhealthy microbes is sometimes called gut dysbiosis, and it may contribute to weight gain.

Some studies have shown that the gut microbiome differed completely between identical twins, one of whom was obese and one of whom was healthy. This demonstrated that differences in the microbiome were not genetic.

Interestingly, in one study, when the microbiome from the obese twin was transferred to mice, they gained more weight than those that had received the microbiome of the lean twin, despite both groups eating the same diet. These studies show that microbiome dysbiosis may play a role in weight gain.

Fortunately, probiotics are good for a healthy microbiome and can help with weight loss, by helping to strengthen our gut health which can fall in line with our weight loss goals. Nevertheless, some studies suggest that the effects of probiotics on weight loss on their own are probably quite small, with people losing less than 2.2 pounds (1 kg). However, probiotics are suggested with The Livy Method as they help with weight loss by improving digestion.

THE MICROBIOME AND IBS AND IBD

The microbiome can also affect gut health and may play a role in intestinal diseases like irritable bowel syndrome (IBS) and inflammatory bowel disease (IBD). The bloating, cramps and abdominal pain that people with IBS experience may be due to gut dysbiosis. This is because the microbes produce a lot of gas and other chemicals, which contribute to the symptoms of intestinal discomfort.

However, certain healthy bacteria in the microbiome can also improve gut health. Certain *Bifidobacteria* and *Lactobacilli*, which are found in probiotics and yoghurt, can help seal gaps between intestinal cells and help heal the intestines. These species can also prevent disease-causing bacteria from sticking to the intestinal wall. In fact, taking certain probiotics that contain *Bifidobacteria* and *Lactobacilli* can reduce symptoms of IBS.

Additionally, lower levels of short-chain fatty acids were linked to worsen ulcerative colitis.

Human studies also suggest that short-chain fatty acids, especially butyrate, can improve symptoms of ulcerative colitis and Crohn's disease. Furthermore, improvements in inflammation were associated with an increase in butyrate production due to its anti-inflammatory properties.

THE MICROBIOME AND THE HEART

Interestingly, the gut microbiome may even affect heart health. A recent study in 1,500 people found that the gut microbiome played an important role in promoting "good" HDL cholesterol and triglycerides. Certain unhealthy species in the gut microbiome may also contribute to heart disease by producing trimethylamine N-oxide (TMAO). TMAO is a chemical that contributes to blocked arteries, which may lead to heart attacks or stroke.

Certain bacteria within the microbiome convert choline and L-carnitine, both of which are nutrients found in red meat and other animal-based food sources, to TMAO, potentially increasing risk factors for heart disease. However, other bacteria within the gut microbiome, particularly *Lactobacilli*, may help reduce cholesterol when taken as a probiotic.

This is in-line with The Livy Method that encourages eating lots of vegetables, heavier carbs in the form of whole grains, darker rices, fruits, legumes, fermented foods, encouraging higher fibre content to feed the microbes in the gut, ultimately encouraging the growth of beneficial microbes. Many of the foods are also prebiotics which feed these flora. Eating foods like dandelion greens, garlic, onions, leeks, asparagus, bananas, barley, oats, apples, cocoa, flax seeds, wheat bran, and seaweed are great for feeding our beneficial bacteria. It is also recommended to go meat free occasionally or when you can, to help support the gut.

THE MICROBIOME AND BLOOD SUGAR

According to Barra et al. (2021) the gut microbiota can also influence blood glucose. Lower bacterial diversity correlates with insulin resistance and higher adiposity (having more fat).

Type 2 diabetes (T2D) is associated with an altered composition of the gut microbiota, where the lower relative abundance of **Firmicutes Clostridia**, but higher **Betaproteobacteria** in diabetic humans was associated with higher blood glucose. There are many correlations between taxonomy (taxonomy is the science of naming, describing and classifying organisms and includes all plants, animals and microorganisms of the world) and possible host functions. For example, the Firmicutes phylum consists predominantly of SCFA butyrate-producing bacteria; specifically, certain *Clostridia* which have anti-inflammatory properties and are less abundant in individuals with T2D.

Faecalibacterium prausnitzii is another butyrate-producing strain that is associated with improvements in glucose tolerance in patients who have undergone gastric bypass surgery, suggesting that bacterial metabolites can also affect glucose homeostasis. In addition, branched-chain amino acids produced by **Bacteroides vulgatus** species positively correlate with insulin resistance. Therefore, short-chain fatty acids seem to help regulate blood sugar levels and improve insulin resistance, especially in people with diabetes or insulin resistance.

Very interestingly, although there are fewer examples of microbes or microbial communities causing changes in blood glucose, the microbiota from obese mice can transmit higher blood glucose into germ-free mice independently of changes in adiposity.

THE MICROBIOME AND THE BRAIN

The gut microbiome may even benefit brain health in a number of ways! Certain species of bacteria can help produce chemicals in the brain called neurotransmitters. An example of this is serotonin. Serotonin is a neurotransmitter which sends signals between your nerve cells. Serotonin is found mostly in the digestive system (stomach and intestines), although it's also in blood platelets and throughout the central nervous system. Serotonin is most commonly known for helping to regulate our mood, but is also involved in digestion, clotting, sleeping, eating, bone health, and libido.

According to Caltech (2015, April), although serotonin is well known as a brain neurotransmitter, it is estimated that 90 percent of the body's serotonin is made in the digestive tract. In fact, altered levels of this peripheral serotonin have been linked to diseases such as irritable bowel syndrome, cardiovascular disease, and osteoporosis. Therefore, it can be seen that if our gut health can influence even this one neurotransmitter, it potentially can influence so many aspects of our health!

Furthermore, the gut is physically connected to the brain through millions of nerves. Thus, the gut microbiome may also affect brain health by helping to influence the messages that are sent to the brain through these nerves. Some studies have shown that people with various psychological disorders have different species of bacteria in their guts, compared to healthy people. This suggests that the gut microbiome may affect brain health. However, it's unclear if this is simply due to different dietary and lifestyle habits.

THE MICROBIOME AND PHASE III DETOXIFICATION

As discussed in the science post Detox, if phase I and II occur effectively, toxins can be eliminated by the kidneys and bowels via urine and stool. Although the liver is thought of as our primary detoxification organ, it requires a large variety of nutrients that must first be absorbed via the digestive system, in order to function optimally. Ironically though, the digestive system is also the initial site of exposure to ingested toxins. Due to these factors, it is recognized that there is an additional third phase of detoxification which occurs primarily in the digestive system.

The third phase of detoxification refers to a highly concentrated anti-porter (transport) system of proteins in the body. There are many anti-porters being researched, particularly P-glycoprotein, an anti-porter in the small intestine that moves toxins from cells into the gut. This transport system ensures the movement of harmful compounds out of the cell and into the detoxification organs.

A healthy diet and microbiome are key to the success of phase III, whereas digestive inflammation leads to the impairment of it. If phase III is compromised, an accumulation of toxins within the cell occurs. Errors in P-glycoprotein expression have been linked to Alzheimer's disease, and suspected to play a role in stress management and inflammatory bowel disease.

ORAL BACTERIA AND THE LINK TO HEALTH

Rheumatoid arthritis and pneumonia are just two diseases that have been linked to gum disease. According to Dominy et al. (2019), bacteria normally present in the mouth can also release toxins that make their way into the brain. Once there, they may contribute to Alzheimer's disease. Maintaining good dental hygiene is not just important for oral health, but can be very important for our overall health, including our brain!

Over 6 billion bacteria, including 700 different species, reside inside your mouth. Some promote health, others provoke disease. It is thought that there are about 15 to 20 harmful strains, but that will continue to evolve over time, and we learn more about how these species interact with each other.

Your mouth, or what scientists refer to as the oral microbiome, is "a complex community with lots of communication between bacteria of the same species as well as across species,". When your teeth feel slimy and in need of a brushing, that is an indication of their presence.

Oral bacteria also thrive inside your cheeks and on your tongue, palate, tonsils, and gums. Your mouth is a great habitat for unicellular (one cell) microorganisms. It's constantly moist, has a fairly neutral pH, and a warm temperature. However, despite this perfect environment to sustain the bacteria, you do end up swallowing bacteria that end up in your gut. As discussed in the science posts on digestion, our acidic stomach acid is a protective mechanism that kills bacteria that may enter the stomach to protect us from getting sick! This is why a healthy digestive system is so important.

Furthermore, there is another portal of entry for bacteria to access our bodies via our mouths. Every time we chew, brush, or floss, these microbes can get pushed into the small vessels in our gums, which gives them access into the bloodstream.

In a healthy mouth, the immune system keeps microbes from entering the body and causing infection. However, when you have chronic gum disease or other oral infections, this system is compromised. When oral bacteria access the bloodstream, they can travel to organs throughout the body, including the brain.

One known organism with the ability to cause harm in other parts of the body is *Porphyromonas gingivalis*, or Pg. Pg has been linked to a number of serious health issues, including pneumonia, rheumatoid arthritis, heart disease, hepatitis, and esophageal cancer.

Researchers now know it can sneak across the blood-brain barrier, a network of dense cells that protects the brain from harmful substances. Once there, Pg can cause pathological changes.

Researchers have observed Pg in the brains of deceased people with Alzheimer's disease. Surprisingly,

Pg major proteins called gingipains, were found in the brains at a level much higher in those that had Alzheimer's disease, than in those with healthy brains of the same age. This supports that Pg may have a large influence on Alzheimer's disease. Currently there is an area of research looking into drugs and possible vaccines to eradicate and limit its spread.

Migration of bacteria from one part of the body to another is a natural process, which can't completely be prevented. However, the number of bacteria that can get into the bloodstream may be reduced by improved oral care. Here's how to do so:

BRUSH AND FLOSS

According to the Canadian Dental Association (CDA), you should brush your teeth for at least 2-3 minutes, ideally, brushing after every meal, because the bacterial attack on teeth begins minutes after eating. At the very least, brush once a day and always before you go to bed.

Flossing removes plaque and bacteria that you cannot reach with your toothbrush. It helps dislodge bits of food that would otherwise collect bacteria and contribute to inflammation and infection on the gums. If you don't floss, you are missing more than one-third of your tooth surface. Plaque is the main cause of gum disease. It is an invisible bacterial film that develops on your teeth every day. Within 24 to 36 hours, plaque hardens into tartar (also called calculus), which can only be removed by professional cleaning. Floss at least once a day, and plaque can be prevented from hardening into tartar.

See this link from the CDA on how to properly brush and floss your teeth.

https://www.cda-adc.ca/en/oral_health/cfyt/dental_care/flossing_brushing.asp

MOUTHWASH

Flossing and brushing are the two main recommendations for teeth care and health.

There is some discussion regarding whether or not mouthwash should be a part of the daily dental routine in a healthy person, and those without gum inflammation. There is some thought that mouthwash may disrupt the oral microbiome to allow for proper growth of good bacteria. It would be like comparing it to using antibiotics, which can wipe out the harmful bacteria that is making us sick, but also the beneficial bacteria. However, this is very individual and it would be important to speak to your dentist if you have any concerns related to your specific dental health and health risks.

EAT MORE FRUITS AND VEGETABLES

Eating high-fibre foods, particularly fruits and vegetables, can reduce the progression of gum disease. Fibre creates more saliva in the mouth, which helps get rid of excess food and offsets harmful acids. Also, these foods keep us healthier in general which is important in preventing disease.

RINSE WITH WATER AFTER MEALS AND CHOOSE WATER AS THE BEVERAGE OF CHOICE

According to the CDA, sugar is one of the main causes of dental problems. Sugary drinks are also a major source of sugars in the diets of pre-teens and teens. As a result, consuming sugary drinks may lead to increased risk of cavities for children, and obesity and type 2 diabetes for the entire population.

Drinking water keeps you hydrated without the added sugars, sodium, and saturated fats, and it helps your body get rid of wastes.

Water also helps to buffer the collection of bacteria in your mouth until you can brush. Rinsing your mouth with water after meals and snacks, then brushing 30 to 45 minutes later, is a great addition to your mouth care.

BE VIGILANT IF YOU ALREADY HAVE A HEALTH ISSUE

People with certain diseases are more at risk for oral disease because they've already experienced a compromise in their immune system. Being vigilant in your oral health care may help lessen the impact.

IMPROVE YOUR GUT HEALTH AND MICROBIOME

There are many ways to improve your gut microbiome, all of which are a perfect compliment to The Livy Method including:

Eat a diverse range of foods: This can lead to a diverse microbiome, which is an indicator of good gut health. These include a source of healthy carbohydrates, good quality protein, and healthy fats.

In particular, legumes, beans and fruit contain lots of fibre and can promote the growth of healthy *Bifidobacteria*. Some high fibre foods that are good for your gut bacteria include:

- raspberries
- artichokes
- green peas
- broccoli
- chickpeas
- lentils
- beans
- whole grains
- bananas
- apples

Apples, artichokes, blueberries, almonds, and pistachios have also all been shown to increase *Bifidobacteria* in humans. *Bifidobacteria* are considered beneficial bacteria, as they can help prevent intestinal inflammation and enhance gut health.

Eat fermented foods and liquids: Fermented foods/liquids can reduce the amounts of disease-causing species in the gut. Fermented foods have undergone fermentation, a process in which the sugars they contain are broken down by yeast or bacteria.

Some examples of fermented foods/liquids are:

- Yogurt
- Kimchi
- Sauerkraut
- Tempeh
- Fermented pickles
- Kefir
- Kombucha

Many of these foods are rich in *lactobacilli*, a type of bacteria that can benefit your health. Research shows that people who eat a lot of yogurt appear to have more *lactobacilli* in their intestines. These people also have less *Enterobacteriaceae*, which is a type of bacteria associated with inflammation and a number of chronic conditions. Similarly, a number of studies have shown that yogurt consumption can improve intestinal bacteria and decrease symptoms of lactose intolerance. What's more, yogurt may also enhance the function and composition of the microbiome.

However, many yogurts, especially flavoured yoghurt, contain high amounts of sugar. Therefore, it's best to opt for plain, unsweetened yoghurt or a flavoured yoghurt with minimal added sugar that is made only of milk and bacteria mixtures, also sometimes called "starter cultures." Additionally, to reap the gut health benefits, make sure the label reads "contains live active cultures".

Furthermore, fermented milk (kefir) may promote the growth of beneficial bacteria, such as *Bifidobacteria* and *lactobacilli*, while decreasing quantities of some other harmful strains of bacteria. Kimchi may also benefit the gut flora.

Limit your intake of artificial sweeteners: Some evidence has shown that artificial sweeteners like aspartame increase blood sugar by stimulating the growth of unhealthy bacteria like *Enterobacteriaceae* in the gut microbiome. Also, there is growing evidence that indicates certain artificial sweeteners like sucralose reduce insulin sensitivity and affect the gut bacteria. Check out the science post on Sugars and the Brain where this is discussed in more detail!

Eat prebiotic foods: As discussed above, prebiotics are a type of fibre that stimulates the growth of healthy bacteria. Taking a prebiotic along with your probiotic if needed as recommended in the Let's Talk Supplements Post can go a long way in building up the good bacteria in your digestive system, and help with the healing process.

Breastfeed for as long as possible: Breastfeeding is very important for the development of the gut microbiome. A baby's microbiome begins to properly develop at birth. However, studies suggest that babies may be exposed to some bacteria even before birth.

During the first 2 years of life, an infant's microbiome is continuously developing and is rich in beneficial *Bifidobacteria*, which can digest the sugars found in breast milk. What's more, breastfeeding is also associated with lower rates of allergies, obesity, and other health conditions that may be due to differences in the gut microbiota.

Eat whole grains: Whole grains contain lots of fibre and beneficial non-digestible carbohydrates like beta-glucan, which are digested by gut bacteria to benefit weight, cancer risk, diabetes and other issues. These carbohydrates are not absorbed in the small intestine and instead make their way to the large intestine to promote the growth of beneficial bacteria in the gut. Research suggests that whole grains can promote the growth of *Bifidobacteria*, *lactobacilli*, and *Bacteroidetes* in humans.

Whole grains can also increase feelings of fullness, reduce inflammation, and certain risk factors for heart disease. However, some people may have some issues with gluten and may have to limit or avoid the intake of it.

While this mostly applies to those with celiac disease or a sensitivity to gluten, more research is needed to determine whether eating grains that contain gluten may also alter the gut microbiome in healthy adults without these conditions.

Eat more plant-based meals: Vegetarian diets may help reduce levels of disease-causing bacteria such as *E. coli*, as well as inflammation and cholesterol. However, it is unclear if the benefits of a vegetarian diet on the gut microbiome are due to a lack of meat intake or if other factors may also play a role.

Eat foods rich in polyphenols: Polyphenols are plant compounds that have many health benefits, including reductions in blood pressure, inflammation, cholesterol levels, and oxidative stress. Human cells can't always digest polyphenols. Because they aren't absorbed efficiently, most polyphenols make their way to the colon, where they are digested by gut bacteria.

Some examples of foods rich in polyphenols are:

- cocoa and dark chocolate
- red wine
- grape skins
- green tea
- almonds
- onions
- blueberries
- broccoli

Polyphenols from cocoa can increase the amount of *Bifidobacteria* and *lactobacilli* in humans and reduce the quantity of *Clostridia*. Furthermore, these changes in the microbiome are associated with lower levels of triglycerides and C-reactive protein, which is a marker of inflammation.

The polyphenols in red wine have similar effects and have even been shown to increase levels of beneficial bacteria in people with metabolic syndrome. However, those that are mindful of supporting their liver may want to only have it on occasion as discussed in the science post Detox.

Take a probiotic supplement: Probiotics are live bacteria that can help restore the gut to a healthy state after dysbiosis. Probiotics may not permanently colonise the intestines; however, they may benefit your health by helping to change the overall composition of the microbiome and supporting your metabolism.

Probiotics may not have a big influence on the gut microbiome composition of healthy people, however, there is some evidence that probiotics may improve the gut microbiome in those with certain diseases.

Interestingly, a Spanish systematic by Álvarez-Arraño, V., & Martín-Peláez, S., (2021) reviewed 27 randomized control trials that met their criteria indicates that both probiotics and synbiotics (a combination of a probiotic and prebiotic), specifically certain strains of Lactobacillus gasseri, L. rhamnosus, L. plantarum, L. curvatus associated with other Lactobacillus species and/or with species from the Bifidobacterium genus, have the potential to aid in weight and fat loss in overweight and obese populations. There is still a need, though, for clinical trials, in order to state more accurate recommendations in terms of strains, doses and intervention times.

Take antibiotics only when necessary: Antibiotics kill many bad and good bacteria in the gut microbiome, possibly contributing to weight gain and antibiotic resistance. Thus, only take antibiotics when medically necessary. If taking Antibiotics, speak to your HCP about taking probiotics to help maintain your good bacterial flora.

As it can be seen, by following all the recommendations of The Livy Method, which facilitates strengthening the health of your microbiome, you may experience not only weight loss, but overall improvements in your health and wellness. Our bodies are not compartmentalised, separate systems. Our bodies are a unique symphony of so many different moving parts, living cells, organisms and systems, that all work together to keep us alive and functioning as best as we can. However, we choose how we fuel, maintain, and take care of it. The better we are able to invest in our health and selves, the more harmonious that symphony of our microbiome is.

Check out these great videos and resources to better understand our microbiome, they have been shared in other Science Posts but are worth watching:

https://www.youtube.com/watch?v=B9RruLkAUm8&t=329s

https://www.youtube.com/watch?v=IDqMB6C1uys

IMPACTT (Canada)

https://www.impactt-microbiome.ca/

link to the Human Microbiome Project

https://hmpdacc.org/ihmp/

https://hmpdacc.org/hmp/

https://hmpdacc.org/

EU Microbiome Support

https://www.microbiomesupport.eu/about/

European Commission food 2030

https://ec.europa.eu/info/research-and-innovation/research-area/environment/bioeconomy/food-systems/food-2030_en#:~:text=Food%202030%20is%20the%20EU's,is%20fit%20for%20the%20future.

Dr. Svetlana U. Perović has personally curated a list of microbiome events that are free and mostly virtual.

https://github.com/SvetlanaUP/Microbiome-conferences-c

https://whatisbiotechnology.org/index.php/science/summary/microbiome/the-human-microbiome-refers-to-the-complete-set-of-genes

This concludes the science series for this round of The Livy Method Program. Hopefully you enjoyed this learning journey that we have embarked on together. Congratulations on still being here and showing up for yourself. It's this kind of self-love and caring, that will truly change your life as well as inspire others. We wish you all the love!

REFERENCES

About. (n.d.). Microbiome Support. https://www.microbiomesupport.eu/about/

Álvarez-Arraño V., Martín-Peláez, S. (2021) Effects of Probiotics and Synbiotics on Weight Loss in Subjects with Overweight or Obesity: A Systematic Review. *Nutrients,* 17;13(10):3627. doi: 10.3390/nu13103627. PMID: 34684633; PMCID: PMC8540110.

Baldi, S., Mundula, T., Nannini, G., & Amedei, A. (2021). Microbiota shaping - the effects of probiotics, prebiotics, and fecal microbiota transplant on cognitive functions: A systematic review. *World journal of Gastroenterology, 27*(39), 6715–6732. https://doi.org/10.3748/wjg.v27.i39.6715

Barra, N. G., Anhê, F. F., Cavallari, J. F., Singh, A. M., Chan, D. Y., & Schertzer, J. D. (2021). Micronutrients impact the gut microbiota and blood glucose, *Journal of Endocrinology, 250*(2), R1-R21.https://doi.org/10.1530/JOE-21-0081

Berg, G., Rybakova, D., Fischer, D., Cernava, T., Vergès, M. C., Charles, T., Chen, X., Cocolin, L., Eversole, K., Corral, G. H., Kazou, M., Kinkel, L., Lange, L., Lima, N., Loy, A., Macklin, J. A., Maguin, E., Mauchline, T., McClure, R., Mitter, B., … Schloter, M. (2020). Microbiome definition re-visited: Old concepts and new challenges. *Microbiome, 8*(1). https://doi.org/10.1186/s40168-020-00875-0

Brown, M.J. (2021, October 11). *How short-chain fatty acids affect health and weight.* Healthline. https://www.healthline.com/nutrition/short-chain-fatty-acids-101

Claus, S. P., Guillou, H., & Ellero-Simatos, S. (2016). The gut microbiota: A major player in the toxicity of environmental pollutants? *NPJ biofilms and microbiomes, 2.* https://doi.org/10.1038/npjbiofilms.2016.3

Deo, P. N., & Deshmukh, R. (2019). Oral microbiome: Unveiling the fundamentals. *Journal of Oral and Maxillofacial Pathology, 23*(1), 122–128. https://doi.org/10.4103/jomfp.JOMFP_304_18

Dobell, C. (1920). The discovery of the intestinal protozoa of man. *Proceedings of the Royal Society of Medicine, 13*(Sect Hist Med), 1–15. https://www.ncbi.nlm.nih.gov/pmc/articles/PMC2151982/

Dominy, S.S., Lynch, C., Ermini, F., Benedyk, M., Marczyk, A., Konradi, A., Nguyen, M., Haditsch, U., Raha, D., Griffin, C., Holsinger, L. J., Arastu-Kapur, S., Kaba, S., Lee, A., Ryder, M. I., Potempa, B., Mydel, P., Hellvard, A., Adamowicz, K., … Potempa, J. (2019). Porphyromonas gingivalis in Alzheimer's disease brains: Evidence for disease causation and treatment with small-molecule inhibitors. *Science Advances, 5*(1). DOI: 10.1126/sciadv.aau3333

Flossing & brushing. (n.d.). Canadian Dental Association. https://www.cda-adc.ca/en/oral_health/cfyt/dental_care/flossing_brushing.asp

Food 2030. (n.d.). European Commision Research and Innovation. https://research-and-innovation.ec.europa.eu/research-area/environment/bioeconomy/food-systems/food-2030_en#:~:text=Food%202030%20is%20the%20EU's,is%20fit%20for%20the%20future.

Gunnars, K. (2019, February 27). *Does all disease begin in your gut? The surprising truth.* Healthline. https://www.healthline.com/nutrition/does-all-disease-begin-in-the-gut

Guo, Y., Zhu, X., Zeng, M., Qi, L., Tang, X., Wang, D., Zhang, M., Xie, Y., Li, H., Yang, X., & Chen, D. (2021). A diet high in sugar and fat influences neurotransmitter metabolism and then affects brain function by altering the gut microbiota. *Translational Psychiatry, 11.* https://doi.org/10.1038/s41398-021-01443-2

How, K. Y., Song, K. P., & Chan, K. G. (2016). Porphyromonas gingivalis: An overview of periodontopathic pathogen below the gum line. *Frontiers in Microbiology, 7.* https://doi.org/10.3389/fmicb.2016.00053

Human microbiome project. (2020, August 20). National Institutes of Health. http://commonfund.nih.gov/hmp/

IMPACTT. (n.d.). Integrated Microbiome Platforms for Advancing Causation Testing and Translation. https://www.impactt-microbiome.ca/

Kristensen, N. B., Bryrup, T., Allin, K. H., Nielsen, T., Hansen, T. H., & Pedersen, O. (2016). Alterations in fecal microbiota composition by probiotic supplementation in healthy adults: A systematic review of randomized controlled trials. *Genome Medicine, 8*(1), 52. https://doi.org/10.1186/s13073-016-0300-5

Microbiome-conferences-etc. (n.d.). Github. https://github.com/SvetlanaUP/Microbiome-conferences-c

NIH human microbiome project. (n.d.). Human Microbiome Project. https://hmpdacc.org/

Scaccia, A. (2020, August 19). *Serotonin: What you need to know.* Healthline. https://www.healthline.com/health/mental-health/serotonin#functions

Sender, R., Fuchs, S., & Milo, R. (2016). Revised estimates for the number of human and bacteria cells in the body. *PLOS Biology, 14*(8). https://doi.org/10.1371/journal.pbio.1002533

Semeco, A., & Kelly, E. (2021, May 11). *The 19 best prebiotic foods you should eat.* Healthline. https://www.healthline.com/nutrition/19-best-prebiotic-foods

Shreiner, A. B., Kao, J. Y., & Young, V. B. (2015). The gut microbiome in health and in disease. *Current Opinion in Gastroenterology, 31*(1), 69–75. https://doi.org/10.1097/MOG.0000000000000139

Stoller-Conrad, J. (2015, April 9). *Microbes help produce serotonin in gut.* Caltech. https://www.caltech.edu/about/news/microbes-help-produce-serotonin-gut-46495

TEDx Talks. (2016, June 27). *Microbiome: Gut bugs and you | Warren Peters | TEDxLaSierraUniversity* [Video]. Youtube. https://www.youtube.com/watch?v=IDqMB6C1uys

TEDx Talks. (2019, December 12). *Your gut microbiome: The most important organ you've never heard of | Erika Ebbel Angle | TEDxFargo* [Video]. Youtube. https://www.youtube.com/watch?v=B9RruLkAUm8

Venegas, D. P., De la Fuente, M. K., Landskron, G., González, M. J., Quera, R., Dijkstra, G., Harmsen, H., Faber, K. N., & Hermoso, M. A. (2019). Short chain fatty acids (SCFAs)-mediated gut epithelial and immune regulation and its relevance for inflammatory bowel diseases. *Frontiers in Immunology, 10.* https://doi.org/10.3389/fimmu.2019.00277

Vijay, A., & Valdes, A.M. (2022). Role of the gut microbiome in chronic diseases: A narrative review. *European Journal of Clinical Nutrition, 76,* 489–501. https://doi.org/10.1038/s41430-021-00991-6

Welcome. (n.d.). Integrative Human Microbiome Project (iHMP). https://hmpdacc.org/ihmp/

What is taxonomy? (2010, April 6). Convention on Biological Diversity. https://www.cbd.int/gti/taxonomy.shtml#:~:text=Taxonomy%20is%20the%20science%20of,and%20microorganisms%20of%20the%20world.

Yano, J.M., Yu, K., Donaldson, G.P., Shastri, G.G., Ann, P., Ma, L., Nagler, C.R., Ismagilov, R.F., Mazmanian, S.K., & Hsiao, E.Y. (2015). Indigenous bacteria from the gut microbiota regulate host serotonin biosynthesis. *Cell, 161*(2), 264-276. DOI: 10.1016/j.cell.2015.02.047

Zheng, D., Liwinski, T., & Elinav, E. (2020). Interaction between microbiota and immunity in health and disease. *Cell Research, 30*(6), 492–506. https://doi.org/10.1038/s41422-020-0332-7

Zoe. (n.d.). https://joinzoe.com/

SPRING/SUMMER 2023 GROUP: TRACKING SHEETS

Use the chart to track your progress throughout the Spring/Summer 2023 Group. This chart can be used to help you pick up on patterns of behaviours and responses and give you a better idea of what weight loss looks like specifically to you. Feel free to fill in all or none of the columns or personalize what types of things you want to track in the notes section.

Use the chart below to track your progress throughout the Spring/Summer 2023 Group. This chart can be used to help you pick up on patterns of behaviours and responses and give you a better idea of what weight loss looks like specifically to you. Feel free to fill in all or none of the columns or personalize what types of things you want to track in the notes section. Happy tracking!

April 2023										
			Meals and Snacks							
Date	Weight	Water	B	S1	L	S2	S3	D	Supplements	Notes (i.e., NSVs, BMs, Exercise, Sleep, Bonus snacks, etc.)
Apr 24			☐	☐	☐	☐	☐	☐	☐	
Apr 25			☐	☐	☐	☐	☐	☐	☐	
Apr 26			☐	☐	☐	☐	☐	☐	☐	
Apr 27			☐	☐	☐	☐	☐	☐	☐	
Apr 28			☐	☐	☐	☐	☐	☐	☐	
Apr 29			☐	☐	☐	☐	☐	☐	☐	
Apr 30			☐	☐	☐	☐	☐	☐	☐	

April Notes:

_____

_____

_____

_____

_____

May 2023

Date	Weight	Water	\ Meals and Snacks						Supplements	Notes (BMs, Exercise, Period, Stress, Bonus snacks, etc.)
			B	S1	L	S2	S3	D		
May 1			☐	☐	☐	☐	☐	☐	☐	
May 2			☐	☐	☐	☐	☐	☐	☐	
May 3			☐	☐	☐	☐	☐	☐	☐	
May 4			☐	☐	☐	☐	☐	☐	☐	
May 5			☐	☐	☐	☐	☐	☐	☐	
May 6			☐	☐	☐	☐	☐	☐	☐	
May 7			☐	☐	☐	☐	☐	☐	☐	
May 8			☐	☐	☐	☐	☐	☐	☐	
May 9			☐	☐	☐	☐	☐	☐	☐	
May 10			☐	☐	☐	☐	☐	☐	☐	
May 11			☐	☐	☐	☐	☐	☐	☐	
May 12			☐	☐	☐	☐	☐	☐	☐	
May 13			☐	☐	☐	☐	☐	☐	☐	
May 14			☐	☐	☐	☐	☐	☐	☐	

Date	Weight	Water	Meals and Snacks						Supplements	Notes (BMs, Exercise, Period, Stress, Bonus snacks, etc.)
			B	S1	L	S2	S3	D		
May 15			☐	☐	☐	☐	☐	☐	☐	
May 16			☐	☐	☐	☐	☐	☐	☐	
May 17			☐	☐	☐	☐	☐	☐	☐	
May 18			☐	☐	☐	☐	☐	☐	☐	
May 19			☐	☐	☐	☐	☐	☐	☐	
May 20			☐	☐	☐	☐	☐	☐	☐	
May 21			☐	☐	☐	☐	☐	☐	☐	
May 22			☐	☐	☐	☐	☐	☐	☐	
May 23			☐	☐	☐	☐	☐	☐	☐	
May 24			☐	☐	☐	☐	☐	☐	☐	
May 25			☐	☐	☐	☐	☐	☐	☐	
May 26			☐	☐	☐	☐	☐	☐	☐	
May 27			☐	☐	☐	☐	☐	☐	☐	
May 28			☐	☐	☐	☐	☐	☐	☐	
May 29			☐	☐	☐	☐	☐	☐	☐	
May 30			☐	☐	☐	☐	☐	☐	☐	

			Meals and Snacks							
Date	Weight	Water	B	S1	L	S2	S3	D	Supplements	Notes (BMs, Exercise, Period, Stress, Bonus snacks, etc.)
May 31			☐	☐	☐	☐	☐	☐	☐	

May Notes:

_____

_____

_____

_____

_____

June 2023

Date	Weight	Water	Meals and Snacks						Supplements	Notes (BMs, Exercise, Period, Stress, Bonus snacks, etc.)
			B	S1	L	S2	S3	D		
Jun 1			☐	☐	☐	☐	☐	☐	☐	
Jun 2			☐	☐	☐	☐	☐	☐	☐	
Jun 3			☐	☐	☐	☐	☐	☐	☐	
Jun 4			☐	☐	☐	☐	☐	☐	☐	
Jun 5			☐	☐	☐	☐	☐	☐	☐	
Jun 6			☐	☐	☐	☐	☐	☐	☐	
Jun 7			☐	☐	☐	☐	☐	☐	☐	
Jun 8			☐	☐	☐	☐	☐	☐	☐	
Jun 9			☐	☐	☐	☐	☐	☐	☐	
Jun 10			☐	☐	☐	☐	☐	☐	☐	
Jun 11			☐	☐	☐	☐	☐	☐	☐	
Jun 12			☐	☐	☐	☐	☐	☐	☐	
Jun 13			☐	☐	☐	☐	☐	☐	☐	
Jun 14			☐	☐	☐	☐	☐	☐	☐	

			Meals and Snacks							
Date	Weight	Water	B	S1	L	S2	S3	D	Supplements	Notes (BMs, Exercise, Period, Stress, Bonus snacks, etc.)
Jun 15			☐ ☐	☐ ☐	☐ ☐	☐ ☐	☐ ☐	☐ ☐	☐	
Jun 16			☐ ☐	☐ ☐	☐ ☐	☐ ☐	☐ ☐	☐ ☐	☐	
Jun 17			☐ ☐	☐ ☐	☐ ☐	☐ ☐	☐ ☐	☐ ☐	☐	
Jun 18			☐ ☐	☐ ☐	☐ ☐	☐ ☐	☐ ☐	☐ ☐	☐	
Jun 19			☐	☐	☐	☐	☐	☐	☐	
Jun 20			☐	☐	☐	☐	☐	☐	☐	
Jun 21			☐	☐	☐	☐	☐	☐	☐	
Jun 22			☐ ☐	☐ ☐	☐ ☐	☐ ☐	☐ ☐	☐ ☐	☐	
Jun 23			☐ ☐	☐ ☐	☐ ☐	☐ ☐	☐ ☐	☐ ☐	☐	
Jun 24			☐ ☐	☐ ☐	☐ ☐	☐ ☐	☐ ☐	☐ ☐	☐	
Jun 25			☐ ☐	☐ ☐	☐ ☐	☐ ☐	☐ ☐	☐ ☐	☐	
Jun 26			☐	☐	☐	☐		☐	☐	
Jun 27			☐	☐	☐	☐		☐	☐	
Jun 28			☐	☐	☐	☐		☐	☐	
Jun 29			☐	☐	☐	☐		☐	☐	

Date	Weight	Water	Meals and Snacks						Supplements	Notes (i.e., NSVs, BMs, Exercise, Sleep, Bonus snacks, etc.)
			B	S1	L	S2	S3	D		
Jun 30			☐	☐	☐	☐	☐	☐	☐	

June Notes:

_____

_____

_____

_____

_____

July 2023

Date	Weight	Water	Meals and Snacks						Supplements	Notes (BMs, Exercise, Period, Stress, Bonus snacks, etc.)
			B	S1	L	S2	S3	D		
July 1			☐	☐	☐	☐		☐	☐	
July 2			☐	☐	☐	☐		☐	☐	
July 3			☐	☐	☐	☐		☐	☐	
July 4			☐	☐	☐	☐		☐	☐	
July 5			☐	☐	☐	☐		☐	☐	
July 6			☐	☐	☐	☐		☐	☐	
July 7			☐	☐	☐	☐		☐	☐	
July 8			☐	☐	☐	☐		☐	☐	
July 9			☐	☐	☐	☐		☐	☐	
July 10			☐	☐	☐	☐	☐	☐	☐	
July 11			☐	☐	☐	☐	☐	☐	☐	
July 12			☐	☐	☐	☐	☐	☐	☐	

Date	Weight	Water	Meals and Snacks						Supplements	Notes (BMs, Exercise, Period, Stress, Bonus snacks, etc.)
			B	S1	L	S2	S3	D		
July 13			☐	☐	☐	☐	☐	☐	☐	
July 14			☐	☐	☐	☐	☐	☐	☐	
July 15			☐	☐	☐	☐	☐	☐	☐	
July 16			☐	☐	☐	☐	☐	☐	☐	
July 17			☐	☐	☐	☐	☐	☐	☐	
July 18			☐	☐	☐	☐	☐	☐	☐	
July 19			☐	☐	☐	☐	☐	☐	☐	
July 20			☐	☐	☐	☐	☐	☐	☐	
July 21			☐	☐	☐	☐	☐	☐	☐	
July 22			☐	☐	☐	☐	☐	☐	☐	
July 23			☐	☐	☐	☐	☐	☐	☐	

July Notes:

_____

_____

_____

_____

_____

Made in United States
Troutdale, OR
08/27/2023

12401757R00263